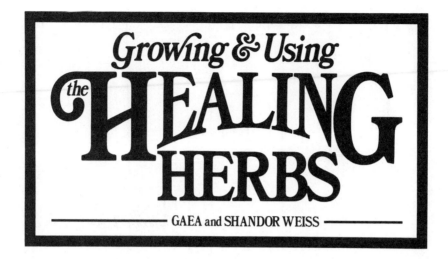

Growing & Using the HEALING HERBS

GAEA and SHANDOR WEISS

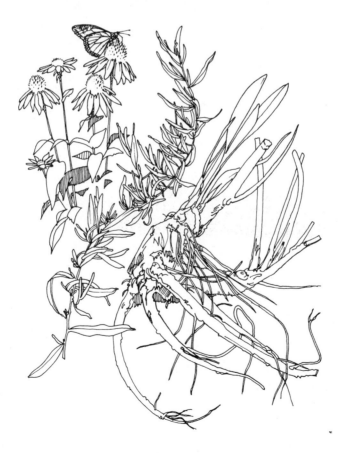

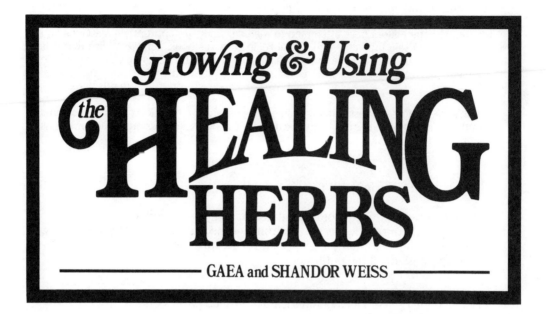

Growing & Using the HEALING HERBS

GAEA and SHANDOR WEISS

Rodale Press, Emmaus, Pennsylvania

This book is meant to be educational in nature and is in no way meant to be used for self-treatment or self-diagnosis. Keep in mind that excess quantities of some herbs can be dangerous. The editors have attempted to include, wherever appropriate, cautions and guidelines for using the herbs and herbal recipes in this book. Yet, we realize that it is impossible for us to anticipate every conceivable use of the herbs and every possible problem any use could cause. Moreover, we cannot know just what kinds of physical reactions or allergies some of you might have to substances discussed in this book.

For this reason, Rodale Press cannot assume responsibility for the effects of using the herbs or other information in this book. And we urge that all potentially serious health problems be managed by a physician.

Printed in the United States of America on recycled paper containing a high percentage of de-inked fiber.

Book design by Anita G. Patterson
Illustrations by Frank Fretz
Art direction by Karen A. Schell
Book layout by Acey Lee

Library of Congress Cataloging in Publication Data
Weiss, Gaea.
    Growing and using the healing herbs.

    Bibliography: p.
    Includes index.
    1. Herbs–Therapeutic use.   2. Herb gardening.
I. Weiss, Shandor. II. Title.
RM666.H33W444   1985   615'.321   84-24827
ISBN 0-87857-533-2   hardcover

2 4 6 8 10 9 7 5 3 1   hardcover

This book is dedicated to our parents, with love and gratitude.

Contents

Acknowledgments

We would like to thank Ven. Chakdud Rinpoche; Ed Smith; Tom Ward; Larry Korn; Ed Alstat, N.D.; Wallace Black Elk; Peter Giffen; Michael Broffman, C.A.; Ven. Shenphen Dawa Rinpoche; Subhuti Dharmananda, Ph.D.; Larry Andrews; Juli Schwartz; Gabriel Howearth; and the many others who shared their vision and knowledge in various areas of herbal healing and gardening. Thanks to our editor, Anne Halpin, for her cheerful and gracious disposition and her skill in bringing out the best. Special thanks to Ven. Gyaltrul Rinpoche for the constant inspiration of his example; and to Philip Kronowitt for his love, generosity, and intellectual scope.

Editor's Note

The editor would like to acknowledge also the contributions of several other people to the book; especially Frank Fretz, artist and herb gardener, whose dedication led him to draw from life the plants in chapter 4. On behalf of the illustrator, thanks to Cyrus Hyde of the Well-Sweep Herb Farm in New Jersey, Eileen Weinsteiger and Mary Anne McCarthy of the Rodale Research Center and Farm, and to Reed and Mary Fretz, all of whom allowed plants in their gardens to be photographed, sketched, and dug up. Also, special thanks to Lila Fretz for her research and organizational assistance. Finally, thanks to Anita G. Patterson and Acey Lee, for their creativity and care in designing and laying out the book.

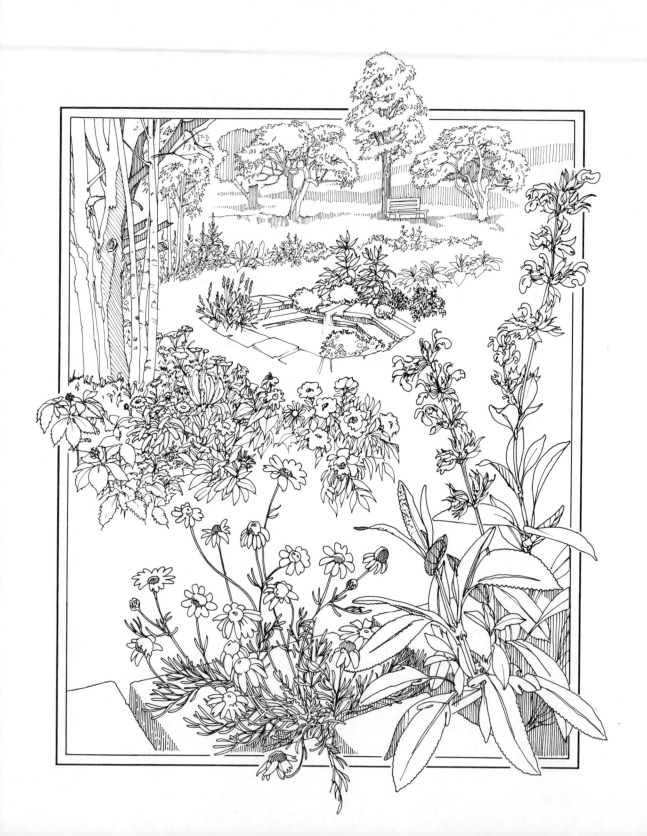

Entering the Healing Garden

*I*magine walking along a backyard path bordered with fragrant flowering herbs. Each plant has been chosen with care; the result is an artful profusion of shapes, sizes, colors, and textures that delights the eye. Near the house, an elegant, spoke-shaped garden of culinary herbs provides rosemary, sage, chives, Egyptian bunch onions, marjoram, savory, basil, oregano, and parsley for the needs of the cooks. The herbs have been set out with half-buried bricks dividing the circle into sections. The rosemary trails from a raised section in the center of the circle. The Egyptian bunch onions, with their elaborate tendrils, form a decorate border around the outside of the circle, looking very much as they did when artists in ancient Egypt employed them in friezes to embellish their frescoes. The circle is pleasing indeed to regard, with spiky chives and frilly parsley forming dense and very contrasting mounds of greenery. The elegant basil's shiny emerald leaves next to the smaller, softly colored foliage of the delicate marjoram provides another appealing partnership.

Nearby, moistened by a fountain, beds of fresh-smelling mints are arranged in a lively composition, their enthusiasm for growing rampant contained with sturdy dividers set into the soil. As we walk farther down the path, several bay laurel trees provide a shady environment, and the gardeners have wisely taken advantage of the shade to plant sweet woodruff on the path itself. Its delightful scent underfoot combines with the heady aromatic smell of the bay laurel. On the other side of the path, ginseng and goldenseal are thriving in the shade of sassafras and birch trees, which fill out the perfume that now captivates us fully.

While taking in the variety of fragrances in this part of the garden, we become aware of a low, steady, soothing sound some way off. Listening, we discern the commingled voices of a great number of bees. We walk farther along the path in the hope of discovering the plant that has so captivated the bees.

The path opens out into sunlight, and the sweet woodruff gives way underfoot to creeping thyme. Here, the gardeners have

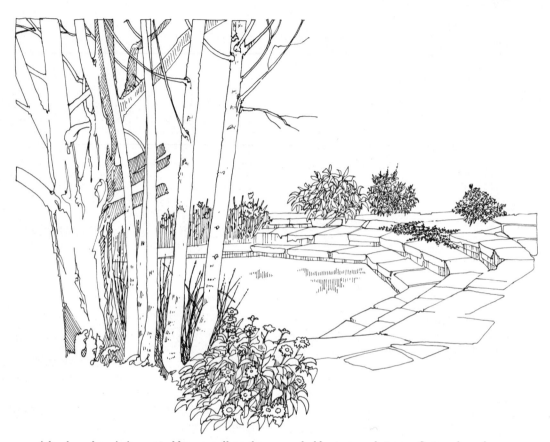

A backyard oasis is created by a small pool surrounded by terraced stones. Spaces have been left between stones, and different kinds of mint flourish there in the moist soil.

constructed a seat made of wood and earth, and planted it with thyme that now covers it completely. What a fragrant chair! Resting there momentarily to appreciate the silver-colored sage planted nearby, we are visited by a hummingbird who slows, hovers, then flies brightly on in the direction of the bee sound.

As we walk farther, the garden opens out into a small meadowlike area. There, in a little orchard of peach, apricot, and apple trees is revealed the secret of the bees. In the midst of the fruit trees stands a single linden tree, towering and graceful, at the height of its flowering, its clusters of creamy blossoms covered with bees. Their sound, once a distant hum, is now a richly textured tone of delight.

What a lovely place! Beneath and among the trees, a "wild garden" of yarrow, fennel, borage, catnip, calendula, dill, coriander, carrots, radishes, burdock, and garlic spills out in apparently random display. The charming disorder, full of color and movement, belies the gardeners' quite deliberate intent to let

Nature take her course, lending the fresh feeling and liveliness of an uncultivated place. Edged by blackberry bushes, this last treasure-store merges gently with the larger landscape beyond it.

This entire yard has been arranged with an attention to the healing qualities of plants. Their bark, roots, flowers, fruit, leaves, oils, and seeds will all find their way into healing teas, salves, foodstuffs, poultices, bath preparations, liniments, and cosmetics.

You are in the midst of our living garden, a wellspring of life, with countless healing aspects. How appropriate that the dominant color of the garden is a calming emerald green, the color that more than any other rests the eyes and calms the mind and body. The silvery blue-green leaves of the borage, the bright-to-forest greens of the various mints, the yellowish green of the fennel, the light gray-green of the lavender harmonize to create a soothing orchestration for our eyes. Greens in the living garden result from the magic of photosynthesis, which changes light into vivid material substance. This rich green color, at the very center of the color spectrum, is the color of balance. It is ornamented and embellished here by every other gorgeous tint the spectrum holds, as the garden brings forth vegetables, flowers, herbs, and fruits. In the midst of blues and violets, which are serene and peaceful, and reds, oranges, and yellows, which are bright and active, greens provide a tone of restful rejuvenation.

Looking out over the garden, we become aware that our walk has brought us to the threshold of a new way of looking at the world. The garden is a doorway to expanding our perceptions of the natural world of which we are a part. In our garden, each living thing can be seen individually, in the fullness of its beauty and usefulness. But the sweetness of the garden is the mixture, the wonderful min-gling and blending of all the plants. It is breathtaking to us. We never realized when we entered this doorway that our attention would be captured so fully by such a fabulous array of scents, flowers, colors, textures, and tastes.

With each plant we have a particular affinity and association. We planted the borage for the beautiful blue flowers it puts forth. And the sage we regard as a crusty plant, strong, like an inveterate mountain man, as different from the borage as a hermit from a businessman. There are the apple trees, with their sweet spring flowering and their delicious harvest. The sturdy comfrey, a dark, thick green in color, which always seems to be exploding into a fountain of the succulent leaves and fleshy stems that we value for their ability to heal wounds and knit bones. The merry parsley. The exhuberant little jungle of mints, each so different from the next. The gentle, clean-scented lavender.

Our garden did not appear overnight, though today it does seem as if it did, quite magically, arrive full-blown in the brilliance of summer. Planning, shaping, and cultivating our garden was an important part of the growing, healing, and learning process we wish to share with you. As we worked in the garden, nature's shape began to reveal itself. Getting our hands into the earth and our minds into the present has taught us a good deal about "investing in simple tasks a sense of their true significance," as Alan Chadwick described the rewarding labor of the gardener in the garden.

The Chinese have a saying about medicines that we believe applies to gardening, too. They say that if a medicine produces noticeable effects immediately, it is not really such a good medicine. If it works within several weeks, it is just mediocre. But if you can take it for your whole lifetime with no visible effects except continuous good health, it is an excellent medicine. So it is with the whole process of gardening–it is a slow activity that fosters an enduring restorative state. One of the healing aspects of gardening is the opportunity to experience the bonds between all things in nature. The awareness that the life-force that moves through the lettuce, the bear, and the oak is the same life-force that moves through us, deepens our respect for nature. It is precisely this recognition of the inherent kinship of all things that is healing to us.

It may very well be that there has never been a gardener whose view and life experience became more narrow from gardening. This was surely true of people such as the poet-scientist Goethe, who studied the process of metamorphosis in plants; of Rudolph Steiner, Sir Albert Howard, and J. I. Rodale, who were pioneers of the modern organic movement; of plant mystics and magicians such as Luther Burbank and George Washington Carver; of Richard St. Barbe-Baker, whose dedication has reforested vast areas of the Sahara Desert, and who has preserved and enhanced forests on many continents; of Alan Chadwick, the unique master gardener who brought biodynamic French-intensive gardening from Europe to the United States; of Masanobu Fukuoka, who has perfected the art of "natural farming" in Japan over the past 30 years; and of Peter and Eileen Caddy, founders of Findhorn, whose lush gardens, grown with spiritual and practical attention, have become world famous.

As Henry David Thoreau wrote in *Walden:*

The indescribable innocence and beneficence of Nature, of sun and wind and rain,

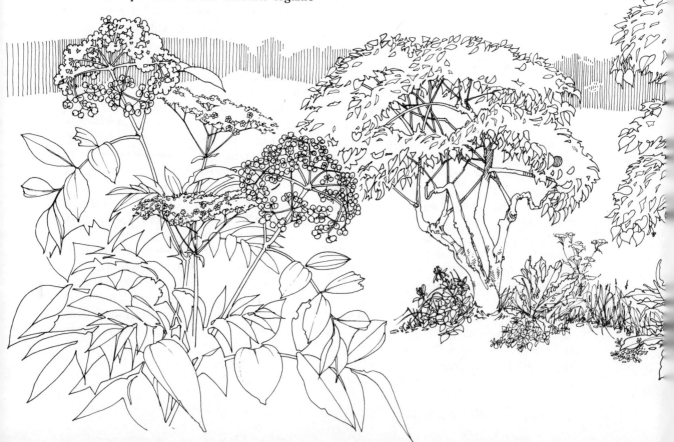

of summer and winter, such health, such cheer they afford forever ... Shall I not have intelligence with the earth? Am I not partly leaves and vegetable mold myself?

The garden is a mirror, and we see ourselves reflected in it. The reflection takes many forms, because gardening cultivates our minds and imaginations as much as it produces a tangible harvest of vegetables or fruits or herbs. We can feel ourselves in the rich and receptive element of earth, the ground of our being. We can see ourselves in the waters of nourishment which come as rain, mist, dew, surface and underground flows, snow, and frost. The sun's warmth, which sets the garden ablaze with greens, is the essence of the warmth and creative powers within us, too.

All around us the infinite forms of plants are arranged in a natural display of beauty.

A small grove of trees can provide healing flowers, leaves, fruits, and bark, as well as a shady spot to sit on a summer day.

Yet this display is really a display of space, which gives all the plant forms their visual definition. This concept is employed in the design of gardens ranging from elaborate Elizabethan mazes to austere Japanese rock gardens, where space is cultured as the expression of natural creativity.

In our healing garden, herbs are the symbol and the literal embodiment of our interest in health. Unlike the botanists, we consider an herb to be any plant or part of a plant which can be used for healing. To us, all plants are herbs. Ralph Waldo Emerson once said that a weed is a plant whose virtues are not yet known to us, and so it is with herbs. Herbs cannot be taken like pills to cure an ailment, of course. And while it is true that many plants cannot be considered medicines in the literal sense of the word—indeed, some are harmful when ingested—in another sense all plants can be thought of as having some value for maintaining health, whether it is to heal a wound or simply to restore the spirit with the sight of a beautiful flower. Our knowledge may be limited, but our view must remain expansive. Just as all metals and minerals have within them crystalline forms, so too do all plants hold restorative qualities.

Although the origin of herbal healing is a subject open to many views, it is generally true and verifiable that in all cultures around the world people have known about and experimented with the curative powers of the plants that grow around them. The Bible lists many herbs that are useful in healing. In Chinese tradition, all medical knowledge is attributed to a mythical hero, the Yellow Emperor. In Buddhist cultures, the Buddha of Medicine gave to man all healing plants and their uses. To the American Indians, the Great Spirit and the Earth Mother revealed their secrets of medicine. In almost all mythologies and cultural epics, there are one or more deities who are credited with the knowledge of healing plants. History, written and oral, supplies further examples.

The fact that modern science is beginning to research and verify herbal remedies has created something of an herbal renaissance in recent years, a resurgence of general interest in the healing uses of plants. It was the movement of science away from the study and use of herbs that has been the anomaly, and it is appropriate that researchers are again focusing their attention on the great natural laboratory of the planet.

Almost all herbal systems are based on knowledge gained through a synthesis of intellect and intuition. European herbalism used the Doctrine of Signatures and the Four Elements to decipher nature's medical codes, while the Chinese system of medicine uses the five elements and alternating yin-yang forces as a map. India's Ayurvedic medicine classified illness and medicine into the three humors, and Tibetan medicine uses a combination of Indian and Chinese systems, though the five elements are labeled differently. American Indians use a system similar to the Doctrine of Signatures, and they also have a system of either four or five elements. In fact, every tribe and healer may have a slightly different version. The variety of systems used for classifying herbs and their uses is an expression of the diversity of human cultures and characters, as developed in a diversity of environments. The similarities among the systems is the expression of the universality of botanic medicines. In the next three chapters we will explore the basic concepts involved in the world's great herbal healing traditions, the sources in which today's uses of healing herbs had their beginnings.

With this background we can all begin to understand the use of herbs in simple ways and to relate them to conditions of harmony or imbalance in our own bodies. An herb with a strong, bitter flavor, we may come to realize, is a plant that an herbalist might use for a person with a weak liver condition. The reasoning goes like this: it is the gall bladder that strengthens the liver's function, and since the taste of bile is extremely bitter, the herbalist would find nature's remedy in the form of bitter herbs. Or, if that herbalist were to look at the Doctrine of Signatures, which is a very old system that relates similar physical characteristics of disease to the physical appearance or parts of plants, he or she might look for an herb that was strongly yellow—the color of human skin when the liver is very weak with jaundice. Oregon grape, for example, has a very bitter taste, a bright yellow root and is considered by herbalists to be one of the most potent herbs for treating liver conditions. In the northwestern part of the United States, you can see this traditional treatment for liver ailments right underfoot, while hiking in the mountains and fields. In other parts of the country, Oregon grape or a close relative is used as an ornamental (it is more commonly known as barberry), and so a liver treatment could grow right in front of a well-landscaped doctor's office!

Similarly, the tastes of many foods have been correlated with the health or illness of our internal organs and functions. The medicine of China and Japan has long identified the use of foods and herbs through their taste. Traditional healers in those countries also classify medicinal plants according to properties such as color, shape, texture, degree of heat or coolness, place of origin, and wetness or dryness. Through the five tastes, salty, sour, sweet, bitter, and pungent, the Chinese correspond plants to five elements. These five elements are both internal and external, relating to the world and to our bodies. By studying this system (which is further explained in chapter 3), or any system of herbal information, we can come to perceive on a deeper level the bond between ourselves and nature. Our bodies are composed of the same elements, minerals, and living compounds that are found in the rest of the natural world. In theory there is no need to take vitamins and minerals in supplement form if you live in the midst of nature and know the properties of healing plants. For every lack or imbalance, there are plants that can supply the missing factors, or that can correct the imbalance.

The healing garden becomes a process in which gardening and the use of medicinal herbs and foods are integral parts of daily living. The natural cycles of gardening and harvesting draw us closer and closer to our own natural rhythms. The herb tea you drink, or the herb bath you soak in has healed you more than once if you have grown the herbs yourself. In fact, every moment in the cycle of planting, growing, harvesting, and using plants is part of a holistic experience with countless harvests of healing moments.

The process of using herbs in simple healing ways need not be a laborious one. Knowing one herb may be enough. In fact, some people have more knowledge of the herbal uses of one favorite plant than many herbalists have for a score of plants. Of course, careful study and research will broaden your herbal experience, but it is not the only way to learn about herbs and it need not be relied on to the exclusion of other forms of learning. Study is good for the indoor winter months and for checking on information, and it is essential to learn which plants can be harmful and should not be used, but the real learning of herbs occurs in direct contact with the plants themselves. Through intimate association, we become familiar with each plant. All of our senses become the medium for exchange. By concentrating, our awareness unfolds deeper and deeper levels of herbal understanding.

The traditional American Indian way of life is a life-style lived in harmony with nature. Native American herbal medicine traditionally has used herbs as instruments of awareness. With prayer and ritual initiation, Indian medicine men and women have used herbs as a way of drawing the healing power from the universe for themselves and their patients.

The fitness and holistic health movements have renewed a similar awareness for us—of food, of our bodies, and of how to care for ourselves preventively. The movement to eat unprocessed, unrefined foods has made people conscious of nutrition and its relationship to total, long-range health. At the same time, there has been a spiritual renaissance, and many environment-related movements. What are these trends but the gradual emergence of a way of life that more harmoniously attunes our lives with nature as a whole?

So for millions of Americans who have become dissatisfied with the quality of life they were leading, nature again has appeared in all of its fullness and variety, as the great life-enhancing garden. It is a healing garden, inviting us to enter and share in a richly rewarding and life-sustaining harvest.

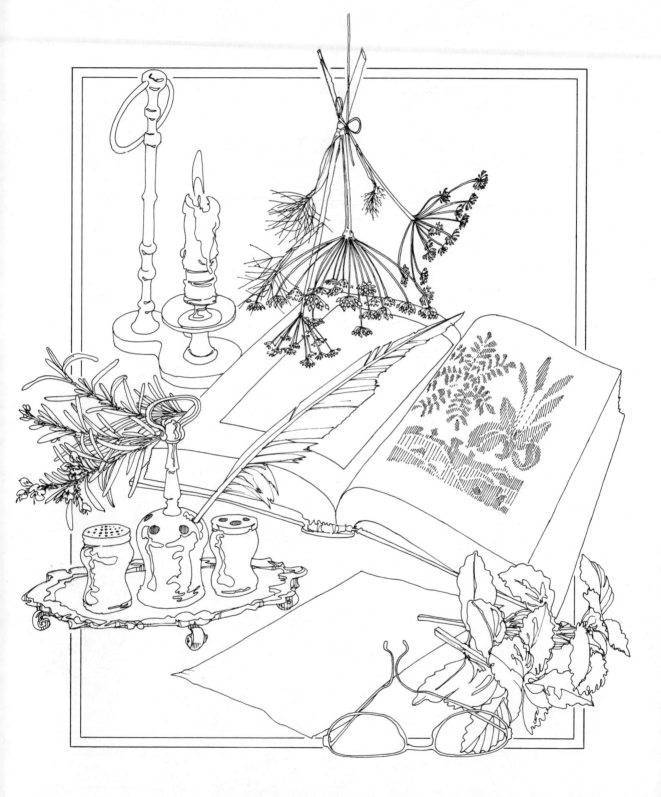

Healing Gardens and Herbal Medicine in History

*T*he garden as a vehicle of nature's perfection and harmony is indeed a rich image. Throughout history and in the mythology of many countries, the image of the garden as a wellspring of spiritual and physical healing power emerges repeatedly. Realizing that herbal and healing gardens have been with us always, since the days when mankind was young, lends richness and depth to our connection with gardens and healing plants today.

The garden myth of Eden described in the Old Testament is the one that most of us know best. Like all of the archetypal gardens, Eden is represented as a place where boundless peace prevailed. Sweet smells filled the air and brilliant flowers shone like precious gems. The great tree at the very center of the garden, an oft-repeated legendary motif, prevailed as the nourisher of all life. This tree was the source of the four great rivers which went out into the four directions. These rivers, in turn, spread the tree's nourishment throughout the garden, or world.

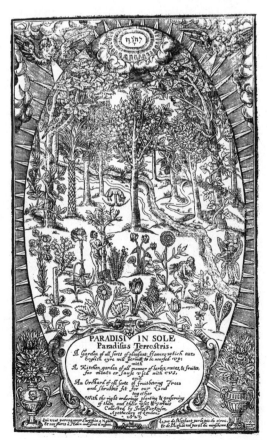

The Garden of Eden as depicted on the title page of a seventeenth century herbal by Parkinson, *Paradisi in Sole.*   (Courtesy of Hunt Institute for Botanical Documentation, Carnegie-Mellon University, Pittsburgh, Pa.)

1

The tree at the center of the garden was a very sacred presence. People in many ancient cultures venerated trees as symbols of longevity, strength, and fruitfulness. Trees embodied the perfect beauty and abundance of the natural world. They represented both the mysteries of change and the solidity of endurance.

The garden in myth and legend was a place of innocence and knowledge, too. In Sumerian and Babylonian garden legends, the serpent, the fruit of the tree, and the woman (symbolizing wisdom) are all accepted as beneficent, positive characters. Humankind's participation in the garden—eating its fruits of wisdom, enjoying its happy qualities—is an intimate and natural participation. As mythologist Joseph Campbell notes in his book, *Masks of God: Occidental Mythology:*

> There is no theme of guilt connected with the garden. The boon of the knowledge of life is there, in the sanctuary of the world, to be culled. And it is yielded willingly to any mortal, male or female, who reached for it with the proper will and readiness to receive.[1]

Here, the mythic garden is seen as a place of complete, natural harmony of body and mind. This view of the garden has prevailed in mythology throughout the ages. The story of the Buddha and the accord prevailing at the "cosmic tree" offers an example of the Eastern view of the garden as a place in which one could attain deep peace and understanding. The legendary gardens in the Pure Lands of the Buddhists were resplendent with jeweled trees and silken nets, redolent of pleasing fragrance, filled with the sounds of delicate bells and birdsongs, and the very earth was transmuted into gold. The gardens of Greek mythology include the Blessed or Fortunate

Isles, far beyond the known world, where Hesperides grew the golden apples of the sun in his garden. Greek legend also embraced the Elysian Fields described by the poet Homer, an earthly paradise and the dwelling place of happy souls after death.

In Tibetan mythology, the goddess of healing brought fragrant healing plants to the world. The gardens she planted, wonderful to behold, were capable of healing those who simply saw them or spent some time in them. The seven paradise gardens of the Mohammedans were also known as places of soothing tranquility. The Mohammedans valued so highly the idea of the garden as a healing beautiful place that they believed that in the afterlife they would dwell in these seven gardens. For them, paradise was a garden.

Ancient Near Eastern cultures combined the beauty and medicinal qualities of plants in their gardens. Around 600 B.C. a famous king, Nebuchadnezzar, confident in the restorative ability of a garden, had three acres of stadiumlike terraces planted with every type of tree, shrub, and flower. The gardens even included simulated mountains like those of his wife's native country. This wonderland was created to cure the queen, who was homesick. A visual extravaganza, it became one of the seven wonders of the world, the Hanging Gardens of Babylon.

In Europe, life in the early monasteries, divested of all frivolity, accorded gardening an indispensable role in the spiritual development of the brothers. The early Christian saints Jerome, Benedict, and Augustine admonished their monks to tend to their gardens as well as to their prayers. Monastery gardens were set in courtyards, surrounded by a cloister. From these simple cloistered gardens, monastery gardens expanded as the buildings of the monastery grew. Fragments of garden plans

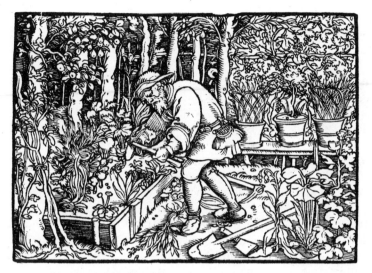

A European herb gardener at work in the sixteenth century. (Courtesy of Hunt Institute for Botanical Documentation, Carnegie-Mellon University, Pittsburgh, Pa.)

from monasteries of that era show physic, or medicinal herb gardens, a cloistered garden of grass and shrubs for the monks to walk in during contemplation, a vegetable or kitchen garden for nourishing the body, and an orchard, which often served also as a burial ground. The abbot himself often drew the garden plans. The monks planted the herbularis, or physic garden, near the infirmary, to be readily available, and so that sick people could enjoy a sort of visual and aroma therapy from its wonderful flowers and fragrances.

From Persia, the gardeners of medieval Europe learned to infuse the garden place with an expansiveness that nourished the spirit. Accustomed to centuries of cramped, protective living, Europeans discovered in the Levant during the Crusades a new open style of gardening. They not only imported wonderful plants such as damask and provence roses, oleanders, and pomegranates, the crusaders also learned to set up elegant tents outdoors on flower-spangled grasses. They enjoyed meals in this lush setting and celebrated games and tourneys in the midst of their garden freedom.

Such rustic scenes were immortalized by painters such as Botticelli.

The Japanese learned to use nature ingeniously as a way to evoke various responses or moods in the viewer. Precisely placed stones, tiny bonsai trees and shrubs, lanterns with the gentle light of candles, graceful bridges, and teahouses were some of the elements that figured in their subtle, complex system of classical landscape gardening. The different types of water basins and fences, sand gardens, rock gardens, and water gardens were more than just aesthetic design elements, they evoked the often understated bond between environment and well-being.

But as time passed, the close integration of nature and people's lives began to break down in many civilizations, and the garden was no longer as revered as it once had been. The coming of the scientific point of view, and in more modern times, of the industrial age, turned people's eyes away from nature as the source of healing power. This distancing can be traced in the history of medicine, too. Over the years, nature came to be regarded as a force to struggle against, not work with. Even in our early American history we encounter only a few opponents to the evolving idea that nature was threatening. Two champions of nature were William Byrd, a Virginia gentleman and scholar, and Estwick Evans, who undertook a wilderness walking tour. These two American intellectuals found the same calming, regenerative power in nature that their gardening forebears had.

In the nineteenth century, Henry David Thoreau and other writers of the transcendental movement gave voice to a deep love and respect for the solitude, beauty and wildness of nature. But their voices were never more than a fashionable overlay on the dominant mood of nineteenth century America, where the urge was to subdue and order wild nature.

Thoreau, like most of the transcendentalists, was ahead of his time, and largely ignored by his contemporaries. In fact, from the beginning of America's settlement by the Pilgrims to the middle of the nineteenth century, natural laws and natural places were not only ignored, they were frowned upon. This cultural bias had a profound influence on the development of medicine and the use of herbs in America.

Herbal Healing through the Ages

Prehistoric records reveal that ancient peoples collected herbs and other rare plants as eagerly as they amassed their more obvious treasures, for in that time plants were the main source of physical medicine. Some of the oldest records of actual medicinal uses for

nature's flora are bones from China. Dating back to 2000 B.C. these "oracle bones" are etched with the names of plants and diseases. Other ancient records include a Chinese herbal from 5000 B.C. which lists herbs still in use today, such as rhubarb, poppy, aconite, and ephedra, (which was used even then to treat asthma). Tablets, papyruses, and other old documents from Egypt, Babylon, Crete, Sumeria, India, and ancient Greece describe the ways in which herbs and plants were used as medicine by healers in those societies.

The oldest known systems of medicine in the world today are those of China and India. Chinese medicine has given us two healing techniques which are still very much in use today—pulse diagnosis and acupuncture. Acupuncture is thought to have originated as early as 2700 B.C. In addition, the system of Chinese polypharmacy, which has survived into modern times, is widely acclaimed as one of the most complete and effective herbal traditions extant today.

The origins of Chinese medicine are associated with three legendary emperors: Fu Hsi, circa 2852 B.C., who formulated the theory of yin and yang; Shen Nung, "the divine farmer," (circa 2697 B.C.) father of both agriculture and of herbal medicine; and Huang Ti, who lived sometime between 2697 and 2595 B.C. He is thought to be the author of *The Nei Ching,* or *Yellow Emperor's Classic of Internal Medicine,* which is still used in China as a medical text.

From the third century B.C. to the seventh century A.D., Chinese medicine was highly influenced by the philosophy and example of Taoist sages who believed in preventing disease through moderation. The Chinese used acupuncture, herbs, massage, diet, and gentle exercises to correct imbalances within the body. They diagnosed through the pulse, and through features of the face, hands, or feet.

The Indian medical system is known as Ayurveda, the "science of life." The origin of Ayurveda is difficult to determine. It is so ancient that it defies the skills of scholars and archeologists alike. In addition, Ayurveda's own account is that the tradition is ageless, like life itself. The explanation for this view goes like this: all things have an instinctive ability to heal themselves. This natural sensitivity forms the basis of Ayurvedic science. Therefore, the essence of Ayurveda has coexisted with life from the very beginning.

According to mythology, the science of Ayurveda came from the realm of the gods. (In Hindu cosmology, gods are a class of beings who have magical powers and live very long lives. They are somewhat similar to the pantheon of classical Greek gods.) The god Brahma was the first one to perceive the principles of Ayurveda. He taught it to the Aswin twins, who became the physicians of the gods. From them the god Indra learned Ayurveda, and he taught it to a small group of human disciples. These physicians then taught the science of life to other physicians of the human realm. Eventually, it spread throughout all of India and much of the ancient world.

Ayurveda was incorporated into most texts of the *Vedas,* the ancient scriptures upon which Hindu culture and religion are based. The *Vedas* are thought to have existed since 10,000 B.C. Although no written records remain from that far back, it is certain that Ayurveda was already highly developed by 1000 B.C. It continued to evolve until about A.D. 1100. By the twelfth century A.D., due to invasions, Ayurveda lost its state patronage and diminished slightly. But it still evolved, particularly along the lines

of mineral and botanical medicine, until well into the sixteenth century.

In the *Rigveda,* over 1,000 medicinal plants are listed, and a special group of sages who knew the secrets of plants is described. These ancient doctors are said to have made artificial limbs, cured wounds, used the soma plant as an anaesthetic (soma is now thought to be a mushroom, *Amanita muscaria*), performed cauterization, and opened obstructed bladders with a surgical instrument.

Indians believe the Vedic works were developed at a time when knowledge, which they view as the masculine principle, and wisdom, the feminine principle, were in balance. In this sense the Indian medical system resembles that of the Chinese, who also feel their medicine developed through intuition and revelation in a distant past Golden Age. The *Charaka Samhita,* one of the most famous Indian medical texts, dating back to preliterate times, was preserved for many generations by oral tradition. Written down at last in the first century A.D., the text mentions 500 herbal drugs. As we will see in chapter 3, Ayurveda had a very strong influence on the herbal healing tradition which developed in Tibet.

The Indian system, like the Chinese system, works to maintain health and prevent disease through a balance of diet, exercise, thought, and environment. Ayurvedic medicine holds the expansive view that "nothing exists in the realm of thought or experience that cannot be used as a medicine." Treatments include not only herbs and other natural substances, diet, and exercise, but also mental and physical practices intended to help the sick person develop positive emotions and qualities. These practices, called yogas, have their parallel in Chinese medicine in the physical and mental exercises of the Taoists, such as Tai Chi, Pa Kua, Chi Kung, and the five animal exercises. All of these disciplines are devoted to changing and regulating the body's vital energies, and to refining the mind.

Dioscorides' famous herbal, written during the first century A.D., contains many references to Indian herbs and treatments. This herbal, which attests to the influence of Indian medicine on the West, is only one example of a continuous flow of medical information from India to the Mediterranean area from Roman times onward.

Like Chinese medicine, Ayurvedic medicine has suffered a decline in modern times. With the British rule of India, Western medicine eclipsed Ayurveda. But now, Indian traditional medicine is experiencing a renaissance and is being explored through modern scientific methods as well as traditional practices. These two great living medical systems, the Chinese and the Ayurvedic, of India and Tibet, allow modern peoples to stay in touch with richly informative traditions. We will learn more about them in chapter 3.

Egyptian and European Medical Systems

Like the ancient medical traditions of China and India, those of Egypt and Greece shared an underlying assumption that nature itself was a healing agent. Each of these systems regarded the human body as a miniature model of the universe and believed that changes in diet and exercise should concur with seasonal changes in the outer world. Behaving according to the dictates of nature could only benefit and increase one's health and well-being, the ancients believed. All of these systems shared a steadfast belief in

plant medicines, the major source of remedies used.

The famous Ebers papyrus, dating back to about 1550 B.C., reveals that the ancient Egyptians knew and used about one-third of the plants in the modern pharmacopoeia. This is an astonishing fact, considering how long ago their culture flourished, and how relatively limited the boundaries of the known world were then. Most of their medicines were of plant origin. Cardamom, garlic, lily, thyme, celandine, juniper, lotus, linseed, fennel, poppy—these and many other plants known today were favored long ago in Egypt. Physicians who were also skilled in the use of mineral medicines contributed to the development of a more refined pharmacy by introducing careful weights and measures. This resulted in standardized doses of medicines.

Egyptian medicine benefited from the trade that by 1500 B.C. linked that country to many other lands. From other parts of Africa, Egyptian travelers brought back plant medicines such as myrrh gum, olibanum, sandalwood, and black alder bark and berries. Sabaean traders from the southwestern tip of the Arabian Desert introduced their own native frankincense to Egypt, as well as exotic plants and plant substances from China and India. These included cinnamon, ginger, the root and bark of the pomegranate tree, and calamus or sweet flag, which were employed according to their prescriptions in Chinese and Indian Ayurvedic medicines. The Cretan civilization of 2000 B.C. also had a strong influence on Egyptian medicine. Saffron, sage, and henna are among the plant medicines that came to Egypt from Crete.

The Egyptians knew how to use herbs as antiseptics and antibiotics. They fed the pyramid builders huge amounts of garlic, radish seeds and juice, and onions to keep them healthy, according to the Greek historian Herodotus. The Egyptians also knew the antibiotic effects both of bread mold and the yeasty lees of beer.

Greek Temple and Rational Medicine

The system of medicine that evolved in ancient Greece, which owed a great deal of its medical knowledge to Egypt, Babylon, and Persia, distinguishes two types of healing, referred to as temple and rational medicine.

As the name suggests, temple medicine was practiced in restful hillside temples. Set in the midst of fragrant groves of sacred trees, temples were natural settings for holistic healing. Carefully planted herb and flower gardens, the clear air, and the sheer beauty of the natural landscape must have been very soothing to the sick. Temple medicine included the use of herbs, massage, exercise, seasonal diet, prayer, and ritual. In fact, these old temples have much in common with our modern holistic health centers, where assorted techniques such as dream therapy, standard Jungian psychology, guided imagery, and "dream" yoga may be used to encourage self-healing. The sick person's environment, diet, level of exercise and relaxation, and inner life were all taken into account in temple medicine, and treatment was designed to balance his system with gentle, integrated methods.

The rational medicine developed by the Greeks had its first great voice in Hippocrates, who remains one of the most enduring influences on the type of medicine which our physicians practice today. It can be argued, as we will see in the next chapter, that Hippocrates had a greater influence than anyone else on the direction in which healing and the use of herbs developed in Europe. His clinical observations of diseases and their stages became a model of Greek science and method. The *Hippocratic Corpus,* a huge body of writings, was a rich source of information for later European healers, although interestingly enough, it was not all written by Hippocrates himself (in fact it shows an Egyptian imprint and style). Hippocrates used herbs to treat his patients, although he did not seem to be aware of as many medicinal plants as the healers of ancient Egypt or India were. Hippocrates' pharmacopoeia included holy thistle, mint, peony, thyme, rosemary, burdock, anise, clove, cinnamon, and violet. Hippocratic medicine popularized the notion first put forth by the great philosopher-mathematician Pythagoras that *nature itself was healing.* In his work entitled *On Epidemics,* Hippocrates tells us, "It is nature itself that finds the way; though untaught and uninstructed, it does what is proper."[2]

The Influence of Galen and Dioscorides

In the first century A.D. lived two Romans, Dioscorides and Galen, who had a lasting influence on Western medicine. Dioscorides wrote five books about medicines from the animal, vegetable, and mineral kingdoms. The works of Dioscorides, as well as those of Galen, were used extensively by healers for the next 1,500 years.

Galen is an early example of the sort of physician who sets himself up as an ultimate authority. Vain and boastful, Galen maintained a very different attitude from the one reflected in Hippocrates' code of ethics. Even in his time the attitude that would ultimately evolve into the separation of "modern" medicine from plant and "natural" forms of medicine was present. Galen created an elaborate system for classifying herbs, but he favored expensive medicines compounded of many ingredients. In the early days of the Christian church, believers were castigated if they had too much faith in Galen's medicine. However, by the Middle Ages, Galen had become the ultimate medical authority. And his influence lasted until the end of the medieval era.

Galenic medicine is characterized by a reliance on theory and scholastic learning, complex, exotic polypharmacy at the expense of simple, native pharmacy, and the supremacy and infallibility of the doctor. Galen was so successful, according to his own report on the matter, that other envious Roman physicians would have liked to take his life.

The Important Role of Monasteries

After the fall of Rome in A.D. 500, agriculture, horticulture, and medicine were preserved only through the monastic system. When Christianity made its way to the British Isles in A.D. 597, along with it came plants and fragments of medical knowledge garnered from the Greek and Roman masters. An extensive herbal and medical folk tradition already existed in Wales through the Druid tradition, which dated back to at least a thousand years before Christ. An Anglo-Saxon medicine began to develop, combining the old Druidic ways with the Greek and Roman influences. It was the duty of monks to care for the sick, and this they did, with the help of what scraps of Greek and Roman herbals reached them, what traditional medical knowledge met them, and

what the experience of their own gardens and patients taught them.

Early in the sixth century A.D., Cassiodorus urged his monks to "study with care the nature of herbs and the compounding of drugs. If you have no knowledge of Greek, you have at hand the Herbarium of Dioscorides, who fully described the flowers of the field and illustrated them with his drawings. After that read Hippocrates and Galen . . ."

During the next 500 years, Anglo-Saxon medicine relied more and more heavily upon fragments of medical knowledge that came from Greece and Rome. *The Leech Book of Bald,* written by a monk in the tenth century, was a compilation of some of the most useful writings that had survived from the Greek and Roman medical traditions.

Exotic Influences from Arabia

Italy's Salerno school of medicine, established in the tenth century A.D., became a vehicle for the learnings of Arab physicians. The Arabian Muslims believed that God, in his wisdom, had provided medicines aplenty in nature (a belief which finds its counterpart in the Old Testament). Arab physicians enthusiastically researched plant medicines and developed a vast amount of information on healing plants from Europe, Persia, India, and the Far East. The Arab businessmen also took an active interest in herbs: they were the first occidental pharmacists and had opened their shops in Baghdad by the early ninth century. Another Arab contribution was the use of astrology in medicine. In Arabic culture, astrology was regarded as a science that could help in the selection of medicines and the treatment of diseases.

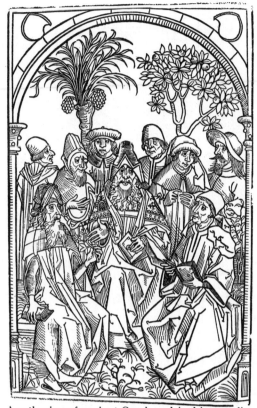

A gathering of ancient Greek and Arabian medical authorities. (Courtesy of Hunt Institute for Botanical Documentation, Carnegie-Mellon University, Pittsburgh, Pa.)

After the Crusades, Arabian pharmaceutical expertise took root in Europe. Highly sweetened and exotically spiced preparations made with plants from faraway lands became popular healing agents. However, the study of native plants still found no favor. Herbalists who had inherited the common sense of the old folk medicine tradition were legally and socially separated from the so-called proper practice of medicine. Folk remedies and the old local traditions of herbal wisdom became more and more of a threat to the medical academies.

Paracelsus

But despite its fall from favor with the medical establishment of the day, the folk tradition of herbal medicine endured. From the latter part of the tenth century onward, herbals, although no model of clarity or accuracy, were written in the native languages of England, Germany, and other European countries. Thus, herbal remedies remained accessible to the common people. Paracelsus, the son of a Swiss chemist and physician, learned about medicinal plants and minerals from his father and was a strong advocate of writing in the common tongue. This was a major departure from the tradition of keeping all herbals and pharmacopoeias in Latin (a practice which effectively kept all the knowl-

(continued on page 12)

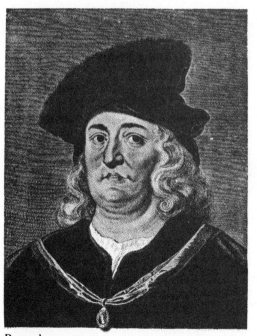

Paracelsus. (Courtesy of Hunt Institute for Botanical Documentation, Carnegie-Mellon University, Pittsburgh, Pa.)

Health Books in the Middle Ages

During the Middle Ages many health books were written to guide lay people. An example of one such book is *The Medieval Health Handbook,* or *Tacuinum Sanitatus In Medicina.* Based on the system of humors and subtle qualities as set forth by Hippocrates, it codified the complexities of the science into simple charts and phrases. The introduction states that it was written in order to "shorten long-winded discourses and synthesize the various ideas," with the intention "not to neglect the advice of the ancients." One entry, placed under a beautiful painting of luxurious fennel plants, reads:

Nature: Warm in the third degree, dry in the second. At other times, warm and dry in the second degree. *Optimum:* The domestic variety, fresh, with a strong taste. *Usefulness:* For the eyes, purifies the eyesight, stimulates milk and urine flow, diminishes flatulence. *Dangers:* It is digested slowly. *Neutralization of the Dangers:* By chewing it well. *Effects:* General bilious humors. It is suitable for cold temperaments, for old people, in Winter when it is possible to find it, in cold regions and in all others in which it grows.

This kind of natural healing knowledge combined empirically discovered physical properties of herbs (for instance, "purifies the eyesight, stimulates milk") with their qualitative or subtle properties (such as, "warm and dry in the second degree").

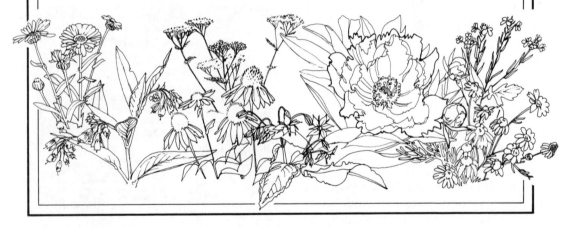

Nicholas Culpeper

One of the most popular herbals of all time is the one written by Nicholas Culpeper in the seventeenth century. Culpeper's herbal is still in print today, and has been published in more than 41 editions over the years. Like Paracelsus, Culpeper wrote in the common tongue. He worked for an apothecary, and he actually taught his master the Latin needed to understand the official pharmacopoeia. Culpeper soon left his job to open his own apothecary shop in a poor section of London, where he treated the common people without prescribing expensive imported medicines.

Culpeper was part of a grassroots movement that threatened both physicians and apothecaries of the day by popularizing simple herbal medicine. Today, parts of Culpeper's *Herbal* are somewhat amusing. It is laced with strange statements, and allusions to the astrological influences of plants. For basil he wrote, "an herb of Mars and under the Scorpion, and therefore called basilicon, it is no marvel if it carry a virulent quality with it." He added that a French physician, "affirms of his own knowledge that an acquaintance of his, by common smelling to it, had a scorpion bred in his brain." But to the people of that time, medical astrology was highly respected. Culpeper treated patients without making a mystery out of medicine, in contrast to physicians of the day who cloaked themselves in a medical mystique.

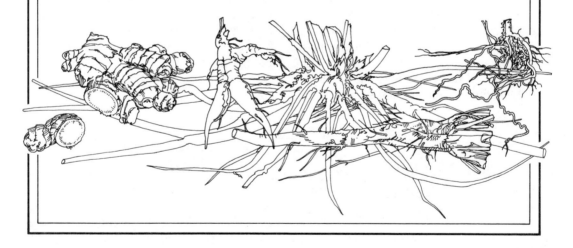

edge, and thus, the practice of medicine, in the hands of college-trained physicians).

Paracelsus, who is remembered by historians primarily as the greatest alchemist (his name means literally, "greater than Celsus"), changed the course of medicine in the western world. He catalyzed the movement toward mineral medicines, a movement that would be taken up much later by chemists of the nineteenth and twentieth centuries. He also predicted the discovery of pharmacologically "active principles" in plants and other substances, but he lacked the research tools to properly isolate and study them.

Paracelsus believed that all medicinal substances, plant or otherwise, contained an essential principle that was pure and entirely beneficial. It was the role of the physician-alchemist, he proclaimed, to discover these subtle secrets of nature and make them available to humanity. To this end he labored long hours in his laboratory, distilling, mixing, shaking, decanting, heating, compounding, rubbing, and otherwise working to effect a "sublimation" of common herbs and minerals.

100 foreign ones, including the first presentation in print of the American corn and pumpkin.

Although few physicians in the sixteenth and seventeenth centuries showed interest in botanic medicine research, some of the most famous herbals have endured from this period. Surgeon John Gerard's *Herbal* was published in 1597. Gerard's love of plants was obvious from the wonderful illustrations that graced his book, and from his enthusiasm for gardening.

Women of the time also contributed to the survival of herbal knowledge. Throughout the history of herbalism, herbalists were often women, sometimes called "wise women." This phenomenon was especially noticeable during the Renaissance. Acting as their family doctors and apothecaries, they prepared or supervised the making of herbal medicines and cosmetics for their families. Often they made carefully compiled notebooks of herbal recipes, which were handed down from mother to daughter.

The Contributions of Botanists and Homemakers

During the Renaissance, botanists began the creation of specimen, or "botanic," gardens. The sixteenth century German physician-botanist Leonhard Fuchs, for whom the fuchsia was named, published in 1542 a landmark book on medicinal plants that set the style for plant description for future botanical writers. He reported 400 native plants, and

Healing Plants in Modern Science

Modern science is no stranger to medicinal plants. More than 25 percent of the medicines commonly used today contain constituents derived directly from plants. Digitalis, one of the modern doctor's most useful drugs for heart disease, came from the lovely foxglove plant. In 1775, Dr. William Withering had discovered its uses in treating angina (which was called dropsy) by following up a lead on an old family remedy. Penicillin, first discovered in soil mold, became a panacea for treating many kinds of infections. Ephedrine, used to treat asthma, was isolated from the ephedra plant, which had long been used in China for the same purpose. Reserpine, a drug used to lower blood pressure, was first extracted in 1947 by the giant Swiss chemical company, Ciba. The company found it in the rauwolfia plant, which was famous as a folk remedy in India. And two drugs used in the treatment of cancer were derived from the alkaloids vincaleukoblastine and leurocristine, which are contained in the Madagascar periwinkle plant.

As these examples show, the healing substances from plants can be extremely powerful.

Herbal Healing— Expression of a Whole System

Throughout all its history, natural medicine has been in many ways a study of the relationship between the entire universe and the individual organism. That is, health and sickness have been seen as the opposite expressions of a single whole system. This view was healing in itself, because antagonism was replaced with openness and acceptance. The healer and patient felt themselves a part of, rather than apart from, the whole of magnificent creation.

The natural healing systems described in chapters 2 and 3 are among the oldest and most popular herbal traditions in the world. The knowledge contained within them represents hundreds—even thousands—of years of empirical research and experimentation. Although these systems of logic may not corre-

spond with those of science, they are valuable, because they have worked for many healers. Modern medicine and science are based only on a theory of gross or measurable elements. Holistic health systems can be more flexible, sensitive, and effective because they work with both the tangible factors of material medicines, as well as with more subtle or immeasurable ones that often affect health.

An example of a subtle element in a natural healing system would be the element of fire. Fire in this context refers to the broad class of natural phenomena that are somehow—in fact or in essence—related to fire. The fire element would include the sun, a burning match, the summer season, midday, a fever, a plant that produces burning (such as cayenne), a person with a hot temper, the heart and blood, a nuclear reactor, and so on. A holistic treatment for someone with a lack of the fire element might include bathing, keeping warm, expressing and/or releasing suppressed anger, moxibustion treatment (see page 50), drinking hot tea, or taking stimulating medicines.

Most healing systems classify universal phenomena into groups of four or five subtle elements such as earth, air, fire, and water (as in the European system) or earth, water, fire, air, and space (as in the Ayurvedic discipline). Factors such as taste, color, sound, direction, season, a person's constitution, diet and activities, former diseases, and so on all affect these subtle elements. Natural healing systems attempt to be all-inclusive, to take into account the wide variety of such internal and external phenomena. It is for this very reason that we can even consider gardening—an external activity that yields fruits for internal satisfaction—as a form of healing.

Every culture has its own ways of interpreting and working with natural healing principles. For example, Europe has Naturopathy, the Chinese have the theory of yin and yang and the five-element system. An overview of these individual healing systems, which all have roots in the ancient world, reveals some of the unifying patterns upon which all are based. In the next two chapters we will explore some of these traditions and the ways in which they have employed herbs to heal.

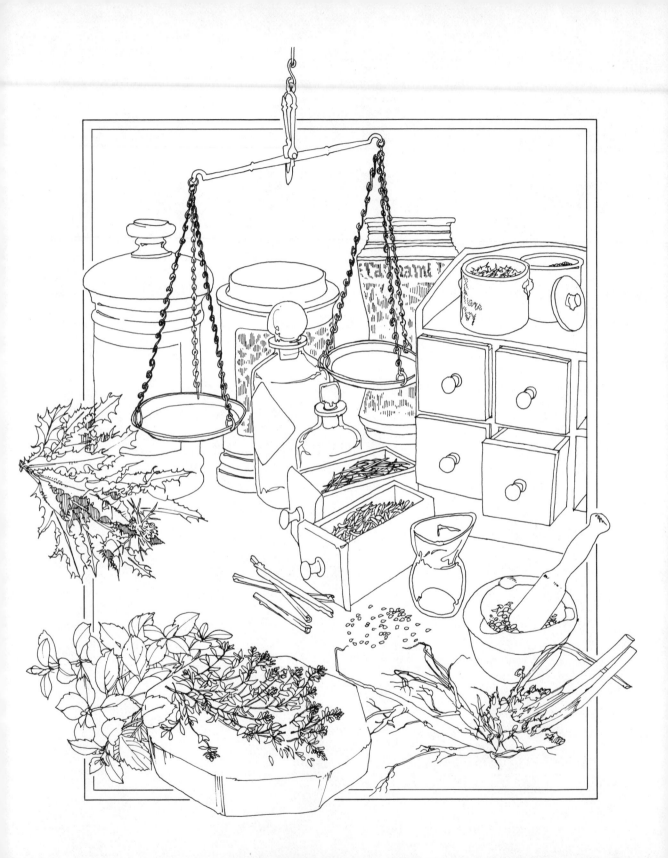

Herbal Healing Traditions in Europe and America

As herbalism developed in Europe, healers began to assign specific properties to the plants they employed. An herb became recognized as cooling or warming, as calming or stimulating. There were numerous ways to discern these herbal properties, perhaps the best known of which was the Doctrine of Signatures, which we will discuss later in this chapter. In treating their patients, early European herbalists selected herbs whose properties would counteract the cause of the ailment. All illnesses were caused, they believed, by an imbalance of "humors" in the body. This theory of humors originated with Hippocrates, known as the Father of Medicine, the one person who has had the greatest impact on the development of natural healing disciplines in Europe.

Hippocrates' Theories of Healing

According to Hippocrates, there are two ways to approach sickness. One is to eliminate the symptoms of disease in the patient, and the other is to restore the patient to health. Hippocrates thus distinguished partial or symptomatic healing from holistic healing. He believed that treating disease as a set of symptoms merely stops the progression of the illness. Even though the "disease" has been treated, a low level of sickness remains in the person because the underlying causes are still there.

In order to explain the holistic approach, Hippocrates introduced the theory of the "healing crisis" to Western medicine. During a crisis, he reasoned, the body goes back through the development of the illness, one stage at a time. One after another, various symptoms of the disease appear as toxins are eliminated from the body. The crisis is a period of regression, meaning a process of returning back to health as the original condition.

Hippocrates taught that a healing crisis should be respected as positive and natural, rather than as something to be eliminated through treatment. When a crisis is stopped, he believed, the body's natural healing pro-

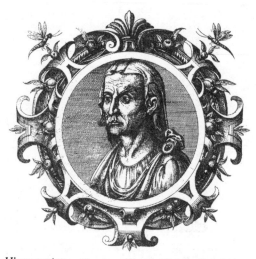

Hippocrates. (Courtesy of Hunt Institute for Botanical Documentation, Carnegie-Mellon University, Pittsburgh, Pa.)

cess is also stopped. Accordingly, the role of the healer is to guide the patient (or oneself) *through* the illness to its natural conclusion, rather than to *stop* the illness.

It is important, however, to know the difference between crisis and sickness. A general guideline is that sickness arises first, and crisis comes after treatment has begun. Hippocrates' "advice" was to let the crisis, or nature, take its course: "When a disease has attained the crisis," he ordered, "or when a crisis has just passed, do not disturb the patient with innovation in treatment either by the administration of drug or by giving stimulants. Let them be."[1]

The Four Humors

Hippocrates' ways of determining the causes of disease were remarkably similar to those being used at the same time (the fifth century B.C.) in India and China. Echoing Indian

Ayurvedic medical theory, Hippocrates described the human body as being composed of:

> . . . blood, phlegm, yellow bile, and black bile. These are the things that make up its constitution and cause its pains and health. Health is primarily that state in which these constituent substances are in the correct proportion to each other.[2]

According to Hippocrates, these humors interact with each other, with a person's diet and activities, and with the environment. The humors correspond to the four elements which the Greeks believed made up all matter (earth, air, fire, and water).

Hippocrates refined and demonstrated the theory of elements and humors with his astute clinical skills. By carefully observing the quantities of bile, phlegm, and blood in his many patients, Hippocrates noted a correlation between changes in the seasons and shifts in the balance of the humors. (The humors were believed to be affected by nonphysical influences but were themselves expressed through physical substances. Hippocrates' measurements were therefore of *quantities* of blood, phlegm, and bile.)

Hippocrates found that in winter, phlegm is predominant. In spring, the blood humor increases and predominates during the summer. During this season phlegm is minimal. Bile increases in autumn. Hippocrates further discovered that an imbalance caused by too much phlegm in winter is naturally cured by the arrival of summer. Similarly, he found that diseases of bile start in fall but subside in spring. And annual cycles of humoral imbalances are corrected naturally with the coming of a new year.

These observations led Hippocrates to formulate a general theory of healing: "treat disease by the principle of opposition to the cause."[3] Accordingly, Hippocrates used foods and herbs as a way of effecting an exchange between the four humors and the four seasons. In order to relate these internal and external factors, Hippocrates used another set of four qualities: hot, cold, dry, and wet. In a discussion in "The Nature of Man," Hippocrates wrote that "the elements, heat, cold, dryness and wetness . . . are all mutually interdependent."[4] According to Hippocrates' theory, then, in winter, when it is very cold and wet outside, we should eat foods that are dry and warming. Conversely, in the summer, foods should be lighter, cooling and with more fluid, to counteract the heat and dryness of that season. Because of its simplicity and commonsense approach, this system found widespread application among early European herbalists and gave rise to the practice of identifying these kinds of general qualities in the herbs they used.

Pharmacological Properties of Herbs

The humoral pathology of Hippocrates is only vaguely referred to by western herbalists today. According to modern science, most of the active effects plants have on the human body are created by a single or a few active components within a mixture of substances found within the plant. Each active component may have one or many effects. The assignation of qualities like hot, dry, cold, and wet may seem simplistic to us today, because we don't understand how they relate to pharmacologically active ingredients. But when the ancients observed a plant with a given quality to be producing an effect on the body, such as inducing perspiration, for instance, they had no way except simple observation to determine if the plant was indeed causing the effect and creating no other side effects at the same time. But although medical research today has become vastly more sophisticated, many herbalists still work with the idea of plants having recognizable qualities. And the idea of humors remains with us in subtle ways we may not notice. We may speak of someone as being in "good humor," without realizing that the concept goes all the way back to Hippocrates and his definition of the humors within us all.

However, the simple assignment of basic properties to herbs is fascinating to read about. After all, these properties formed the basis of a long tradition of folk healing that persisted in Europe for thousands of years, and that grew up in America, too. Some herbalists still define herbs in terms of these simple qualities, and we will refer to them in our discussions of individual plants in chapter 4. So let us trace a bit of the development of Hippocrates' system and its applications in European herbal healing.

A key to the use of these subtle qualities in herbology is to recognize that they are understood to complement basic pharmacological science. For example, herbalists say that ginger is drying and warming because they believe that it increases urination and causes perspiration. Therefore it is called, among other things, a "diuretic" and a "diaphoretic" (these terms are all defined in the glossary at the back of this book). These are the herb's pharmacological properties—the effect on a person's body—which herbalists have traditionally observed in their patients.

In herbology, plants are perceived to have varying combinations of qualities and degrees of each quality, too. A plant can be both heating and drying, or heating and moistening. It can be cooling and drying, or cooling and moistening. One herb can be very warming, while another may be just slightly warming. But both are considered heating herbs.

The way in which these qualities are assigned to plants is really very simple. Heating herbs are believed to produce warmth in the body. Generally speaking, all of the aromatic herbs, such as anise and caraway, are considered warming. Many of the bitter herbs, such as Oregon grape, are also classified as heating.

Cooling herbs, on the other hand, are those which healers believe take heat away

Interview with Dr. Ed Alstat:
Naturopathic Medicine

QUESTION: Dr. Alstat, could you describe how you got interested in naturopathic medicine?
ANSWER: Well, I graduated from pharmacy school in 1969, and then spent seven years working as a retail and hospital pharmacist. But something wasn't right. After awhile I saw that the people I was dispensing medicines to weren't being cured by them. I began to wonder if I could even help myself if I got sick. So I decided to take some time off and examine it. Someone gave me a copy of *Organic Gardening,* and I started a garden. I had always been interested in medicinal plants, and I started to grow some of them in my little garden. The combination of a new life-style and a little more research convinced me of herbal healing's validity. So I went back to school to become a naturopathic doctor.

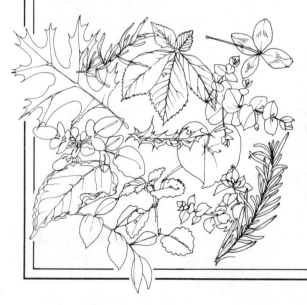

QUESTION: Dr. Alstat, you were trained as a pharmacist and as a naturopath. Can you describe how you integrate the different disciplines in your practice?
ANSWER: From my studies as a pharmacist I've learned that generally, plants have a pharmacological principle that is their guiding mechanism. But in a lot of herbal books the list of symptoms that an herb cures is endless. When most laypersons read that, they wonder how one plant can treat so many conditions. And there seems to be twelve plants that you can use for the same problem, too. Often, they try one and maybe it works and maybe it doesn't.

For example, you may see an herb that is basically for the nervous system which is also "for coughs." But if you have a cough with a sinus drainage, then you wouldn't use an herb that would supress the nervous system. If you understand what's causing the cough initially, and if you understand the mechanism of the herb, then you can apply an herb that is simply an expectorant, and will keep the mucus loose and out of the lungs.

From the naturopath's point of view, each person is an individual. It's good to know the pharmacology of the plant, too. But what may work for one person, even on a pharmacological principle, may not be as effective in the same dosage for another person. [Different people have varying degrees of sensitivity to the active principles in herbs and medicines.] Because of this, the textbook description of a lot of herbal properties won't be of so much value. You will have to approach each person in a completely different way. When using a holistic approach, it's hard to define a simple herb remedy in most cases.

QUESTION: It seems that you're saying it isn't enough to just read books and learn what's in them.

from the body, or from some part of the body. Often, plants that contain highly volatile oils (like wintergreen or spearmint) are categorized as cooling. Cooling herbs (borage is another example) are known as refrigerants. To get an idea of what a refrigerant is, think of a hot summer day, and then imagine eating a slice of watermelon or cucumber. These are two of the best-known refrigerant foods.

Whether an herb is classified as moistening or drying depends on its individual properties, also. An herb that has been observed

---

ANSWER: Yes. It takes a lot of knowledge to use an herb correctly. It's my opinion that people nowadays have been misled by the popular attitude of "Well, just take this herb and use it for this. . . ." Back in the early 1900s and before that, when herbalism was used a lot more than it is today, I believe people knew a great deal more about herbs. There were things that were not taught, but were simply taken for granted. Not all of this information has been transferred to the general public.

But there are herbs that can be used without a great deal of learning, also. They are applied, not so much as a treatment for a disease or condition, but as an overall strengthener of the body, or for a nutritive value. They are commonly called "alteratives," implying that they are nutritionally effective for many different conditions.

QUESTION: What are some of your favorite and safe herbs that you would recommend?
ANSWER: Well, if I had to choose, garlic would be number one, as far as a very common herb that's easy to grow and store. It probably has more therapeutic value than half of the rest of the herbs. And then, I would also keep calendula, which is safe enough and is very good for surface problems, scrapes and so on. Hypericum (St. John's wort) is a good safe plant; the flowers especially, as an infusion in oil, are good for bruises and injuries. The echinacea is probably the most valuable plant in the naturopathic repertoire. It is pretty safe in normal dosage, but like any plant, if you use it for too long you may begin to have side effects. If you use *anything* for too long you will experience side effects. Even chamomile, if used too often can create the same symptoms that it was intended to treat. In this respect, using herbs is very similar to the principles of homeopathy.

And then, there's a lot of value in dandelion, and burdock, which are both safe. Also, yellow dock. All these give you a pretty broad therapeutic range.

QUESTION: What are some herbs you would recommend the novice herbalist to stay away from?
ANSWER: Well, you should probably stay away from poke, which is a very good herb but is potentially dangerous, and then the obvious ones like aconite, tansy, poison oak, foxglove. There *are* herbs that will get you in trouble pretty quickly. But there are so many safe herbs that are easy to find and are more popular.

QUESTION: What would you recommend to the person who has read a few books about herbs and is interested in gardening? How would you recommend they proceed in using plants for health and the prevention of disease?
ANSWER: It's good to start working with the safe herbs, learning as you go. The culinary herbs, which have a lot of medicinal properties, are a good place to begin. And learn the herbs in your backyard. Don't get carried away in the beginning with some of the more exotic herbs.

You should definitely learn the identification of the plants. If you're going to experiment or try to use herbs for therapy, make sure that you've got the right herb. For example, a person who's first beginning to learn about herbs might go to the nursery and look for calendula. Well, calendula is commonly called marigold, too. But that particular marigold in the nursery may not be the correct one, but a completely different species. The names are often interchanged. And when we're looking into nursery stock, the plant names are often confused.

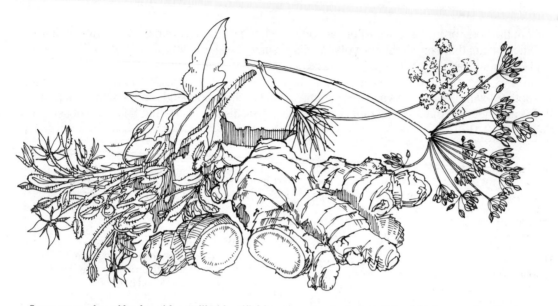

Some examples of herbs with readily identifiable properties include, left to right, borage (cooling), ginger (warming and drying), and fennel (moistening).

to increase urination, such as bearberry, is considered drying. Any astringent herb, such as oak bark or sage, is also called drying. Usually the aromatics (like anise or caraway) are thought of as drying. But there are exceptions: fennel, for example, is regarded as moistening (it is said to increase milk in lactating women). An herb is also considered to be moistening if it is mucilaginous or demulcent (soothing). Flax seed, marshmallow, licorice, and slippery elm are good examples of this latter type of moistening herb.

Traditional Functions of Herbs in the Body

One way European herbalists began to develop a better understanding of herbal properties was to think in terms of parts of the body that they thought were influenced by each herb. That is, they began to define for

each herb specific "centers of activity" in the body. For example, cayenne pepper, classified as a heating herb, was designated as affecting the circulatory system because it was observed to increase the flow of blood, especially to the capillaries near the surface of the skin. Perhaps this explains why people who live in very hot climates use hot peppers in their cooking. The peppers may actually help them to dissipate body heat by circulating it to the skin surface, where it then causes cooling as perspiration evaporates and heat radiates into the surrounding air.

Ginger is another heating herb that is assigned properties similar to those of cayenne. But ginger's center of activity is defined as lying primarily in the internal organs. In the traditional European system, it is thought to create a type of heat that stays inside the body. Ginger is therefore used by herbalists in the winter and in more northern climates. They employ it as a remedy for colds and to "strengthen" the kidneys and bladder. These differences between cayenne and ginger are due to the body's different centers of activity for each herb.

To make matters more complex, herbs are not limited to just one center of activity, either. There are many herbs that are used to treat several diverse problems at once, such as acne, constipation, headaches, lethargy, and indigestion, for example. The primary center of action for such an herb could theoretically be the liver and gall bladder, where it would be thought to cause an increase in bile secretion. The theory goes like this: Increased bile secretion improves digestion of fats and oils, which in turn improves complexion. An increase of bile will also help alleviate chronic constipation. Cleansing the colon is an important function. The accumulation of toxins in the bowels, due to poor food decomposition and elimination, contributes toward a generally toxic condition which can result in many of the symptoms listed above. Toxins in the colon are absorbed by the blood, therefore, the cleaner the colon is, the cleaner the blood will be. And the liver helps filter toxins from the blood. If the liver's rate of activity is increased, then the blood will contain fewer toxins. Many gall bladder/liver-centered herbs —such as Oregon grape—are described as affecting the body in all these ways. Such theories are simplistic in modern medical terms, and largely unsubstantiated by medical research. But traditional herbology does not approach healing from the perspective of laboratory analysis. It has always been based on empirical observation of individual people.

Types of Activity in Herbs

In addition to their properties and centers of activity, herbalists recognize three "types of activity" in herbs. An herb can be designated eliminating, building, and/or neutralizing. Very basically, eliminators are herbs that are seen to cause the body to urinate, perspire, defecate, sneeze, cough, salivate, expectorate, vomit, dissipate (nervous energy), or excrete (waste matter from the blood or tissues). In holistic healing terminology, eliminators are said to cause a loss of energy. Their use is based on the assumption that to begin with, there is an excess of something in the body. For example, according to this theory, when the pathways of elimination from the body are blocked by constipation, waste products and toxins accumulate and can eventually cause serious illness. Eliminating herbs are used to correct this problem. On the other hand, if there is no excess to begin with, the use of eliminating herbs can cause a deficiency. Some examples of herbs that have traditionally been called eliminators include:

Butternut	Because the bark is traditionally used as a laxative.
Ginger	A heating herb that is considered diaphoretic and slightly diuretic.
Mustard	Mustard seeds are famous as an emetic.
Peppermint	One of its traditional functions is to dispel gas.
Sage	One of its uses has been as a mild nervine which is reputed to reduce excess nervous energy.
Thyme	It is sometimes used as an expectorant to clear the lungs and nose.

Building herbs perform the reverse function of eliminators in traditional herbology. Herbalists believe they help the body conserve or increase energy in a variety of ways. This property makes building herbs valuable for preventive health maintenance, and they have also been employed in treating chronic deficiency diseases. The gentlest type of building herb supplies valuable minerals, vitamins, hormones, sugars, and other substances that nourish the body. Others are thought to exert a mild stimulating effect on specific organs, glands or metabolic processes. The concept of a building herb is foreign to most modern pharmacognosists and allopathic doctors, and to others of a similar scientific bent. "What does a building herb build?" they would ask. "And by what mechanism does it work?" But herbalists who use plants as builders or eliminators or neutralizers view things differently. To the herbalist, the empirical knowledge that a particular herb has worked in a particular way for many people over many years is enough. From this point of view there is no need to isolate in the laboratory the active substances in the herb or the particular mechanism through which it produces its effects in the body. Here, then, is a list of some of the traditional building herbs and their properties:

Dandelion	The leaves are rich in vitamins and minerals. Dandelion roots are considered a builder for the pancreas.
Licorice	With its sweet flavor and demulcent properties, licorice is considered in herbal tradition to be a builder for the stomach, spleen, and pancreas. Licorice encourages water retention, the opposite effect of an eliminating diuretic.

Nettle	The leaves and stems are rich in nutrients, especially iron, and are considered a builder for the blood and also the liver.
Raspberry	Raspberry leaves are a well-known builder for the uterus. They contain magnesium, which is used to help the uterine muscles relax and work smoothly.
Slippery elm	The bark is said to be building to the nerves because of its nutrients.

Neutralizing herbs work by maintaining the status of an organ or system. In this sense they are considered tonics, which promote an enduring condition of health. Perhaps the most famous herb designated a neutral tonic is ginseng. Ginseng has a strengthening effect on the nervous system, and it has been found to contain adaptogenic principles (ginsenosides) which protect the body against stress if taken properly and at the right dosage for long enough periods of time. Herbalists say that ginseng has neither a positive (building) nor negative (eliminating) factor. The net effect is one of generally improved health, rather than a change in the balance of bodily functions. Some other traditional neutral herbs include:

Apple	The bark of apple trees is one of the better known tonics for the spleen.
Dock	The root serves as an astringent tonic for the colon.
Holy thistle	Regarded as a neutral tonic to the liver and to the female reproductive system.

The Dynamics of Herbs and Centers of Activity

The next step in understanding the dynamics of herbal healing, as it has been defined in European tradition, is to look at the relationship between the types of herbs and their activity centers. Herbs can be builders, eliminators, and/or neutrals all at the same time, in different centers of activity of the body. In the examples we gave above, we described the chief type of activity that has been associated with several herbs. Here we will fill out other secondary and tertiary properties for some of the same herbs:

Butternut	The bark is classified as an eliminator to the colon but is also considered a builder for the liver and a neutral for the spleen.
Dock	Dock is considered a builder to the blood and neutral to the colon.
Holy thistle	Neutral to the liver, female reproductive system, and blood, the holy thistle is also regarded as an eliminator to the spleen.
Licorice	Licorice is considered to act as a builder for the kidneys, female reproductive system, stomach, spleen, and pancreas and neutral to the liver.
Oregon grape	Traditionally this herb has been called an eliminator to the blood, liver, colon, and spleen. In other words, it is believed to have four *centers* of activity but only one *type* of activity.

Uses of Herbs in European Traditions

Herbalists in Europe, or anywhere else for that matter, have been able to use herbs either individually or in combination with each other to treat illness or promote general good health. In Europe, the traditional use of a single herb to treat an illness was called "simpling." Simpling was a local art, practiced by villagers and peasants as well as healers. Different plants were used as simples in different parts of Europe, according to which species were found in each locality.

The Art of Simpling— Healing with a Single Herb

Simpling was a very basic way of using herbs for healing once their properties were understood by the herbalist. This old theory stated that for each disorder within the human body, there was one plant that contained the perfect combination of antidotes. Such a plant was called a simple. Simples usually met three criteria: they were very mild herbs and harmless even in large doses, they were consumed in relatively large amounts for several days or more, and they were native and/or local species in the places where they were given as treatments.

Different traditions of simpling developed in each region of Europe as inhabitants recognized the local simples and used them century after century. This idea paralleled the practice of following an uncomplicated diet based on local crops, which was common in traditional agrarian societies. In the context of simpling there was a special reason for this, though. People have an innate sensitivity to the needs of their bodies, and this "homeostatic" instinct is enhanced by a basic diet. According to the philosophy behind simpling, when a person ate and drank the local food and water, and ate moderately and

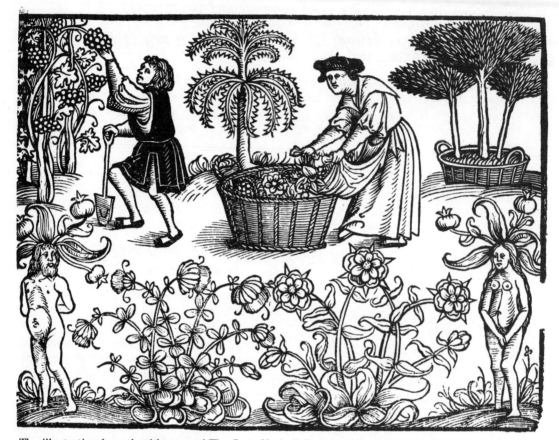

The illustration from the title page of *The Grete Herball* shows herb gathering in sixteenth century England.   (Courtesy of Hunt Institute for Botanical Documentation, Carnegie-Mellon University, Pittsburgh, Pa.)

plainly according to the seasons, he was more easily satisfied. Desires for unhealthy or exotic foods did not arise, and health problems tended to be uncomplicated. Any slight imbalances that developed in the body from one season to the next could be helped by using one of the local healing plants as a simple.

Today, herbalists generally consider that more herbs must be used to match the increased complexity of our modern diets. For someone who eats apples from New Zealand, tomatoes from Mexico, cashews from Brazil, and miso from Japan, herbalists believe that it is not inconsistent to use medicinal plants from distant places, also.

Polypharmacy— *Using Herbs in Combination*

Traditionally, herbalists responded to more complex health problems by combining herbs to complement and enhance their individual properties. This art is known as polypharmacy, and it is probably almost as old as simpling. Throughout the history of western herbalism, the use of single or mixed herbs has been a choice of individual style and need. But today there are unprecedented health problems that favor the practice of polypharmacy.

In simpling, the selection of an herb is based on its specific pharmacological properties and its subtle general properties. Beyond that, particular choices often have to do with personal preference or affinity. In polypharmacy, individual herbs may be selected in much the same way, but the combination of these herbs in a formula is where simpling and polypharmacy diverge. Whereas a single herb used as a simple *may* embody one or two, or perhaps three functions ('eliminating, building, and neutralizing), a formula should definitely contain *all three* of these functions to have a balanced effect.

One of polypharmacy's guidelines is to use the smallest number of herbs possible in order to achieve the desired result. The more herbs that are used, the more difficult it becomes to balance their many different properties. This is because each herb acts both on its own and in relation to the activity of the other herbs. So in order to combine herbs, it becomes more important to know

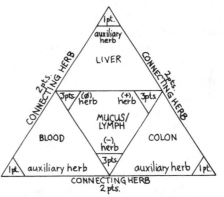

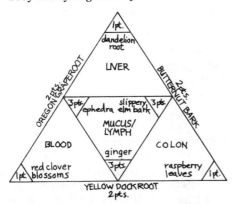

This type of diagram might be used by herbalists to design a formula for a "spring tonic" intended to affect several parts of the body in a synergistic way.

There are 18 parts (unit measures) to the whole formula. The diagram shows how they are apportioned in order to emphasize primary (shown in central triangle) and secondary centers of activity. Note how building, eliminating, and neutralizing functions are balanced in the center.

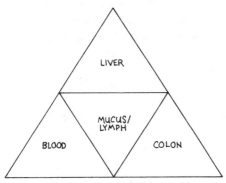

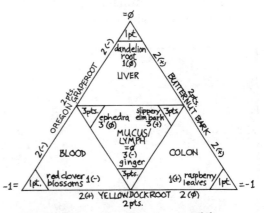

Ginger is used as the primary eliminator, slippery elm bark as the builder, and ephedra as the neutralizer. Together they make up 9 parts, half the formula.

The numbers at the outer corners of the triangle represent a summation of the values of the connecting and auxiliary herbs.

their strengths and properties relative to one another.

Selecting Herbs for a Formula   An example might help illustrate how herbalists synthesize these ideas. In designing a formula for chest congestion, an herbalist might choose elimination as the most important herbal function. Therefore, he or she might choose ginger, thyme, or eucalyptus as an eliminator, because each of those herbs is credited with expectorant properties. But when phlegm and mucus are eliminated, there will be some irritation to the throat. So the formula needs a building herb, one that is soothing and moistening instead of drying. Slippery elm bark is often used for this purpose. So is licorice. Then, to balance the formula, the herbalist might choose a neutral herb on the basis that it would serve as a tonic that gives tone to the lungs and throat. The neutral tonic would be something that helps keep the system resilient when faced with the extremes of eliminating and building. Sage would perhaps be a good choice to play this role in the formula.

There is a great amount of flexibility in determining the relative amounts of each herb in these sorts of simple formulas. A general guideline followed by many herbalists goes like this: If all the herbs are about equal in strength, then the herb with the primary function should make up one-half of the formula. Each of the other two functions will then constitute one-quarter of the formula. In the example formula above, there are three herbs. If we divide the quantities into four parts, then ginger makes up two parts of the formula, and slippery elm bark and sage each make up one part.

Formulas that contain more than three herbs, but which still have one center of activity, are also not too difficult for herbalists to design. In the example above, if ginger is not chosen as the eliminator, eucalyptus and thyme could both be added, one part of each, as eliminating herbs.

Herbalists feel there can be a distinct advantage in using a formula that has more than one center of activity. A blend of herbs working together can replenish many interdependent bodily functions simultaneously, which better enhances the holistic healing process. For example, an herb formula designated a "spring tonic" could equally affect the liver, colon, blood, and kidneys. A spring tonic is taken to correct the effects of heavier eating over the winter months, which has

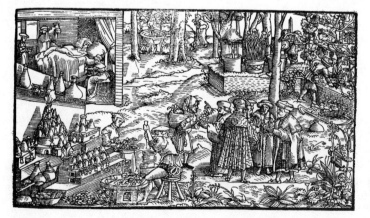

This plate from a German herbal published in 1536 shows herbs being distilled and used to treat a patient.   (Courtesy of Hunt Institute for Botanical Documentation, Carnegie-Mellon University, Pittsburgh, Pa.)

placed more strain on the liver and caused the entire eliminative system to become "sluggish" or congested. This traditional view would conflict with the position taken by most allopathic physicians, who would find the idea of a spring tonic simplistic.

The Doctrine of Signatures

Another famous method European herbalists used to designate the healing properties of herbs was the Doctrine of Signatures. A concept which may sound outlandish, the Doctrine of Signatures stated that every medicinal herb revealed its therapeutic properties by a "sign." Of course this sign was subject to interpretation, and medieval herbology abounded with interpretations. For example burdock, by its signature, was said to be good for one's hair, because its burs clung naturally to the hair of passersby. And dandelions were said to be good for disorders of the bile, because their yellow flowers were the color of a jaundiced person's skin. Undoubtedly,

many signs were ascribed to plants *after* their properties had already been discovered by other means.

Another Doctrine of Signatures related plants to people, from head to toe. Flowers and fruits were the plant's head; leaves and branches were hands and arms; the trunk was its abdomen, and the base and roots were its legs and feet. According to this system, parts of plants were chosen for their healing powers according to the part of their structure that corresponded to the anatomy of the ailing human. For example, to stop bleeding from an abdominal cut, yarrow leaves would be gathered from the middle of the stem, while leaves from the base would be used for cuts on the feet.

A slightly different version of this principle related the regions of a plant to the four elements. Thus, the fruit and seeds, ripening through the influence of the sun, were related to the element of fire. The leaves were akin to air, and the trunk, which transports water, embodied that element. And of course, the roots represented the element earth. In this

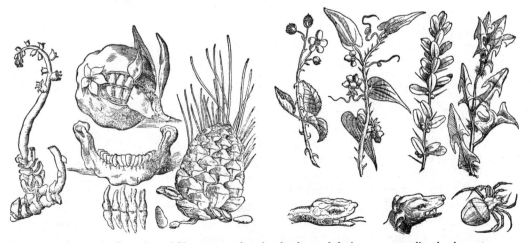

Two examples of the Doctrine of Signatures, showing herbs and their corresponding body parts. Both examples are from *Phytogonomica* by J. B. Porta, published in Naples in 1588. (Courtesy of Hunt Institute for Botanical Documentation, Carnegie-Mellon University, Pittsburgh, Pa.)

Walnuts: Signature of the Head

Some of the old explanations for the signs of plants according to the Doctrine of Signatures are particularly complete and exceedingly odd to us today. One of the best we've come across was written by William Cole in *Adam In Eden,* 1657:

> Wall-nuts have the perfect Signature of the Head: The outer husk or green Covering, represent the Pericranium, or outward skin of the skull, whereon the hair groweth, and therefore salt made of those husks or barks, are exceeding good for wounds in the head. The inner woody shell hath the Signature of the Skull, and the little yellow skin, or Peel, that covereth the Kernell, of the hard Meninga and Pia-mater, which are the thin scarfes that envelope the brain. The Kernel hath the very figure of the Brain, and therefore it is very profitable for the Brain, and resists poysons; For if the Kernel be bruised, and moystened with the quintessence of Wine, and laid upon the Crown of the Head, it comforts the brain and head mightily.

Perhaps it is something to think about, next time you shell some walnuts while drinking wine (if indeed you ever find yourself in this situation). Does this signature, so perfectly described, have any relation to the reality of walnuts' healing properties? Well, in ancient times, walnuts were used for hair tonics and poison antidotes and to prevent madness. But are they still useful in these ways? Perhaps there are some brave readers out there who will keep bruised walnut kernels moistened with wine on the crown of their heads to see if it does prevent madness!

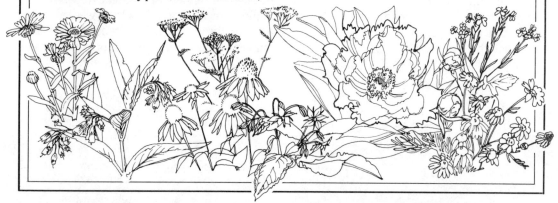

system, specific parts of herbs were used to oppose or support corresponding elemental balances within individuals. For example, if a person was found to be very light and airy, then root herbs were used. If a person was too earthy, then leaves were used instead of roots.

The selection of herbs based on their signatures followed one of two methods—opposition or similarity. A signature could represent some force that would oppose an unhealthy condition, following Hippocrates' idea of treating disease by opposition to the cause. Or, as in homeopathy, which we'll discuss next, it could represent a similarity to a disease symptom, as in the case of dandelion flowers and jaundice.

Throughout most of its history, European herbology relied on the four-element system of the ancient Greeks, the humoral pathology of Hippocrates, and on the Doctrine of Signatures.

Herbal Healing Developments in the New World

Natural healing in America during the nineteenth century developed along several major lines. But three disciplines—Native American medicine, used mainly by settlers in the frontier states, a system called Thomsonian medicine after its founder, and a new system from Germany, called homeopathy—had the most influence.

Homeopathy

In 1825, the first homeopathic physician in the New World opened his practice in New York. Homeopathy had been developed in Germany by the physician and chemist, Samuel Hahnemann, who lived from 1755 to 1843. It was based on the principles of *vis medicatrix naturae* (the healing power of nature) and *similia similibus curantur* (like is cured by like). This idea had been common in German folk healing and was also found in early Greek theories. Hahnemann became convinced of its validity by testing many herbs and minerals on himself and others and observing the results. He noticed for example that cinchona bark, which was used to treat malaria, produced the symptoms of that disease when given to a healthy person. This observation led him to theorize that medicinal substances gave the body a similar, curable version of the disease itself. The principle behind homeopathy is the same one on which our modern immunization procedures are based. Homeopathic remedies are intended to stimulate the body's own natural healing abilities.

Hahnemann also discovered that the smaller the doses of his remedies were, the more effective they seemed to be. Eventually he developed a process of dilution in which the original substance was not actually present in the final dose. Hahnemann explained that the "pattern" of the medicine had been imparted to the medium (such as water), and it was this pattern that produced a result.

Homeopaths paid close attention to their patients' thoughts, feelings, moods, habits, and psychology, as well as to their complete physical condition. All of this information was used to match the patient with the proper herb or mineral medicine, which had been tested for its effects on a healthy person.

Although the public was receptive to homeopathy, the medical establishment, along with herbalists who endorsed the use of very powerful herbs, looked upon such intangible medicine with skepticism. But even many regular physicians suspected that homeopathy worked. They used homeopathic camphor water in the administration of their calomel pills, when Hahnemann prescribed that treatment for the various Asiatic cholera epidemics that raced through the United States from 1831 to 1849.[5]

Although the number of homeopathic doctors has declined greatly (there are approximately 1,500 of them in the United States today), homeopathy has had a profound impact on herbal medicine in America. Homeopaths were the first to actively research native American plants for their healing properties. This inspired a renewed search among orthodox physicians in America into the native medicinal flora. Homeopathy's success with minute, pleasant doses inspired herbal practitioners and orthodox physicians alike to adopt more subtle treatments with their traditional herbs or drugs. As a result, herbal medicine became popular as a safe, gentle form of health care in the second half of the nineteenth century. Americans began to feel equally comfortable with the homeopath, the herbalist, and the allopathic doctor.

Native American Herbal Traditions

The Native American tradition of Good Medicine means living in harmony with nature. Nature's harmony itself is Good Medicine. To Native Americans, health and healing are part of a way of relating to the entire world.

American Indian healers feel that they are responsible for the welfare of the Earth and all her creatures. The Indians call the Earth's creator the Great Spirit (also the Great Mystery, Grandfather Sky, the Holy Mystery, and various other names). They call creation Great Mother, or Grandmother Earth.

This Native American view of the interdependence between human beings and all of Earth's creatures parallels the principles of ecology in modern science. But the Native American tradition of Good Medicine is not as theoretical or factual a science. Rather, it is based on direct perceptions, and the knowledge that the medicine man or woman accumulates.

Thus, a Native American healer gathers herbs with a genuine feeling of exchange from one aspect of Creation to another. The Good Medicine healer views plants not merely as chemical combinations that help the human body but also as part of the whole of Creation. They are infused with the same spirit, power, and life-forces that animate and flow through all the universe. Believing this, the healer regards plants as relatives, calling them "medicine people."

Native American herbalists had established a vast pharmacopoeia of indigenous medicinal plants. Some of the more common ones (included in chapter 4) are basswood, bearberry, beech, birch, blackberry, butternut, corn, echinacea, garlic, ginseng, goldenseal, gravelroot, horsetail, mints, oak, onion, Oregon grape, poplar, and wild ginger. In addition, virtually every herb introduced from Europe was quickly adopted by the Native American healers. Among these, alfalfa, burdock, comfrey, dock, mullein, and plantain became very popular.

There are two main sources of knowledge about plants and their healing uses in the Native American tradition. One is cultural and the other personal. Cultural knowledge simply refers to information that has been handed down from one generation to the next.

The other method of learning about "medicine people," personal exploration, developed because of the Indians' nomadic life-style and geographic migrations. For example, when the Sioux left the Great Lakes area for a home on the Plains, they went through changes such as riding horses instead of rowing canoes, experiencing intense sun, wind, and sand, instead of water and shade, and a vastly different diet of animal and vegetable foods prompted new health needs. Such drastic changes occurred in such relatively short periods of time that the people responsible for the health of their tribe had to find and learn about healing plants through personal exploration. They did not have centuries of accumulated written records to draw on, as did healers in the established cultures of China, India, Tibet, Persia, and even Europe. And so, the task of the medicine man or medicine woman was (and still is) to interpret nature in a way that led to the tribe's harmony with her.

Although each tribe and each totem uses varying symbols, virtually all Native Americans follow a system of subtle elements that corresponds to the four directions of the compass: north, south, east, and west. In addition, two other directions (or powers) complete the mandala (a graphic symbol of the universe) of natural healing. These are "up," representing Grandfather, the Great Spirit, and "down," representing Grandmother, the Earth. The Great Spirit embodies the Fire element, while the Grandmother, naturally, represents the Earth element. The East represents the light of wisdom, illumination, freshness, spring, peace, and understanding. From the South comes the power of life, fertility, growth, and warmth. The West represents maturity, autumn, rain, thunder, and also death or the quality of things coming to an end. And from the North comes the cold purifying winds, the cleansing of austerity, the strength of endurance, and the white snows and hairs of old age. The Native American healer classifies herbs and medicines according to the Four Directions and Two Powers. Native Americans often apply a type of Doctrine of Signatures (see page 29) in assigning such qualities to their "medicine people."

Native Americans also use the totem symbolism of animals and other natural phenomena to classify healing properties of plants. These vary widely from tribe to tribe, and from individual to individual. Members of tribal clans may share a totem, such as the snake or antelope societies of the Hopis, or individuals may have their own totems. The bear, the eagle, the turtle, the bison, the coyote, the badger, thunder, lightning, rain, and wind are all used as totems, and each is considered to represent varying qualities and meanings. For example, the well known Cherokee medicine man, Rolling Thunder, embodies the qualities of his name; like thunder he is powerful, deep, and strong. In fact, it has been observed that wherever Rolling Thunder travels, he is often accompanied by rain, thunder, and lightning storms.

The Four Directions and Two Powers (as Grandfather and Grandmother are also called) represent a complete system for analyzing the physical, psychological, and spiritual needs of individuals. For example, a person's constitution may be predominantly of the northern direction (cold, austere, enduring). If such a person becomes too "isolated" in that element, or set of qualities, he or she needs an influence from the southern direction for balancing. The balancing influence can come from a medicine, an activity, or a food.

Because the use of healing plants is so personalized in the Native American tradition, it is difficult, and perhaps wrong, to simply describe certain uses. The essential gift of this tradition is its emphasis on direct experience and relationship with nature as the healing force.

The mystical process of discovering an herb's healing uses is illustrated well in the life story of the famous healer Black Elk. Black Elk had a powerful vision at the age of nine, and he believed that his life's work was to unravel its meaning, so that through understanding, the vision could work for his people. Part of that vision was of a four-petaled flower which would help the weak people of his nation. The four petals represented the powers of the Four Directions coming to heal and strengthen. But, like other aspects of a medicine man or woman's vision, it could not be used to help until it was acted out in physical reality. As Black Elk recalls the event:

> I knew that I must have this herb for curing, and I thought I could recognize the place where I had seen it growing that night when I lamented.

> After One Side and I had eaten, I told him there was an herb I must find, and I wanted him to help me hunt for it. Of course I did not tell him I had seen it in a vision. He was willing to help, so we got on our horses and rode over to Grass Creek. . . .

(continued on page 36)

Interview with Wallace Black Elk

Black Elk's vision was one of restoring his people's balance with nature. The remarkable tales he told were recorded by John Neihardt *(Black Elk Speaks)* in 1932 and by Joseph Epes Brown *(The Sacred Pipe)* in 1950. In 1952, Black Elk's life came to an end. Through these books, though, Black Elk touched the hearts of many Americans who came after him. Even more importantly, the living tradition he worked so hard to preserve was carried on by his spiritual heir and grandson, Wallace Black Elk. Like his grandfather before him, Wallace Black Elk is a medicine man of the Sioux tribe. He is also an astute observer of our modern culture. With a foot in both worlds, he converses with the Great Spirit as well as with the scientist and medical doctor. Knowing that this interview would reach many people, he decided to tell "the secret and the sacred" part of his healing tradition.

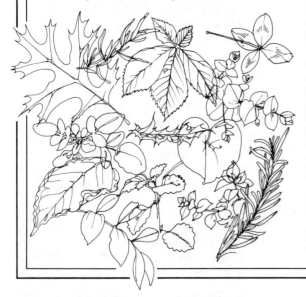

QUESTION: Black Elk, what is the primary cause of sickness and disease?
ANSWER: Pollution of the mind comes first. Then, the physical part comes later.

QUESTION: How does this relate to the use of herbs in your tradition?
ANSWER: When we talk about the herbal plants, we begin to talk about the spiritual food people and medicine people. Pollution begins in our minds. There was a time, once, when there was no pollution of the mind. A long time ago, before even Columbus thought the world was round. Then people started thinking about how they could do good, and how they could do bad. [That is, the act of thinking "good or bad" is a fall from the grace of simply *being* naturally good.] And then sickness came. Tunkashala (Grandfather Spirit) warned us, through prophecies. He knew it would happen. So, Tunkashala infused his power into the fire, into the green, into the rock, and into the water, and then disappeared. But he's still there, like this air, he's there but you can't see it with your naked eye. But we believe he is there.

So, when this creation formed—we call it Grandmother, the Earth, she became pregnant. So she gave birth to all creatures. It's like a seed, planted. Then a next seed. It keeps going from generation to generation. Every plant—these flowers here—they flower and make seeds, and then they grow some more like that. It's continuous life. So, it's the same with all the animals that live in water, and the creepy-crawlies, and the four-legged, and the winged, and us two-legged. So, we all relate. That's why when we say, "To all my relations," the power is still there. From the original creation. So people pray, talk to those powers.

This may seem strange to some people. But I know what I'm talking about. We talk about how there is power in everything. All the creatures dance, they sing songs, the stone people dancin', the water, everything: power. In fact, from the water, vibrations and sounds come. We understand all this.

But now, the whole universe is contaminated. The mammals and creepy-crawlies and winged and two-legged are all contaminated. That's why Tunkashala infused his power into the green and the medicine people.

See, these herbs are medicine people, because each one has a part in the human structure. When a person takes this medicine, the virus or enemy that is in you can be fought by the body. So, the medicine goes inside you and arrests the bacteria, what we call "enemy." Then it expels, out. The he [the medicine] reconstructs any part that had damage, the red cells, the white cells, the platelets, or he builds calcium, the frame or bone structure. Or, that little fiber [collagen] that builds tissues: if the enemy breaks it, then he goes there and mends it, and patches it so it be a fiber again. So any part that is broken off, the spirit, that medicine, goes there and reconstructs that damage.

And then, within four days he disappears. So that was the power of Tunkashala. He infused his power into those plants so they became a medicine. They are *creators,* they reconstruct, they re-create that heart or liver or kidney, or wherever the enemy does damage. He goes and repairs.

QUESTION: Black Elk, how do you learn about the different uses—the powers—of the plants, in your tradition?
ANSWER: Through a vision quest. It takes years. If you want to carry the power, you make your commitment. And then you carry this pipe and go up to the mountain. Then you have to humble yourself. You will be blessed, and the power of the Four Winds will show you the plant.

QUESTION: Black Elk, what plants do you use according to these ways of learning about them?
ANSWER: Oh, as I say, the pharmaceutical department is out there . . . [Black Elk says this as he laughs and waves his hand toward the nearby mountains.] But maybe perhaps I'm going too fast.

These plants are food, spiritual food, and they are medicine. And these are our home. So, the trees are our home. The forest is our home. Where all the creatures live, in the forest. And it holds water and all the herbs, plants, and medicine, the grass. Each one has a part. And each creature knows the herbal plants. So when they are sick, they could nibble on, and drink water, and lay down, and they be all right. And man learned from those creatures. So we know what to eat.

So, our leading food is springwater. Springwater is a medicine. *Medicine.* It *is* a medicine. We call it that. Springwater is a medicine. It could clear, rinse off your mind. Crystal clear your mind. Get all the pollution washed away . . . rinsed, and give you encouragement, healing, comforting . . . everything comes with it.

Then, of all the food, our leading is corn. There are many kinds of corn, but to us the calico is best. Of fruits, the cherry is the leading.

The old people used to tell us that the Tree of Life (represented by the cherry tree) was, *once.* But it withered and fell over. From the root, its white sprout came out and it got a little green, and pretty soon it turned green and bloomed. And inside there's a flower, and that grew, and then two leaves flowered, and then inside is another flower. So it kept branching until it was the Tree of Life. So the Tree of Life will once again grow here and it will bloom and flourish again. So, that is the definition of life. My grandpa talks about this. He saw it in a vision.

I looked down towards the west, and yonder at a certain point beside the creek were crows and magpies, chicken hawks and spotted eagles circling around and around.

Then I knew, and I said to One Side, "Friend, right there is where the herb is growing." … As we neared the spot the birds all flew away, and it was a place where four or five dry gulches came together. There right on the side of the bank the herb was growing, and I knew it, although I had never seen one like it before, except in my vision.

It had a root about as long as my elbow, and this was a little thicker than my thumb. It was flowering in four colors, blue, white, red, and yellow.

Something must have told me to find the herb just then, for the next evening I needed it and could have done nothing without it.[6]

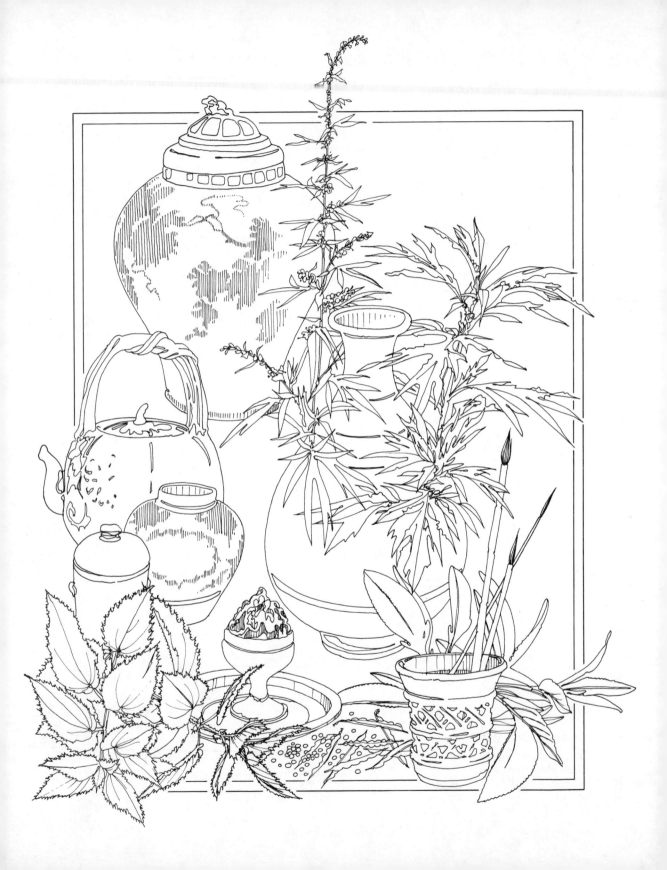

Herbal Healing Traditions in the East

*A*lthough it is the European and American traditions that are most in evidence among herbalists in the United States today, the influence of eastern herbologies is being increasingly felt. In this chapter we will look at the use of herbs in Chinese and Tibetan medicine.

Chinese Healing: The Medicine of Harmony

China's knowledge of herbs goes back to ancient times when Shen Nung's *Classic of Herbs,* the first known Chinese herbal, was compiled. In the latter Han Dynasty, Chang Chun Ching established the Chinese method of making herbal formulas. The time-tested practice of polypharmacy in Chinese herbology is one of its most distinguishing features today. Almost all Chinese herbs are used exclusively in formulas that combine four to twelve or even more ingredients.

The variety of herbs and other substances used in Chinese medicine is another of its distinguishing characteristics. The most recent

Chinese pharmacopoeia contains over 5,700 entries that include common and uncommon herbs as well as medicinal minerals and animal parts. Today there are more than 500 herbal formulas in use in Chinese medicine, of which about 200 are the most important or commonly used.

The great herbalist Tao Hung Ching added commentaries to Shen Nung's classic that presented a system for analyzing 365 herbs according to their use as superior, general, or inferior drugs. Superior drugs are those tonics and herbs (like ginseng) that can be taken for a long time with no ill side effects. General herbs (like ephedra) are used to treat diseases, and their use is discontinued with remission of the disease. Inferior drugs (like aconite) are actually poisons that are used in a medicinal way for brief periods of time, and in small amounts. The establishment of these guidelines—superior, general, and inferior—greatly contributed to the well-known safety feature of Chinese herbology. By categorizing medicines in this way, Tao Hung Ching and succeeding herbalists more easily determined the proper amounts of ingredients to use in their formulas.

Adaptations of the Chinese methods of using herbs for health care and prevention of disease can be found in many other eastern countries. One reason Chinese herbal medicine is so popular is because of its emphasis on prevention as a healing method, an approach that stems from an ancient cultural view. Chinese herbology applies the principle of prevention by emphasizing the use of tonics and "adaptogens," or herbs that strengthen the whole body. In particular, the Chinese healers pay special attention to herbs that strengthen or regulate the body's immune system. This kind of therapy is known today as biological response modification.

To Chinese philosophers and physicians, nature itself is the model, the unifying principle, and the source of understanding. This source or principle is called "Tao" in Chinese. The concept of Tao probably has been present in Chinese culture for many thousands of years, and certainly for at least 2,500 years. It is itself a way of being, a way of preserving life and health by living in harmony with nature's principles. But Tao is more than achieving a naturally healthy life through harmony. Tao is the harmony of life itself.

Chinese physicians use five diagnostic methods in order to find a patient's pattern of "disharmony." These include visual observation, listening (to the person's voice, coughs, etc.), smelling body odors, questioning the patient's medical history, and wrist palpation or pulse diagnosis. Eight external principles or factors are used in assessing patterns of disharmony, including yin and yang.

The Tao of Yin and Yang

The determination of harmony in Chinese medicine is based on the universal theory of yin and yang. Originally, the Chinese character for yang meant the sunny side of a mountain. Its qualities are associated with heat, stimulation, movement, activity, excitement, vigor, and light. The original character for yin meant the shaded side of a mountain. Yin's qualities are associated with cold, passivity, inaction, darkness, and responsiveness.

There are five principles of yin and yang that are used in the Chinese medical system. They are:

All things are composed of both yin and yang.

The yin and yang aspects can each be further divided into yin and yang.

Yin and yang are polar pairs that cannot exist without each other.

Yin and yang control or balance each other.

Yin and yang change or transform into each other.

In the external world, a balance of yin and yang indicates a healthy environment. In the human body, a balance of these two forces represents a state of health. The Chinese healer must learn many aspects of yin and yang as manifested in seasonal cycles, properties of food and medicine, variations in the constitutions of patients, types and stages of sickness, and techniques of treatment. Each subject mentioned above is complex and elaborate, as one might suspect from examining these five principles of yin and yang.

There are some basic principles of yin-yang that can be easily applied to any form of natural healing. For example, the functions of building and eliminating described in the discussion of European natural healing in chapter 2 can be related to conditions of yin or yang. A person who is too yin is made more yang with a building therapy. A person who is

YIN AND YANG PHYSIOGNOMY OF THE BODY

Characteristic	Yin	Yang
body height	tall	short
body size	fat, thin	slightly heavy, well developed
muscle tone	loose	tight
orientation of feet while walking	pointing out	pointed in
weight distribution while walking	on heels	on toes
posture	slumped over	erect
knees	pointed in	bowed out
head size	large	small
face shape	large forehead, pointed chin	wide chin, jaws &/or cleft chin
hair on head	straight, thick, yellow	curly, wavy, red, black
skin color	light	dark
shape of ears	small, pointed, sticking out	large, large lobes, flat, low on head
position of eyes	wide apart	close together
orientation of iris	toward ears	toward nose
white of eyes	exposed below iris	exposed above iris
shape of eyes	big, round	small, thin
color under eyes	blue, white, purple	dark brown
eyebrows	thin, pointed downward	thick, pointed upward
nose	large	small
distance between mouth and nose	small	large
mouth	large	small
teeth	angled out	angled in
shape of hands and fingers	long, thin	short, thick
hand temperature/moisture	cold, or warm and wet	hot and dry
nail shape	flat, concave	bulging, convex
body hair	not much	profuse
voice	soft	loud
speech	reserved	talkative
body odor	slight	strong
perspiration	very little	copious

too yang is made more yin with an eliminating therapy. Herbs that are hot, warm, sharp, sweet, bland, light, or of weak fragrance are considered yang. They are used to balance a yin condition. Herbs that are cold, cool, sour, bitter, salty, strong, heavy and strongly fragrant are yin, and they are used to balance a yang condition. An herb can also contain both yin and yang characteristics. For example, licorice root tastes sweet at first, but after a few moments it also tastes bitter. Ginseng root is a very yang herb, but it also has a slight bitter taste. And the ginseng leaf has a yin quality: it is used to decrease fire energy,

(continued on page 44)

An Interview with Michael Broffman, C.A.

Michael Broffman, a holistic health practitioner in Marin County, California, grew up in New York City. As he was growing up, he and his friends were occasionally involved in gang fights. Since many of Michael's friends were Chinese anyone who was injured, whether they were Chinese or not, was taken to Chinatown for doctoring by a traditional herbalist. Michael became the neighborhood guide and escort for anyone in need of these health services. Over the years, he developed an interest in Chinese medicine, and eventually he went to Taiwan to study more formally for several years. Now he maintains a traditional Chinese medical clinic in San Anselmo, complete with treatment rooms, a large kitchen, and a pharmacy with over

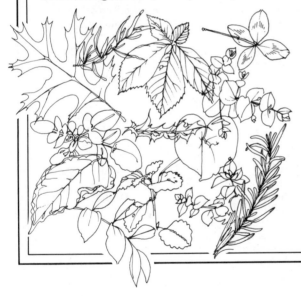

300 Chinese herbs and formulas. We visited Michael to learn more about how he applies traditional Chinese techniques in contemporary California.

QUESTION: Michael, how were you trained as a practitioner of Chinese medicine?
ANSWER: My training was part of an apprenticeship system.
    In the study of herbs, we would experiment with the plant, using it in a variety of ways and forms, noting its effects. After all of this we would compare our experimental information with the standard literature.

QUESTION: Many people in the West have heard that traditionally, in Chinese medicine, the doctor was paid to keep people well. If the patient got sick, the doctor's fee was withheld. Could you comment on the Chinese view of health and healing and the idea of natural or preventive medicine?
ANSWER: In the tradition in which I am trained it is commonly felt that a practitioner is simply a mirror for the patient. But what we would *really* like to create, if possible, is no reflection: a situation in which the patient doesn't see himself in a narcissistic way. Health, healing, and natural are reflective terms, capable of containing a value judgment. Even though we judge the values to be positive, many patients can, through fear and self-cherishing, easily place a negative value on their opposite terms, on sickness, destruction, and unnatural. By concentrating on that, actual health and healing is diminished. It is with great reluctance and reservation that we treat in Chinese medicine. Even to say to the patient, "How are you feeling today?" has already (albeit subtly) manipulated

the patient's response: they are either feeling (and hence, they could be good or bad), or they are not feeling. In Chinese medicine, we want to maintain a neutral position; we want to simply observe rather than interpret. [It is a common practice of Chinese doctors to say very little while treating their patients. The correct advice or treatment is given, but information that might feed a patient's hypochondria tendencies is withheld.]

QUESTION: How do Chinese herbalists regard the use of plants in the healing process?
ANSWER: There is nothing that cannot be used medicinally. A person knowingly or unknowingly is constantly interacting with the natural environment in, let us say, a medicinal way. Sometimes it is formal, like having your pulse read and herbs prescribed. And sometimes it is informal, like strolling beneath the eucalyptus trees. Therefore the role of herbs is no different than the role of anything in our environment. All phenomena create an experience, a feeling, for us that promotes the movement of our energy through life. When we categorize things into good or bad, we generally close ourselves to those things labeled bad, and they don't further our healing or growth process. For example, most people don't like to think about impermanence, death. But really, such contemplation can be one of the best medicines [in the sense that it can help us to cope with upsetting concepts that create worry and thus, ill health in us].

We have no system of ranking plants or other medicines in an order of importance. This is a Western idea. It is a mistake to think that ginseng is more valuable than the old soot that collects on the inside of your stove pipe. Each herb, and each phenomenon, has its own profound quality. So how can anything be more or less than this?

QUESTION: Are Chinese herbs inherently different than American herbs? What do you think about the use and cultivation of Chinese herbs in America?
ANSWER: A "Chinese" herb transplanted from China to California becomes an overseas Chinese herb, with all the immigration problems—acceptance, prejudice, restrictions, language difficulties, and assimilation—you might perhaps expect. Several generations of Chinese herbs here in California become American-born Chinese herbs, which are much different in usage and attitude than overseas Chinese herbs. We are really dealing with a "melting pot" effect here.

Keep in mind the idea of context. There are three basic contexts for an herb. They are its growing environment, the other herbs in a prescription in which it will be combined, and its interaction with the person. The value of an herb can be altered by any or all of these factors.

QUESTION: Do you think the Chinese and Western systems of medicine can be integrated successfully?
ANSWER: Yes, they can—but the end product will not be Chinese or Western. To retain the "essence" of the Chinese system, it cannot be meshed with Western science, because fundamentally they are operating with different views of the world. The value of Chinese medicine to the West is its foundation in wholeness and gentleness and the feeling of completeness that can come from its openness.

which is yang. In general, roots are considered the most yang part of the plant, while fruits and flowers are the most yin. Compared to its root, a plant's leaves are yin; but compared to its flowers, they are yang.

There is a yin and yang relationship between plants (and people) and their environment, too. A yin environment often produces more yang herbs, and a yang environment creates more yin herbs. We can take ginseng as an example again. Ginseng naturally grows in damp, cold, shady places, often high in the mountains on northern slopes. These are all yin conditions which attract their opposite, yang, in the ginseng root. In the tropics there is a much greater yang force due to a greater amount of solar radiation. This great yang power produces plants which are more yin. Tropical plants are generally larger, leafier, juicier, and more fragrant than plants native to cooler climates. Even cactus plants are yin; growing as they do in hot, dry environments, they are full of water. Because of these ecological factors of yin and yang, the foods and herbs that grow in one's own region are considered the best medicine. They are thought to be naturally balanced to the local harmonies of yin and yang that affect people as well.

Other factors also affect the degree of yin or yang in herbal medicines. Fresh herbs are more yin than dried herbs (they contain more moisture). An herb can be made more yang by drying it in the sun or more yin by drying it in the shade (remember the shady side of a mountain?). The degree of heat used in preparing an herbal infusion also has a relative yin or yang influence. Sun tea, for example, which is simply steeped in a glass jar in the sun, is a very yin method of preparation (it is a passive method). Correspond-

ingly, sun tea is usually made in the summer to balance that season's yang quality. Boiling herbs in water for a short period of time and making an infusion are also yin methods, but they are more yang than making sun tea. Simmering herbs for a long time is an even more yang method, and it is applied most often to roots. Drinking an herb tea that has cooled maximizes its yin quality, while drinking it hot is more "yang-izing." Alcohol extraction produces a very yang product; the yin alcohol attracts the yang qualities of the herbs.

Generally, Chinese methods of preparation aim at maximizing the herb's basic qualities. A yang herb is simmered a long time to bring out its yang qualities, which are then used to balance a person's yin condition. Yin herbs are prepared to maintain their yin qualities (such as volatile oils), and are usually given as an infusion. Enhancing the yin in yin herbs is supposed to make them more effective in treating a yang condition. In formulas, though, herbs which embody a strong emphasis of yin or yang are most often balanced with herbs having only a slight emphasis of the opposite value. This reflects the emphasis on harmony, which is so highly valued in Chinese medicine.

In order to make their herbal remedies even more harmonious, Chinese physicians recommend taking them at varying times of the day, depending on the part of the body being treated. If the sickness is in the upper part of the body, teas or medicines are taken one hour after eating. If the tea is for the arms or legs, it is taken one hour before breakfast. Medicines for the bones are taken one hour after dinner or before retiring. Tonics and supplements are taken on an empty stomach, and the patient is advised to remain calm and move slowly afterward.

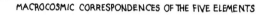

MACROCOSMIC CORRESPONDENCES OF THE FIVE ELEMENTS

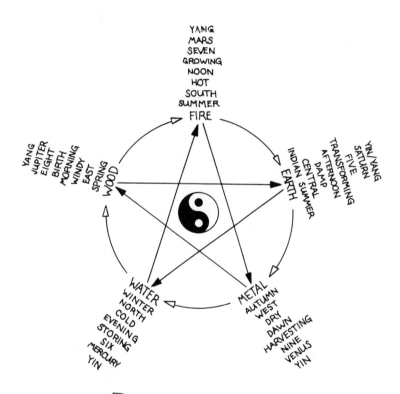

KEY: = NURTURING CYCLE ➤=INJURING CYCLE

MEANING OF LEVELS, USING FIRE AS AN EXAMPLE:

FIRE - ELEMENT
SUMMER - SEASON IN WHICH ELEMENT IS STRONGEST
SOUTH - DIRECTION OF ORIGIN OF SEASON / ELEMENT
HOT - TYPE OF WEATHER OR CLIMATE
NOON - TIME OF DAY
GROWING - TYPE OF ACTIVITY IN NATURAL CYCLES SUCH AS PLANT AND HUMAN LIFE
SEVEN - SPECIFIC NUMBER
MARS - PLANET
YANG - BASIC QUALITY

This diagram shows how the Chinese five elements refer to qualities
present in the outside world.

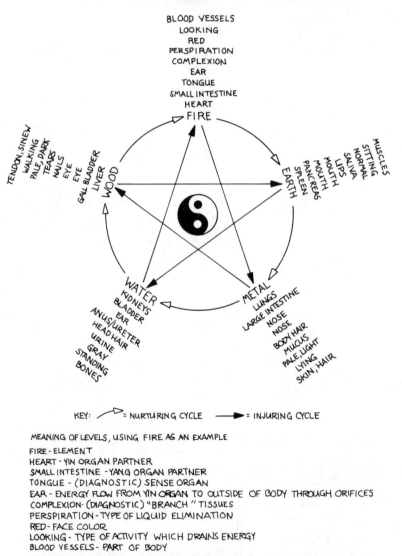

MICROCOSMIC CORRESPONDENCES OF THE FIVE ELEMENTS

KEY: = NURTURING CYCLE   = INJURING CYCLE

MEANING OF LEVELS, USING FIRE AS AN EXAMPLE

FIRE - ELEMENT
HEART - YIN ORGAN PARTNER
SMALL INTESTINE - YANG ORGAN PARTNER
TONGUE - (DIAGNOSTIC) SENSE ORGAN
EAR - ENERGY FLOW FROM YIN ORGAN TO OUTSIDE OF BODY THROUGH ORIFICES
COMPLEXION - (DIAGNOSTIC) "BRANCH" TISSUES
PERSPIRATION - TYPE OF LIQUID ELIMINATION
RED - FACE COLOR
LOOKING - TYPE OF ACTIVITY WHICH DRAINS ENERGY
BLOOD VESSELS - PART OF BODY

This diagram shows the relationships between the five elements and the corresponding parts of the human body.

FOOD AND FLAVOR CORRESPONDENCES OF THE FIVE ELEMENTS

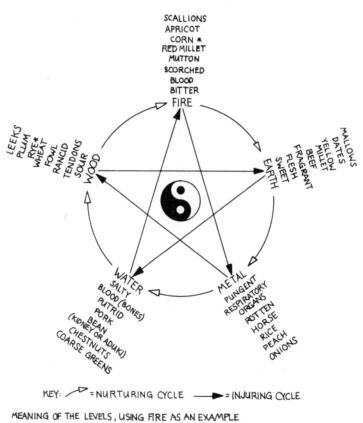

KEY: ↗ = NURTURING CYCLE ——▶ = INJURING CYCLE

MEANING OF THE LEVELS, USING FIRE AS AN EXAMPLE

FIRE - ELEMENT
BITTER - FLAVOR
BLOOD - TISSUE MOST AFFECTED BY THE FLAVOR
SCORCHED - ODOR
MUTTON - MEAT
RED MILLET/CORN - GRAIN
APRICOT - FRUIT
SCALLIONS - VEGETABLE

* THESE ARE WESTERN OR MODERN EQUIVALENTS

This diagram relates the five elements to foods and flavors.

The Mandala of Five Elements

As useful and prevalent as yin-yang theory is in Chinese medicine, there is another system that augments it. This is the Chinese system of the five elements—wood, fire, earth, metal, and water. As with the system of four elements developed by Hippocrates (and discussed in chapter 2), the Chinese five elements are classes of qualities that correspond to each other. The diagrams included here list many of these correspondences. They are often drawn in the way you see them here or in the form of a chart. We have grouped them here according to major categories, in

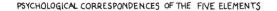

PSYCHOLOGICAL CORRESPONDENCES OF THE FIVE ELEMENTS

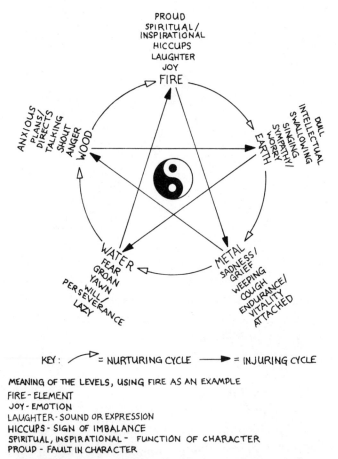

KEY: ⟋▷ = NURTURING CYCLE ——▶ = INJURING CYCLE

MEANING OF THE LEVELS, USING FIRE AS AN EXAMPLE
FIRE - ELEMENT
JOY - EMOTION
LAUGHTER - SOUND OR EXPRESSION
HICCUPS - SIGN OF IMBALANCE
SPIRITUAL, INSPIRATIONAL - FUNCTION OF CHARACTER
PROUD - FAULT IN CHARACTER

This diagram shows how the five elements relate to psychological qualities.

order to make it easier to understand the principles of the system.

In a strictly medical sense, the elements refer to the organ systems in the human body. There are two organs, a yin and a yang organ, for each element. These represent an interdependent relationship in which the health of one organ is inseparable from the health of the other. Generally it is the yin organ that is referred to—and treated—according to the five-element system. However, in Chinese medicine, there are no clear boundaries to the organs. Within the body, the organs also include channels and points (such as those used in acupuncture), tissues, diagnostic areas on the face and body, emotions, thoughts, and character traits. Outside of the body, the organs interact with outer phenomena such as the seasons, climates, colors, and times of the day. The body's organs are viewed together as a vast comprehensive function relating to the entire mandala of five elements.

Here is a simplified example of how the internal organs relate to the outside world in the Chinese five-element system: sour is the taste associated with the liver. The sour taste and the liver organ are both part of the wood element. Wind is the climatic factor of wood, and it is associated with spring, the season of wood. Spring is the time of year when liver ailments are most likely to develop, and it is the best time of year to treat the liver. Spring is like a doorway to the liver, and all wood element factors will influence the liver more directly at this time. In the most basic application of the system, the Chinese physician checks the relative balance of elements in a person and treats the one *preceding* the weakest element. For example, in order to strengthen the liver (wood), it is important to increase or strengthen kidney energy (water). A slightly more complex treatment would address the liver and kidney functions simultaneously.

The dynamics of this nurturing cycle indicate that an imbalance in the season of one element will lead to an imbalance in the season of the next element. In other words, a weakness of the kidneys in winter will manifest in spring as a liver disorder; a liver weakness

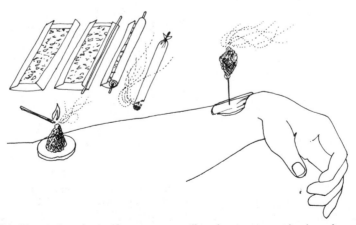

This illustration shows three ways moxibustion treatment is given: by indirect heating, by rolling and use of a moxa wick, and by heating through a needle.

in spring will turn up in summer as a heart disorder; a heart weakness in summer will appear as a spleen disorder during Indian summer; and a weakness in the spleen during Indian summer will manifest as a lung disorder in autumn.

The Art of Moxibustion

Moxibustion is a modern word referring to the burning of moxa, an ancient term meaning a substance used to transfer heat. That substance is almost always mugwort (*Artemisia sinensis* or *A. vulgaris*). Moxibustion is the nonintrusive partner of acupuncture therapy. It consists of burning cones, wicks, or sticks of compressed mugwort fibers over specific acupuncture points. Moxibustion, like acupuncture, is an intricate art which must be studied and learned before it can be used effectively. It is one of the most interesting herbal therapies in Chinese medicine.

Moxibustion is considered a very stimulating therapy, and it is used for people who are weak, tired, cold, or deficient in some way. "The mugwort from which moxas are made has the power of extracting the yang energy from the yin," states *Yellow Emperor's Classic of Internal Medicine* (the *Nei Ching*). Traditionally, proper moxibustion starts when the mugwort is first harvested. The plants are gathered and dried in full sun each summer successively for seven to nine years. Then the plants are rubbed until the downy fibers on the underside of the leaves come off. This "down" is then sifted to remove stems and packed for use as moxa.

Although the mugwort dries rather quickly, the moxa is prepared in this traditional way in order to absorb the sun's fire element, which makes the dried plant fibers

extremely yang. This yang fire power is then imparted to the patient during moxibustion treatment. In recent times, however, it is rare to find moxa processed in this laborious way. Like finely aged wines, moxa has succumbed to the accelerated pace of our age.

Herbs from the Rooftop of the World: Tibet's Medical Tradition

The Tibetan system of medicine is one of the more subtle and sophisticated healing systems surviving in the world today. Throughout its history Tibet's isolation, harsh climate, and often dangerous terrain demanded from its inhabitants an intimate knowledge of nature. Most of the people living in the Land of Snows, as Tibet is sometimes called, were nomads moving with the seasons from lowland meadows to high mountain pastures with their herds. The knowledge accumulated by Tibetan healers over centuries from the study of wild plants and ancient medical texts has remained largely undisturbed, protected by the country's inaccessibility and strong isolationism.

As we mentioned in chapter 1, the healing traditions of Tibet have been greatly influenced by the Indian system of Ayurvedic medicine. It was in the sixth century A.D. that Ayurveda first came to the Land of Snows. At that time, two medical sages of the Ayurvedic system traveled to the court of Tibet's first king. They were quickly accepted, and their knowledge was propagated through a lineage of oral transmission from teacher to student. During the eighth century A.D., Buddhism came to Tibet, producing a great flowering of religious, artistic, cultural, and scientific disciplines. It was during this era that many of the ancient Sanskrit medical texts from India were first translated into written Tibetan.

The influence of Buddhism in Tibet greatly accelerated the adoption of India's medical science there, for two reasons. Buddhism emphasized service to humanity as practiced by the medical community. Accordingly, the study of medicine was one of the five basic Buddhist scholastic pursuits. Additionally, Ayurveda was considered to be the teaching of the Buddha himself. Hindu mythology states that Ayurveda was first taught by Brahma. But according to Buddhist doctrine, Brahma first learned Ayurveda from a prehistorical Buddha named Kasyapa.

In the early period of Tibetan medicine, medical scholars from China, Persia, Mongolia, Pakistan, and Nepal joined practitioners of native Tibetan medicine and medical doctors from India in debates and conferences in the royal court. From this, a synthesis emerged which is not just Ayurveda, not simply Chinese or Mongolian medicine. Yet it includes elements from these systems. Although this unusual blend is particularly Tibetan, it is actually very similar to Ayurveda. As the well-known Ayurvedic scholar, Bhagwan Dash, says:

Even though physicians from other parts of the world were invited, and medical texts of those countries were translated into Tibetan, they were all molded into the fundamental principles of Ayurveda. Therefore, in the current practice, the Tibetan system has a close resemblance with Ayurveda.[1]

Some scholars of Ayurveda, including Bhagwan Dash, even consider the Tibetan tradition to be the most authentic representation of Ayurvedic medicine. Many of the Sanskrit texts, having been translated into Tibetan, were then lost or destroyed in their native country of India. Today they survive only in the Tibetan version. In addition, many native Tibetans became respected scholars and practitioners of these medical arts and sciences. They advanced the science with further research and study and wrote innumerable texts and commentaries of their own. Thus the tradition grew in its depth and comprehension.

Some of the herbs used in the Tibetan pharmacopoeia today are rare and unique to that part of the world, but many of them are the same as, or similar to, plants found growing in other places. For example, plants such as white oak, mustard, nettles, sage, mugwort, and alfalfa are found in both California and Tibet.

Plants form the basis of almost all Tibetan medicines, but herbal formulas often include at least one nonvegetable ingredient as well. Pharmaceutical materials are categorized into eight types: metallic drugs, minerals, medicinal stones, decoctions from fruits and flowers, leaves of medicinal plants, stems of plants, roots of plants, and medicines made from various animal parts. Tibetan physicians claim that medicine can be made from any substance on Earth.

Medicinal plants are categorized and described according to the five-element system found in the Ayurvedic medicine of India (see page 5). These elements—earth, water, fire, air, and space function in the growth of plants in that earth forms the foundation on which to grow, water provides the necessary moisture, fire gives heat for growth, air creates movement around and within the plants for

(continued on page 54)

An Interview with Chakdud Tulku Rinpoche

The following interview is with Ven. Chakdud Tulku Rinpoche, a Tibetan Lama (teacher), trained from the age of five in the Buddhist monastic tradition.

In 1959, Rinpoche fled the Communist Chinese takeover of Tibet. He spent the next 20 years teaching other Buddhists in India and Nepal, in addition to caring for many sick fellow refugees. In 1979, he came to the United States at the request of some of his Western students. Since 1980, he has been living near Eugene, Oregon, where he is the resident Lama of a Yeshe Nyingpo Dharma center. Rinpoche also maintains a regular schedule at a medical doctor's clinic in Eugene, where he consults the doctor on difficult cases. He has also been teaching medical seminars to Western health practitioners in many cities on the West Coast.

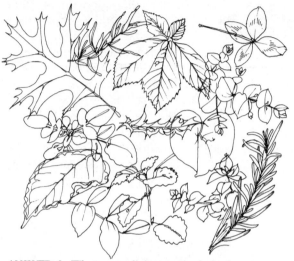

QUESTION: Rinpoche, what is the meaning of medicine and healing in the Tibetan tradition?

ANSWER: When one is learning and practicing (the medicine), this is inner medicine. When doing things on the outside, then this is outer medicine. Herbal substances temporarily cure sickness. All the causes, conditions, and results of healing ultimately lead to the Medicine Buddha [in other words, enlightenment].

QUESTION: Rinpoche, how are plants used for healing in Tibetan medicine?

ANSWER: In Tibetan medicine, not only herbs are used. Herbs, animal parts, earth, rocks, and salts are used, too. There are many different ways of making medicines. With herbs, sometimes we use the trunk, sometimes the root, sometimes the leaf, sometimes the flower, and sometimes the food. There are different times and different ways for different sicknesses. It is not the same all the time.

The times for taking the parts of the plants are different, also. Leaves are picked when they are just coming out. If only the flower is used, it is picked when it comes into maturity. If a food part is being used, then it is picked when the flower turns into that food. For roots, when all the flowers fall is the time to take them.

With some plants, only the root is used, with others only the trunk, and still others only the leaves. It's different for each plant and sickness.

QUESTION: Rinpoche, one thing that distinguishes Tibetan medicine from other herbal systems is the idea that the same type of plant from different environments will have different healing qualities. Can you describe why this is so?

ANSWER: Most sicknesses are from heat or cold. Someone who has a heat disease needs plants from a very high mountain where it is very cold. For a cold disease plants from a low warm place where the sun is shining are used.

Taste is also important. Almost all bile diseases are heat diseases and almost all medicines used to treat them taste very bitter. But sometimes we mix in something with a slight sweet taste for a bile disease. For air diseases, we would use some kind of plant with oil, something sticky, or milky. With phlegm diseases, usually we need plants with a salty taste, and sometimes with a sour taste. For an air disease, whatever we use, whether it is root, trunk, leaf, and so on, we taste to see if it is sweet.

But not only taste is used. There are also many different things to learn. How the land is—high or low, if it is a cold place or a hot place. How is the plant growing? Is it big or small? Does it touch a spring? In what way does it get its water? When all this knowledge is connected, then a good understanding will come.

QUESTION: How are these qualities discovered in Tibetan medicine?

ANSWER: Most of Tibetan medicine comes from what the Buddha learned, from his wise eyes looking at plants to see what kinds would benefit different kinds of sicknesses. This is how it is taught in Buddhist medicine.

QUESTION: In the Tibetan system, were herbs ever grown in the garden?

ANSWER: No.

QUESTION: They were always collected in the wild?

ANSWER: Ah, yes, yes. Why? Because of different places and different conditions. There are many different lands. The earth's conditions are not the same everywhere. The water's conditions are different. Heat, and so on—these things cannot be brought into a garden . . . But it *may* be possible to do it. I don't know. *May*be . . .

growth, and space provides the area for the plants' growth.

These are the parameters of what might be called Ayurvedic ecology. The proportion of these elements in plants varies according to climate, altitude, exposure, season, and specific local conditions. And it is the elemental makeup of a plant that often determines its use in Tibetan medicine. According to this tradition, the actual healing qualities of different specimens within a species will change according to the elemental balance of the plant's environment and processing.

The Tibetan physician sees each plant as a microcosmic reflection of the conditions of the environment in which it grows. The doctor notes these environmental conditions as he gathers plants. He then processes each plant according to the way he plans to use it in future preparations.

For example, if a plant is to be used for its cooling properties, it will be collected from a shady and windy place and dried in the shade and wind, rather than in the sun or indoors. Plants growing in places exposed to regular or strong winds contain a greater proportion of the air element than their relatives in more sheltered spots. It is principally the light and cool properties of air that are, in this example, being maximized in the plant. (Air is also associated with qualities of motility, bitterness, instability, and a whitish color.)

All plants grow in earth, but some grow in thin, rocky soils while others are found in deep, heavy soils. Plants that grow where the element earth is stronger generally embody more intensely that element's properties, which are heaviness, strength, smoothness, firmness, and the capability of increasing pungency. Plants growing where the water element predominates tend to be more like

water: heavy, cool, smooth, soft, moist, oily, and without a pungent aroma.

Exposed areas and the southern slopes of hills receive more sunlight, and thus the element of fire is strong in plants growing there. If a plant is to be used for heating (such as the mugwort used in moxa, page 186), it will be gathered from a sunny place and dried in the sun. Herbs with the qualities of fire are sharp, light, hot, rough, oily, and without a pungent smell or taste.

As in other surviving ancient healing systems, herbs in Tibetan medicine are considered more effective when their habitat is related to the home of the patient. The belief is that people, like plants, also contain varying proportions of the five elements. Generally, Tibetan doctors like to use plants from high places for people who live in high places, and vice versa. And in certain cases, they maintain that the herb should even be administered in the place where it naturally grows. If the plant is moved from a high place to a low place, for example, the air element, being light and unstable, will diminish in its effect on a person who needs more of that element.

Balance of the Humors

In the Ayurvedic system, health and sickness are viewed as the balance—or lack of balance—between three body humors: phlegm, bile, and air. The three humors are a condensation of the five elements. Water and earth combine to make phlegm, while space pervades all three humors.

When a humor's influence is in excess of a normal balance, a "disease" of that humor can develop. Deficiency symptoms can appear, also. Diseases may be caused by any combination of two or three humoral imbalances.

The five elements determine the tastes and other properties of the herbs which are administered to correct imbalances of the humors. An herb's taste quality is an especially good indicator of its predominant elements. In general the following patterns are defined:

> The taste is sweet if earth and water predominate.
>
> The taste is sour if earth and fire predominate.
>
> The taste is salty if water and fire predominate.
>
> The taste is bitter if water and air predominate.
>
> The taste is acrid if fire and air predominate.
>
> The taste is astringent if air and earth predominate.

The Tibetan healer uses taste and other properties of an herb as a guide in concocting medicines to correct specific humoral imbalances. The table, How Flavors Balance Humors, gives an idea how the flavors and humors correspond.

Spiritual Imbalances

Besides humoral imbalances, the Tibetan healing system accords (as do most Eastern medical philosophies) a corresponding spiritual imbalance to each physical one. It is chronic behavior patterns, they believe, that gradually upset the physical balance of humors in a person's body, which in turn leads to disease. According to Buddhist philosophy, for example, the basic cause of each illness is one of the "Three Poisons." Ignorance will cause a phlegm imbalance; anger, a bile imbalance; and excessive desire, an air imbalance. The Buddhists also define a relationship between the five elements and the "Five Poisons": earth-pride, water-anger, fire-desire, air-jealousy, space-ignorance. The space-ignorance relationship is considered

---

HOW FLAVORS BALANCE HUMORS

Humor	decreased by substances that are:	increased by substances that are:
PHLEGM	sour, salty, astringent, light, rough, acrid, sharp	sweet, bitter, cool, soft
BILE	bitter, astringent, cool, soft	sour, salty, acrid, warm, sharp, smooth
AIR	sweet, sour, smooth, heavy	bitter, acrid, light, cool, rough

the source of all poisons. A healer using this system would prescribe character improvement in the deficient area and medicine corresponding to its element counterpart.

Tibetan Polypharmacy

Tibetans generally make compounded formulas out of their herbs, as the Chinese do. In fact, the Tibetans are famous for their skill in polypharmacy. Their herbal formulas are designed to perform three functions in the patient's body: the main therapeutic action, a supportive action, and a safety or neutralizing action. Although a skilled physician can make up medicinal combinations on an individual basis, very often Tibetan doctors rely on traditional formulas that have been in use for many centuries.

Although there has not in the past been much contact between Tibetan doctors and their herbalist counterparts in Western countries, in recent years a dialogue has begun. Information has begun to be exchanged, and more people in the West are starting to study Tibetan healing techniques. In Switzerland, for example, a preparation called Padma 28, which is based on a traditional Tibetan herbal formula, has been popular for some years. In the United States, schools such as the Institute for Traditional Medicine and Preventive Health Care, in California, and the Arura Institute of Buddhist Medicine, in Oregon, are offering instruction abut the medicine of Tibet. A growing number of herbalists are expressing interest in traditional healing techniques from the East and in exploring what can be learned, adapted, and applied here in the West.

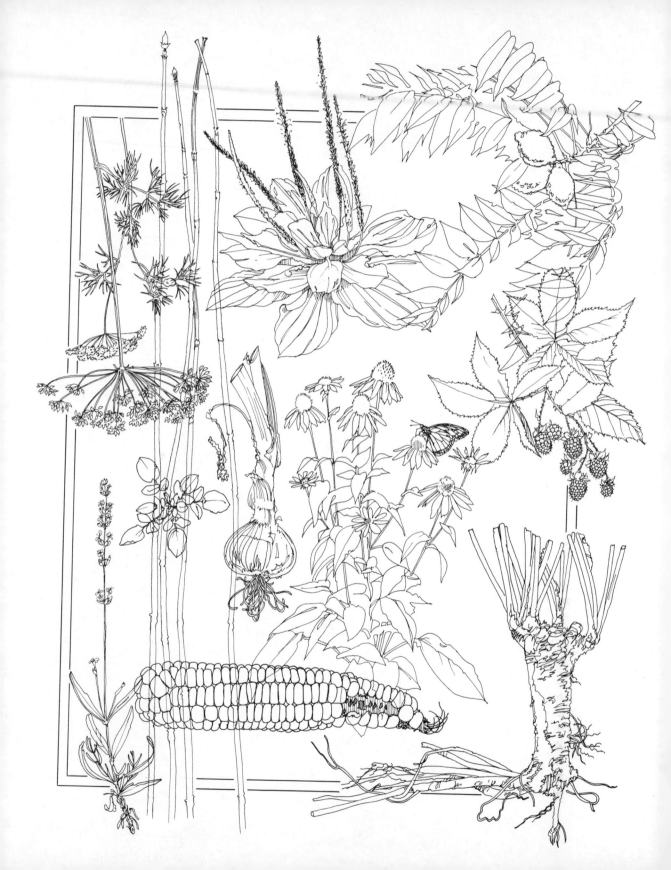

An Illustrated Guide to Healing Plants

This illustrated guide contains only a tiny number of the plants available in the mountains, valleys, plains, stream banks, and fields of nature's pharmacopoeia. How did we choose the plants for this guide? We looked for plants which have a long, respected history of use in at least one system of traditional herbal medicine. Many of the plants we chose are used in two or more systems. Many are being investigated by modern researchers, and when available, we have included information on their findings. Generally, the plants we selected are found and used for healing in many countries. Alfalfa, for instance, is used in many European countries, as well as in Chinese herbal medicine. So are yellow dock, garlic, rosemary, mugwort, bearberry, sage, and licorice. Most of the plants we chose are adaptable to a variety of growing conditions, but we did select some plants with limited or special growing conditions, because we feel strongly that they are very good healing herbs. Ginger and cayenne, for instance, are both tropical plants, and in more temperate regions must be grown in greenhouses. Goldenseal and ginseng both are rather difficult to culti- vate and require special lath houses or semiwild cultivation in woodland settings.

Some of the plants included in the guide are vegetables, fruits, flowers, and berries, which you may not have considered part of the herb world. In the broadest sense, however, a healing herb is any plant or part of a plant that can be used to increase health and alleviate distress. Apples, blackberries, peony blossoms, lavender flowers, and cabbage are all herbs, using this definition.

Finally, we chose the plants for this guide because we know them and enjoy growing them and using them ourselves. Because there is such an immense number of healing plants all around the world, and even in our own backyards, we had to leave out many plants that we know to be useful and effective for healing. We hope that this guide will serve as an introduction, however, and will provide a glimpse into the marvelous world of healing herbs.

The Resource Guide in the back of the book lists books, schools, and teachers which can help you to continue your studies, in both growing and using herbs as medicine.

In this chapter, we have included some instructions for harvesting, drying, and storing specific herbs, but for a more complete discussion of these subjects, please refer to chapter 6. The guide also includes some information on making herbal preparations from the herbs listed, but more detailed information on making medicinal preparations, cosmetics, salves, compresses, and so forth is also included in chapter 6. Chapter 5 contains more detailed information on the cultivation of healing herbs, which augments the growing tips given for each plant in this chapter.

With a few exceptions, the plants in this chapter have been drawn to scale. Plants shown by themselves are one-half life size; plants shown with roots are one-quarter life size, and the roots are one-half life size.

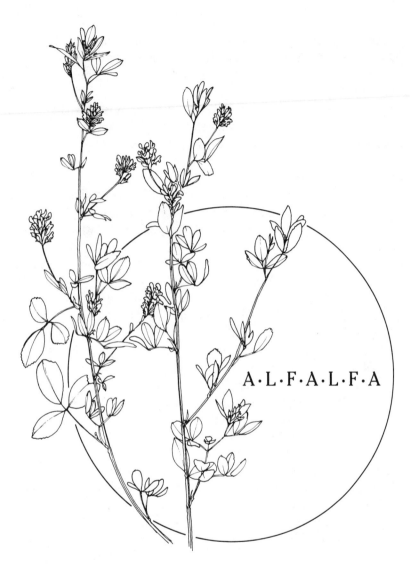

ALFALFA (Lucerne, Buffalo Grass)
Botanical: *Medicago sativa*

Although today alfalfa is best known as a forage crop, it is a time-honored medicine in many cultures. European herbalists knew about its soothing and strengthening qualities centuries ago. When alfalfa was brought to the United States around 1850, its nutritive and medicinal qualities quickly established its value with folks in the Great Plains region where it was referred to as Buffalo Grass. Native Americans collected the plant's seeds and ground them into flour to thicken and enrich gruel and to enhance bread. They introduced the plant's young shoots and leaves to their diet as tasty greens. Known as *Mu-Su* in Chinese medicine, alfalfa made its way to China during the late Han Dynasty (around 200 A.D.) from its original home in Persia. One of its most common uses in Chinese medicine is for treatment of ulcers. It is also used in Chinese medicine to strengthen the digestive tract and stimulate appetite.

Alfalfa grows from Maine as far south as Virginia and then westward to the Pacific coast. It reaches 1½ to 3 feet in height when fully grown. Alfalfa is a succulent perennial plant which sends up 15 to 30 stems from its crown. Its leaves are trifoliate, like clover leaves, but alfalfa leaves are longer than clover leaves and have a blunt tip. The blossoms, which grow on upright spikes, range in color from purple to pale blue or lavender. Alfalfa is a legume, like peas and beans, and after flowering the plant develops hairy, spirally contorted pods.

The alfalfa plant gives a visual impression of great vigor, and that impression is certainly not a mistaken one. Alfalfa is a healing plant in many ways. It begins by healing the soil in which it grows. It sends down impressive roots (alfalfa roots have been recorded reaching down to depths of 68 feet and more!) that break up heavy clay and hardpan and bring up valuable nutrients from the subsoil. Like other legumes, it fixes nitrogen in the soil. Its ability to break up and enrich the soil makes alfalfa a very beneficial plant. Mixed with clover, it creates a soil-replenishing ground cover. Because of its high mineral and vitamin content, it makes an excellent fodder for livestock. And for those same reasons, alfalfa is a fine green manure.

Alfalfa does best in a loamy soil. It can, however, be planted in heavy clay soils after a planting of clover has helped to aerate and loosen the soil. It does better in clay soil than it does in sandy soils, because it is a heavy feeder and clay is generally richer in nutrients. Seeds are usually sown in the autumn, so that the plant has an opportunity to establish itself before the winter cold sets in and causes it to go dormant. Before planting, manure and rock phosphate can be dug into the planting area to prepare the soil and to help establish the stand. Seeds can be broadcast over large plots, or planted in rows, about 18 inches apart. Although alfalfa is somewhat resistant to drought, it does require watering, especially in its early stages of growth. A young stand of alfalfa should be thoroughly irrigated every two weeks. Each year, irrigation can be decreased as the plant takes hold and sends its penetrating roots down into the subsoil.

A crop of alfalfa planted in fall will produce its first flowers late the following spring. If it is cut and harvested promptly, the plant will usually achieve a second flowering during the growing season. Alfalfa is harvested for use as animal fodder when 10 percent of the plants are in bloom. For medicinal uses, the plant should also be harvested at flowering time. Cut back the plants to within 3 inches of the crown. Then dry them for storage according to the directions given in chapter 6.

Alfalfa is rich is some important nutrients, including calcium, phosphorus, iron, potassium, magnesium, essential enzymes, choline, sodium, and silicon, as well as vitamins A, B$_6$, D, K, and P. Herbalists have long used alfalfa to treat ulcers with surprisingly good results.

The vitamin P, or rutin, that alfalfa contains builds capillary strength and reduces inflammation of the stomach lining, the vitamin A helps maintain the stomach's health, and enzymes present in alfalfa aid in food assimilation. Alfalfa tea aids in the digestion of proteins, starches, fats, and sugars.

The part of the alfalfa plant used is the flowering top and leaves, which are dried and made into a tea. Western herbalists make the tea with the whole leaves and flowers and then strain off the plant parts. Chinese herbalists make a fine powder of the dried plant parts by grinding them with a mortar and pestle. They then add the powder to water to make a tea.

Alfalfa must be afforded a prominent place in the healing garden, both for its restorative qualities to the soil and the ecosystem in general, and for its traditional healing uses.

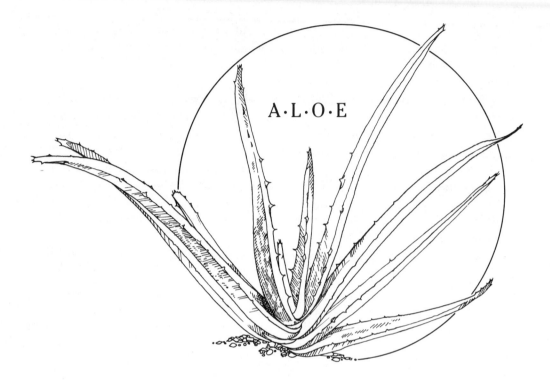

ALOE (Burn Plant)
Botanical: *Aloe vera*

Aloe is an unusually striking plant. Its long, fleshy and succulent leaves radiate upward and outward from its crown. A member of the Lily family, aloe is native to East and South Africa, where it grows to heights of 30 feet or more. It has been transported to the West Indies and other tropical countries, and it will even grow well in some Mediterranean countries. In both the southwestern and southeastern United States, aloe thrives outdoors. It is often planted as an ornamental and reaches heights of 6 to 8 feet.

Throughout the less tropical parts of the country, aloe can be successfully cultivated indoors or in greenhouses where the plant can be exposed to southern, southeastern, or eastern sun. Medium-size potted aloes, about a foot tall, are commonly available in nurseries and the plant sections of department stores. They thrive best in light, well-drained soil and do not require frequent watering. A healthy plant potted in a wide, shallow pot continuously sends up offshoots. You can remove these shoots and pot them separately when they are only 1 to 2 inches tall. The easiest way to remove offshoots is to unpot the plant, brush away the dirt, and separate the babies from the mother plant. Then return the mother plant to its pot, adding fresh soil as needed.

Every garden or household should contain several of these beautiful, useful plants. They are absolutely the best external remedy for minor burns and skin inflammations. Aloe can also soothe insect bites, mild cases of poison oak, ivy, or sumac, diaper rash, heat rash, or sunburn. In most cases, the fresh juice of the plant affords prompt relief when applied immediately to a new burn. Even if you apply it some time later, the healing properties of aloe will have positive effects on burns and other skin problems.

The easiest way to use a fresh aloe leaf is to cut off as much of one of the succulent leaves as you need for treating a problem. The plant will heal the cut section of its leaf, and you can use the rest of the leaf at some other time. Slice open the cut leaf, and dab its juice or gel directly on the skin problem. The gel, which is thick, translucent, and very pale green in color, can be scraped off large leaves with a spoon, but take care not to include any of the "bitters of aloe" from the rind of the plant. Minor burns and rashes heal best if the area is left open to the air for some time. If more protection is needed, you can cover the area with a light gauze bandage.

Aloe is a popular plant—over one *million* gallons of lotions and other aloe products are sold annually in the United States. About 80 percent of the aloe products sold are manufactured to be taken internally. Traditionally, herbalists crystallized aloe vera extract to use as a powerful laxative and cleanser for the liver, kidneys, and spleen. Medical authorities now question the use of aloe as an internal medicine because a substance called anthraquinone, which it contains, is believed to have caused gastrointestinal cramping in some people.

In 1972, a group of 30 manufacturers of aloe products formed a trade association called the National Aloe Science Council. The council told the Food and Drug Administration (FDA) it planned to establish standards for the production of aloe vera products, along with a code of ethics for the manufacturers of aloe juices, drinks, and other food products. The group is also planning scientific studies to "confirm or dispel folktales" concerning the plant, whose internal use has attracted controversy because of the lack of scientific testing and because of lax industry standards in extraction of its gel.

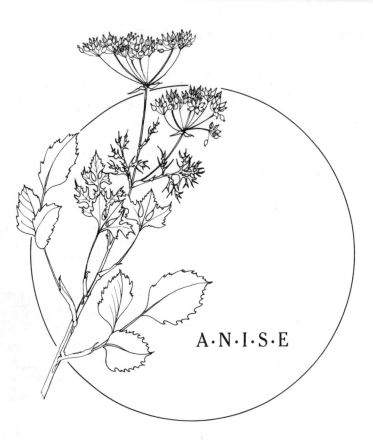

A·N·I·S·E

ANISE

Botanical: *Pimpinella anisum*

    Because it is gentle, safe, and delicious, anise is a very good addition to the herb garden. The ancient Egyptians cultivated anise, as did the Greeks and Romans. The Romans made an anise-laced cake, a forerunner of our modern wedding cake. This *mustaceum* was a delicious way to end a long feast, and the digestion-aiding properties of the anise seed in it balanced the otherwise rich ingredients. Anise leaves and stalks are an ancient salad herb, popular even today in France and Italy. They have a sweet, licoricelike taste and are delicious served fresh, or steamed and sautéed with a bit of olive oil, garlic, and lemon juice.

    Sweet anise with its succulent, hollow stalk, and feathery, fernlike leaves is a member of the Umbellifer family. Displayed against its vibrant light green foliage are the plant's white flowers in the umbrellalike shape characteristic of the group, which also includes angelica, coriander, and fennel. Anise has a perennial root except in cold climates, where the plant is an annual herb. It grows from 1½ to 2 feet tall in moist, fairly rich soil and full sun.

Plant anise seeds when the danger of frost is over and cover with about ⅛ inch of topsoil. The seeds will germinate in 7 to 14 days, depending on the air and soil temperature. Because it has a long taproot, anise can only be transplanted in the seedling stage. By late summer, the plants will be ready for harvest, although you can gather small amounts of the feathery leaves before then.

Anise's healing properties emanate from its seeds. Gather the seeds when they have turned from green to grayish brown. Cut the entire umbel along with a length of stalk when the seeds are ripe. Then hang the anise stalks with their seed clusters upside down in a paper bag, as described in Drying Herbs, in chapter 6.

Medicinally, sweet anise has warming and moistening properties. It is also slightly diuretic and has been used traditionally in European herbal medicine to treat flatulence and indigestion, to sweeten the breath, and to increase mother's milk. Mildly expectorant and helpful in the relief of cough and congestion symptoms, anise appears frequently as a flavoring and active ingredient in cough syrups and lozenges.

Star anise is the star-shaped pod of a tree (*Illicium anisatum* or *Illicium verum*), and in Chinese medicine enjoys some of the same uses as sweet anise does in European medicine. The star anise tree is native to China but also grows in Japan and North Vietnam. Star anise is a tender evergreen tree or shrub which grows up to 18 feet in height. It has alternate, shiny, aromatic leaves, and yellow, unscented flowers with many petals which appear in solitary fashion. These are followed by the starlike fruit, with eight rays, each containing a shiny, flat, oblong seed. The star-shaped fruits are collected when they are green and then sun-dried until they become woody and reddish brown. The star anise tree was imported to Central America, and now it grows wild in Yucatan, Mexico, and Costa Rica. The tree likes well-drained, fairly rich soil, and adequate moisture. It can be grown in climates where the temperature does not drop below freezing. Gardeners in colder areas can cultivate it indoors or in a greenhouse.

Star anise is found in many recipes traditional to Chinese and Japanese cuisine and medicine. Unlike sweet anise, the star anise has warming and drying qualities. The Chinese often chew on a ray of star anise after meals to sweeten the breath and relieve flatulence. Japanese people plant the tree in temple courtyards and pound its bark to make one of the ingredients for their temple incense.

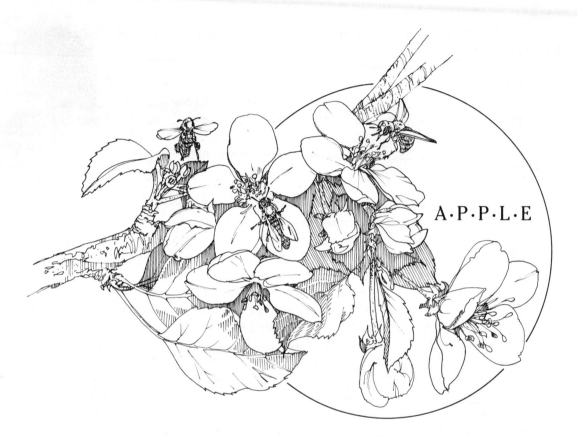

A·P·P·L·E

APPLE

Botanical: *Malus* species

Apple is called the "king of fruits," but the entire apple tree is also a noteworthy agent of natural health maintenance. The old saying about apples could well be changed to an apple *tree* keeps the doctor away. The tree's fruit, flowers, buds, leaves, twigs, and bark all impart health-giving properties. The only part you shouldn't use is the seeds. They are toxic and should not be consumed in quantities greater than the number of seeds in the apple being eaten at the moment. Several years ago a man died from eating a cup of apple seeds. He had saved them and eaten them all at once, thinking they were a delicacy.

Today, approximately 2,000 varieties of apple trees are known or cultivated around the world. All of these are descended from the wild crab apple, a member of the Rose family believed by many to be a native of central Asia. The crab apple itself has countless varieties, since each tree seems to develop fruits of varying shape, color, texture, and flavor. The fantastic diversity of apples is in itself a healing characteristic, reminding us of nature's own vigor and creativity. Although modern marketing trends have limited popular awareness to 4 or 5 apple varieties, it wasn't long ago that 20 to 25 different kinds could be found in the same market during a growing season.

In recent years, renewed interest in the culture of old apple varieties has made it easier to find and grow some of the traditional types. This is important because the modern commercial apples were not bred for resistance to pests and diseases or for old-fashioned home storage. Now, however, plant breeders are working to develop new varieties that can withstand some of the more troublesome diseases. Also, more variety means a greater selection of tasty, fresh, in-season fruit throughout the growing season. These days apple trees come in all sizes, from dwarf types that are 5 or 6 feet tall to standard varieties that reach 30 feet or more in height. There are apples for cold regions such as Maine and Minnesota, and there are even apples for warm places such as Florida. Generally, apples thrive best in temperate climates with a moderate, but recognizable winter. They prefer rich, loamy soils with plenty of moisture and good drainage. The best place to get details on individual apple varieties and growing conditions in your area is your local nursery or USDA Cooperative Extension Service Office. You will also find some information on incorporating trees in the herb garden in chapter 5, and some recommended sources of more information on growing fruit trees in the Resource Guide at the back of the book.

The apple tree's first healing component, its inner bark, is collectible in springtime, when the tree's nutrients are flowing in the cambium layer to meet the coming needs of buds and leaves. Generally, herbalists favor the inner bark of apple tree roots over the inner bark of the trunk (which is more effective than the inner bark of the branches). Trees in an old apple orchard that are being removed provide a good source of root or trunk bark (as well as fine firewood). Be sure to get permission from the owner before you do any collecting, though, and also make certain the trees were grown organically. If you don't know of any apple trees that are being chopped down, the bark can be collected from sucker shoots or pruned branches. It is also possible to dig and cut out a small piece of root from a well-established tree, but you must make sure you do not sever a main root branch. Follow the directions in chapter 6 under General Guidelines for Harvesting, for removing and processing the inner bark of trees.

The buds, blossoms, and leaves of apple trees are also used medicinally. Gather them in the spring, just before each of them reaches maturity, and dry completely in the shade where it is not too hot (see chapter 6 also).

Apples themselves translate into many good things in the kitchen. You can dry or can them, make apple jelly, sauce or butter, cider, and many other products. The best way to store apples is in their fresh state. For best results, handpick apples when ripe, leaving the stem intact, taking care not to bruise them, either. Pick only the most perfect apples; they will keep best. Pack layers of apples in boxes, crates, or barrels, alternating layers of apples with layers of straw, sawdust, or dry maple leaves. Do not let the apples touch each other. Place the containers in a root cellar, dry basement, garage, or cool pantry or closet. Any place is good for apple storage if it stays relatively dry and cool without freezing. Check the apples now and then, and take out any that may be rotting. Stored this way, the apples should keep until the spring.

The Japanese consider apples the most yang fruit, suitable for people who want to continue eating fruit while maintaining a yang dietary balance. This yang quality of apples also makes them more appropriate for people living in northern climates, which is where apples grow best. Apples contain malic and tartaric acids, and salts of potassium, sodium, magnesium, and iron. They are slightly laxative, calming, and purging. In herbal medicine tradition, they are regarded as having a cleansing influence on the liver, colon, spleen, and kidneys.

Apples have been used in traditional cuisine for centuries as a tasty way to enhance health and as a foil for rich foods. Applesauce was often served with pork or goose to aid digestion of the fatty meat. Apples can also be paired with slices of cheese or with cheese in a pie to serve as a digestive aid. Fresh, unsweetened apple cider is a healthy beverage and a pleasant way to decrease stomach acidity. In her classic book, *A Modern Herbal,* Maude Grieve reported that in Normandy, where apple cider was one of the most popular beverages, the occurrence of kidney stones or gallstones was almost unheard of. New England folk medicine also prescribes the apple to dissolve stones. Although there is no scientific evidence that apples really do work this way, the tradition is a long-standing one, and modern day naturopaths still prescribe apples to help patients pass stones from the gallbladder. For therapeutic effects, tart apple varieties such as McIntosh, Pippin, Granny Smith, or Newton are the best. People with sensitive stomachs should always eat their apples cooked.

In early spring, the sight of apple trees in bloom is one of the most picturesque country scenes. Apple blossoms are widely admired for their beautiful white and pink hues and their spicy sweet fragrance, but not many people know that the blossoms have medicinal properties as well. The world-famous French herbalist Maurice Mességué uses an infusion of apple blossoms to treat sore throats and colds, and as a diuretic.

Perhaps the most famous part of the apple tree, as far as herbalists are concerned, is the bark of the inner root or trunk. It is considered a superior neutral or astringent tonic for the colon, kidneys, bladder, and spleen. In Chinese medicine, apple tree bark is used to treat what they call "wet" or "soggy" spleen disorders such as diabetes, hypoglycemia, or blood toxicity. Other traditional uses for apple tree bark have included the treatment of nausea, fever, and vomiting, all common symptoms of flu. The inner bark of wild crab apple trees is considered the best for use in herbal therapy.

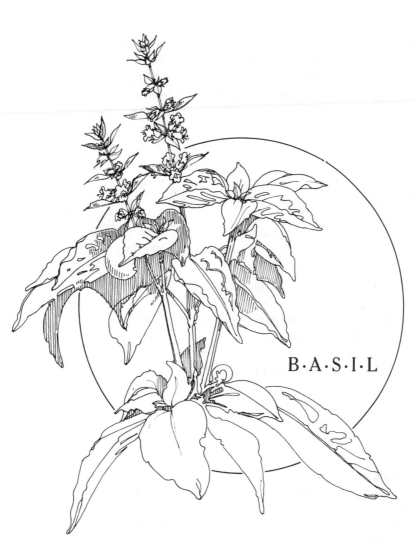

B·A·S·I·L

BASIL

Botanical: *Ocimum basilicum*

Ancient lore seems to have accorded basil somewhat mixed attributes. In Italy basil signified love; in Greece it meant hate. And in Jewish lore, basil was said to bring strength during long fasting. In India basil was sacred to the gods Krishna and Vishnu and pots of the herb appeared in many gardens in their honor. The French called basil the *herbe royale,* or royal herb. Though no one knows exactly why, basil has also been called the "king of herbs." One possible origin of its name is the Greek word for king, *basileus.* But another origin cited is *basilicus,* an old name for serpent (perhaps the name derived from basil's use as an antidote for poisonous insect bites).

Nicholas Culpeper, the English herbalist, opined on the astrological nature of basil. He declared that as "an herb of Mars and under the Scorpion . . . it is no marvel if it [basil] carry a virulent quality with it." The venerable herbalist further proclaimed that according to a French doctor named Hilarius (no pun intended) basil bred a scorpion in the brain of one man who merely sniffed the plant!

Basil is a tender annual herb found growing wild in many countries including India, Africa, Japan, Persia, and Malaysia. Its leaves are oval, but the edges tip inward toward the central spine, giving a slight appearance of ruffles. Basil is usually brilliant green but can range from yellow-green to deep green, depending on the soil in which it is grown. There are many varieties of the plant, including one that is deep purple-red, but all of them share the sweetly pungent minty-licorice aroma and taste.

Basil is easy to grow and makes a delightful addition to the herb, flower, or vegetable garden. Besides its elegant and aromatic contributions to the garden, basil is a beneficial companion plant to tomatoes—it is believed to enhance their flavor and growth and protect them from harmful insects. Planted as an edging in a more traditional herbaceous border or in an informally arranged herb garden, basil makes a lovely visual statement, too.

Wait until the danger of frost is past before planting outdoors, as this herb is very sensitive to frost. Sow the seeds in rows, ¼ inch deep and 12 inches apart. Another way to protect against frost damage is to start the seed indoors and transplant the seedlings 12 inches apart when the danger of frost is over and the soil has warmed. Basil likes rich, well-drained soil and plenty of sun. It will thrive best if you enrich the soil with well-rotted compost or manure.

Pinching back the tips of the herb before it flowers will produce a bushier plant with a longer growing season. Use the freshly pinched tips of the plant and leaves gathered selectively during the growing season to season sauces, soups, stews, and many Italian and Mediterranean dishes. As the summer progresses, harvest the mature plant before it flowers and dry it in a warm, shady place on screens or muslin. For culinary purposes, you can use basil leaves fresh or dry, or preserve them by storing them in a glass jar, covering the leaves carefully with olive oil. The leaves turn dark, but their flavor is fully preserved.

Traditionally classified as a warming and moistening herb, basil is regarded as slightly antiseptic, a mild nervine, and emmenagogue. Imbibed as an infusion by nursing mothers, basil is considered a safe, gentle tonic that helps expel gas in the infant and increase lactation in the mother. It has also been used to relieve nausea and headaches. Basil is so fragrant and gentle that we might tend to overlook its healing qualities. That would certainly be our loss, for it is precisely the simple qualities of basil, and its gentle effects, that make it a reliable medicinal plant.

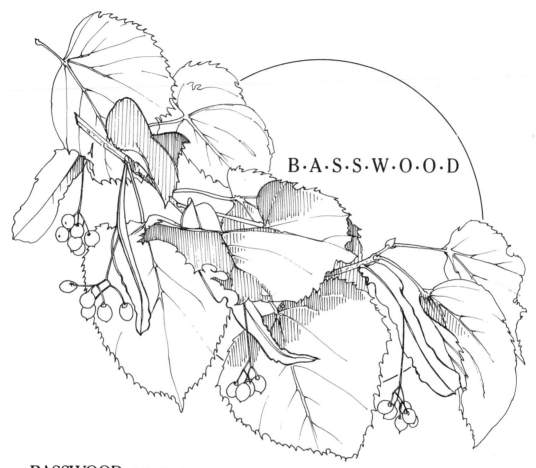

B·A·S·S·W·O·O·D

BASSWOOD (Linden)
Botanical: *Tilia americana, Tilia europaea*

The majestic basswood, known in Europe as the linden or lime tree, may reach a height of 100 feet or more. Landscapers have great esteem for its elegant, symmetrical shape, as witnessed in European parks where the stately uniformity of linden trees provides delightfully shady avenues along promenades. The European tree's chartreuse-tinted flowers enjoy a memorable association in the minds of the literati. They are responsible for the famous *tilleul* tisane whose scent and flavor, along with a madeleine cookie, aroused tomes of forgotten childhood memories for the French author Marcel Proust.

John Gerard, the sixteenth century English herbalist, eloquently praised the beauty of the basswood when he wrote, "It yieldeth a most pleasant shadow, under and within whose boughs may be made brave summer houses and banqueting arbors...." During the medieval era of Europe, basswood was often "pleached," the tender branches of trees from opposite sides of an avenue or path woven overhead into magical arbors and long green tunnels.

Basswood is also native to eastern North America, from the New England states south to the Carolinas and west to the Mississippi River. The European variety of the tree is nearly identical to the American variety, but it is usually smaller and bears smaller leaves. Basswood leaves are heart-shaped, occasionally lopsided, around 5 inches long, and slightly serrated. They are a lovely dark green on top and light green on the underside. The tree produces clusters of attractive creamy white or pale yellow pendant blossoms.

Basswood trees thrive in rich soil and require a moderate amount of moisture. They can be propagated from seeds, which take two years to germinate. If that is too slow for your taste, try making a cutting or layering, as described in chapter 5. The linden tree suffers from dryness and excessive heat. When summer droughts or hot spells occur, cover the ground under the tree with a loose, 6-inch-thick mulch of straw or leaves to slow the evaporation of moisture from the ground around the tree's roots.

A linden in bloom will often be buzzing with a very loud, distinct hum of the honeybees who love this tree. Europeans consider the honey made from the linden tree to have the finest flavor of any honey in the world. These same flowers so beloved by bees are the part of the tree most often used medicinally. Linden flower tea is a popular beverage in Europe, where it can be found at cafés and restaurants. Medicinally, European herbalists recommend it for nervousness, insomnia, cramps, and indigestion, which arises from an inability to relax while eating. Many Europeans also use the flowers in a medicinal infusion at the onset of cold symptoms, especially in combination with other cold-preventive herbs such as yarrow flowers and sage.

Linden flower baths have been used in Europe for centuries to treat insomnia, hyperactivity, and anxiety. It is said that linden flower baths can calm irritable or restless children, too. To make a bath with these lovely blossoms, follow the instructions given in Herbal Bath for Gentle Healing in chapter 6.

The basswood tree bears both fruit and flowers throughout most of the summer. The small, slightly sweet flowers ripen into yellowish green fruits about the size of a pea. During the warm summer months fresh basswood flowers can be enjoyed right from the tree. But for use during the winter, when they are most often needed, the flowers should be picked just before their full bloom and dried according to the directions in chapter 6. Collecting the flowers can be fun, especially for people who like climbing trees. One of the most effective methods for collecting quantities of these flowers is to spread some old bed sheets on the ground below the tree. Then climb the tree and gently shake the branches. Mature flowers will fall onto the sheets below. This technique works best after a few days without strong winds. Right after a windy day most of the mature flowers have already been blown away.

Basswood flowers can also be preserved in a tincture, by packing a jar with fresh blossoms and covering them with brandy (see Tinctures, chapter 6). You do not need to remove the flowers, but you can strain them off if you prefer. A tablespoon of this mixture added to a cup of hot water makes a good nightcap when you feel a cold coming on.

Native Americans used a decoction of the inner bark of the basswood to wash and treat burns. Indians and Europeans as well have also used the inner bark to make strong rope. The light weight, close grain, and softness of the linden tree's wood have made it a popular carving material.

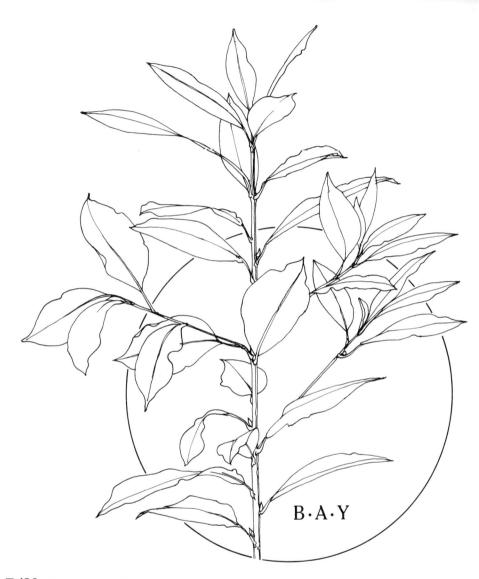

BAY (Bay laurel, Sweet bay)
Botanical: *Laurus nobilis*

The stately, fragrant bay tree has always symbolized glory and honor. It was sacred to Apollo, the Greek sun god, and when the ancient Greek civilization flourished, bay branches from the sacred groves near the healing temples were gathered and woven into wreaths to honor great artistic figures, heroes, and athletes. To wear the laurel wreath was a mark of tremendous esteem.

The lovely bay tree, which is native to the shores of the Mediterranean, reaches heights of up to 60 feet in its native habitat. Sweet bay, as it is often called, is a highly aromatic, smooth-barked tree, with dark green, shiny leaves that merits a place in your landscape design if you live where the climate is mild. The leaves are lance-shaped with wavy edges. Crushing one between your fingers releases the heady, invigorating scent and flavor characteristic of the plant.

One of the most beautiful and aromatic of all trees, sweet bay is notoriously difficult to propagate. Seeds almost invariably grow moldy; cuttings are very difficult to root and take up to six months when they are successful. With this in mind, you might simply prefer to purchase a young tree from a reputable nursery.

Bay trees can be grown outdoors in moderate climates, where the temperature does not fall below freezing. Freezing temperatures or icy winds endanger the tree, and it must be protected from these conditions. In northern climates, sweet bay trees can be grown in containers and taken indoors for the winter. A large container with wheels on the bottom makes it easy to move the tree outside during the warm weather and back inside when the weather becomes cold. Sweet bay trees need a moderate soil with good drainage and plenty of sun. Indoors, trees will grow between 3 and 6 feet tall.

Today the leaves of the bay are best known as a culinary herb. You can pick and use the leaves fresh all year-round or dry them (see chapter 6). Medicinally, bay has a gentle tonic effect and is considered warming and drying. Europeans use a simple infusion of the dried or fresh leaves as a general tonic, especially to help the digestive organs. Infusions of bay leaves have been used also to expel gas from the stomach and bowels. The California bay laurel and Oregon myrtle are related species, whose leaves the Native Americans and early settlers used to treat headaches, stomachaches, and rheumatism, although the effectiveness of these treatments hasn't been verified by current studies.

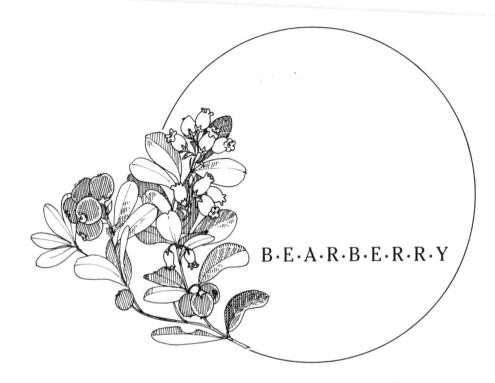

BEARBERRY (Bear Grape, Uva Ursi)

Botanical: *Arctostaphylos uva-ursi*

Heads of state and diplomats of the world might do well to follow an old custom of Native Americans, regarding bearberry. The American Indians made it a practice to add bearberry leaves (which they called kinnickinnick) to the peace pipe they smoked during tribal councils. The herb's calming and mentally clarifying influence promoted great accord among the tribes.

European herbalists considered bearberry a "kidney" herb under the astrological influence of Libra, encouraging balance and harmony. Chinese medicine also connects this kidney herb with the peaceful condition of the element water.

Bearberry is a perennial shrub with long, fibrous roots and trailing stems that often form a tangled mass of ground cover up to 18 inches high. The leaves are small, oval, and leathery in texture, and fringed with short hairs. They are a rich, deep forest green color, which occasionally turns slightly orange or mahogany-colored with age. The tough stems and branches also have a mahogany color. Pink or white flowers bloom in early summer and develop into clusters of small, dry, reddish berries by early autumn. These berries are a favorite food of bears, a characteristic which is alluded to by the fact that this plant's name means the same thing in English, Latin, and Greek—bear grape.

Bearberry is happiest on dry, sandy soils throughout Great Britain, northern Europe, and northern central Asia. In North America, its range extends from Canada south to New Jersey, Wisconsin, and northern California. It can often be found growing on the most precipitous sand banks, cliffs, and ledges, checking erosion in these otherwise barren places. In the higher alpine forests, bearberry can be found as a beautiful ground cover, rambling among majestic specimens of fir, pine, or spruce. Another natural placement for bearberry is in low-maintenance, drought-resistant landscaping. Landscape designers love to use bearberry as a ground cover to hold sandy and easily eroded soils in place, just as it does in its natural environment.

Bearberry can be transplanted (with some difficulty) by layering one or more branches of well-established wild plant into an earthenware pot set into the ground. Allow the layer to set roots for at least one full growing season before separating it from the parent plant and taking the new plant home.

You can also obtain bearberry plants from nurseries. The plants thrive in light, sandy, rather poor soil that is *not* rich in humus. Once established, the plant will spread slowly and make a lasting, attractive ground cover. In a landscape design, bearberry also does well when planted in between taller members of the Heath family such as blueberries or huckleberries.

It's best to collect bearberry leaves in the autumn, before the first frost. Because of their thick, leathery texture, they are difficult to dry. Be sure to spread them thinly; avoid piling them into deep layers, or they will ferment before they are dry.

The Doctrine of Signatures (which is explained in chapter 2) assigned bearberry the quality of being useful in removing "sand" and "gravel" from the kidneys. This parallels the plant's affinity for sandy terrains. And in the various herbal traditions in countries where bearberry grows, it is actually regarded as an excellent herb for the kidneys. It has a history of use in formulas for removing sand and gravel from the kidneys. Besides being employed as a urinary tract disinfectant, bearberry is regarded as a diuretic and a neutral tonic that reduces infection and swelling. Both European and American herbalists have used bearberry leaf tea to treat infections in the kidneys, bladder, ureter, uterus, prostate gland, and vagina.

In Chinese medicine, bearberry tea is used to treat incontinence, as it is thought to contract the sphincter muscle. It has been used to treat leukorrhea, uterine ulcers, excessive menstruation, and vaginal infections, too. The treatment consists of a tea that is drunk as a beverage and also used as a douche. Women in labor sometimes drink the tea to strengthen contractions.

Among its active constituents, which include tannin and gallic acid, bearberry contains a glucoside called arbutin. This sugar complex is metabolized only in the urinary tract. Here, it is broken down into glucose and hydrokinone. Hydrokinone is very similar to the powerful antiseptic, phenol. So bearberry actually releases a potent antiseptic chemical right where it is needed to clear up kidney and bladder infections.

Herbalists have long been impressed with bearberry's medicinal usefulness, even if it lacks significant scientific backing. And we can relate an anecdote from our own experience. One of our mothers experienced the return of a very painful bladder infection while she was visiting us. We persuaded her to chew on a bearberry leaf until she could consult her doctor. Her pain, and her skepticism, lessened within minutes.

Manzanita (*Arctostaphylos columbiana* and *A. glauca*) is another plant of the same genus, with almost identical medicinal qualities. This beautiful shrub, which displays pale gray-green leaves and dark red bark, can be found growing abundantly on the dry hills and plains throughout California. Manzanita's sweet red berries can be powdered and mixed with water for a refreshing summer drink. The American Indians gathered large quantities of manzanita berries, which are high in vitamin C, and dried them for winter use. Herbalists in southern areas sometimes substitute manzanita leaves for bearberry leaves.

Trailing arbutus (*Epigaea repens*), a common woodland ground cover, also contains arbutin and also has served as a replacement for bearberry. Trailing arbutus grows on moist, sandy soils under the shade of low pines, hemlocks, and scrub oaks throughout the eastern half of North America. Like bearberry, it is a member of the Ericaceae.

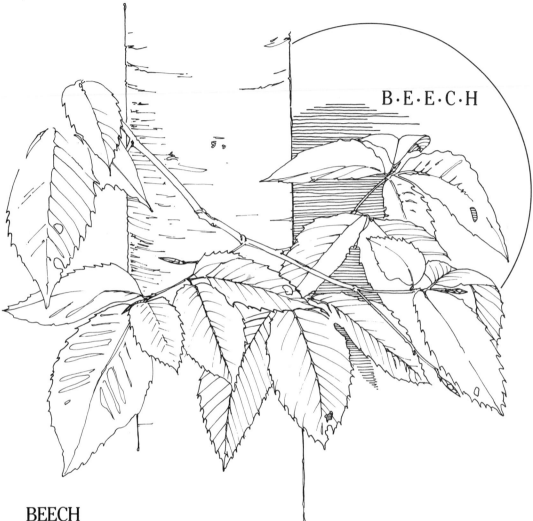

BEECH
Botanical: *Fagus grandifolia, F. sylvatica*

The beechnut is one of the sweetest nuts from the northern forests, and until not very long ago, it was available in country groceries in the eastern United States. In Europe these small triangular nuts are used as fodder for swine, but in America the beechnut has long been popular as a food for people. The authors of *Edible Wild Plants of Eastern North America,* Merritt L. Fernald and Charles A. Kinsey, describe the old method of gathering beechnuts:

> *Then all was bustle to get out blankets, spreads, old sheets and other large cloths to spread carefully beneath the heaviest-fruiting trees to catch the abundant harvest of nuts which fell from the opening burs.*[1]

With its smooth silvery gray bark, blue-green leaves and symmetrical round canopy, the beech is one of the most beautiful trees found in North America or Europe. The American beech (*Fagus grandifolia*) usually reaches heights of about 60 feet, while the European species (*F. sylvatica*) can grow as tall as 80 feet. Beech trees can be seen in mixed stands of hardwoods and conifers, growing in the rich, moist but well-drained soils found on gently rolling hills and at the bases of mountains. The beech also grows in the woods of coastal plains along the East Coast of the United States. The tree does well in any of these environments from New England westward to Ohio, Illinois, and Missouri, and southward to northern Florida and Texas. In the southern extremities of its range, beech is more common in the mountain ridges and highland woods.

Beech trees provide dense shade when they mature. Young trees should be planted in a soil with amendments of well-rotted compost or manure and should be frequently watered. See chapter 5 for some basic information on tree-planting procedures. Harvest and dry the beech tree's leaves and bark according to the directions given in chapter 6.

In his *Herbal,* the English herbalist Gerard described some sixteenth century uses for this beautiful tree:

> *The leaves of the beech are very profitably applied unto hot swellings, blisters, and excoriations; and being chewed they are good for chapped lips, and paine of the gums. The kernals or mast are reported to ease the paine of the kidneys if they are eaten . . . the water that is found in the hollownesse of beeches cureth the naughty scurfe, tetters, and scabs of men, horses, kine, and sheepe, if they be washed therewith.*

Although they probably didn't know what the "naughty scurfe" was, Native Americans used beech for purposes similar to those Gerard lists. They steeped a handful of fresh beech bark in a cupful or two of water and used the tea for skin rashes, especially poison ivy. Early American settlers applied bruised beech leaves directly to burns and also made the leaves into a decoction, which they used to treat both scalds and frostbite. According to the Doctrine of Signatures, these uses of beech for skin problems correspond to the tree's smooth, tight and elastic skin, or bark. Both American and European herbalists have used the infusion of beech bark and leaves to bathe sores, swellings, and wounds.

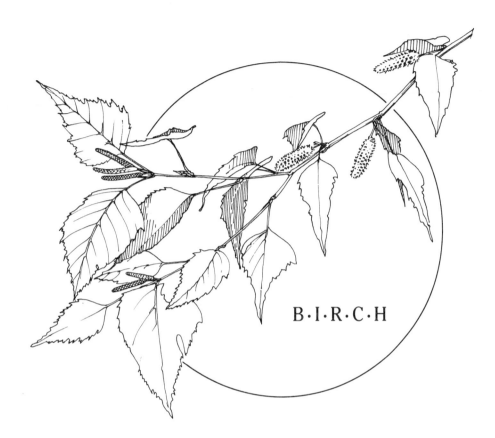

BIRCH (Sweet or black birch; paper, canoe, or silver birch)
Botanical: *Betula lenta* and *B. papyrifera* (also called *B. alba*)

The numerous species of *Betula* all possess a membranous outer bark that peels off readily in paperlike strips. In fact, an old sanskrit word, *bhurga,* from which our word birch may have derived, means "that which is written upon." The many varieties of birch trees can generally be divided into white, black, and yellow birches. The white birch grows throughout Europe from Sicily north to Iceland, and eastward to Asia. A larger variety of the white birch, commonly called the paper birch, grows in eastern North America from the New England states to the Great Lakes region, in northern areas of the Pacific Northwest, and north of these areas, throughout Canada.

The distinctive charm of the white birch is reflected in its silvery white bark, pretty, ovate, serrated leaves which are fuzzy on the underside, and in the tiny, graceful catkins which dangle from its branches. The catkins usually persist over the winter and help to identify the tree in the spring. The paper birch is a tall tree—it can reach 100 feet in height—and can be found growing in mixed coniferous hardwood forests, and at the borders of lakes, streams, and swamps. It has been a highly popular landscape tree for the past several decades. As an ornamental, however, silver birches often fall prey to borer attacks when planted outside their normal range. All the birches prefer light, moist soil and do well when planted near streams and lakes.

The black birch, also called sweet birch (*Betula lenta*), can be found growing in eastern North America from Maine to Tennessee and west to Iowa. It grows up to 75 feet in height and has dark brown bark which resembles that of a cherry tree. Another "black" birch, also known as river birch (*B. nigra*) has thin, shaggy bark of a terra-cotta color and grows in swamps and river lowlands in the South, north as far as New Jersey. Yellow birch (*B. lutea*) has lustrous yellowish gray, shaggy bark.

Wherever birch trees grow, they have been used by native people for a large variety of healing purposes. The active principle contained in birch oil, methyl salicylate, is related to aspirin and has been found useful in treating rheumatism. It is a local analgesic that is effective in topical applications. Among European herbalists, the birch is best known as a remedy for kidney disorders; it is used in the form of a simple infusion taken in cupfuls three times daily. European and American herbalists also use a hot poultice made from the leaves, bark, and catkins of the birch tree to treat open wounds and skin irritations. Native Americans used birch leaves, buds, catkins, and inner bark in these very same ways—as a diuretic, detergent, and antiseptic. Birch leaf tea can be added to a bath as a refreshing skin tonic and is an effective scalp wash that discourages dandruff and hair loss. You can harvest all these parts of the birch tree in the spring and dry them for year-round use, according to directions in chapter 6.

When making an infusion (from leaves and buds) or a decoction (from twigs and harder parts), remember that the plant's volatile oil quickly dissipates with heat. Do not boil or even simmer the tea, but simply allow it to steep in warm water until the water cools. Keep the container tightly covered. When you dry birch parts to store for later use, dry them only at room temperature, no hotter, to preserve the oil.

The bark, young buds, leaves, and twigs of the sweet or black birch contain a highly aromatic oil which is used to make the flavoring agent, oil of wintergreen. A few drops of this oil adds a refreshing note to bath water or cosmetic preparations such as after-shave and massage oil. Birch oil is also considered beneficial to boils and sores when applied externally. General guidelines for extracting essential oils and making after-shave lotion and massage oil are given in chapter 6.

In the spring, the black birch circulates a copious amount of sap, which can be tapped in much the same way as the sap from sugar maples. The sap can then be boiled down to make a syrup. The very diluted taste of the unboiled sap is similar to that of pure water, and people sometimes use it instead of water when local water supplies are contaminated. You can also substitute the sap for water when making birch tea with the buds, leaves, or twigs.

Birch beer is made from the twigs and inner bark of the sweet birch. To make it, place 4 quarts of finely cut twigs or inner bark into a 5-gallon stoneware crock. Add 4 gallons of water or birch sap and bring to a boil. Mix in 1 gallon of honey, and remove the crock from the heat. When the solution has cooled, strain and discard the solid parts. Then place one cake of soft yeast on a piece of toast and float it on top of the brew. Cover the crock (but not too tightly) and let the mixture ferment until the solution begins to settle, about one week. Then, the "beer" can be bottled, capped tightly, and stored in a cool, dry place. Unopened bottles can be stored for several months to a year, depending on how complete the fermentation process was before bottling, and other variables such as storage conditions and the tightness of the bottles' seal. Once opened, you can store the birch beer in the refrigerator for about a month.

The white or paper birch does not contain the same aromatic oil as does the sweet birch, but Native Americans used its sap to make a sweet syrup, or boiled down the sap into birch sugar. They also boiled the bark of the white birch to use for purposes similar to that of the sweet birch—to treat wounds, bruises, and burns. White birchbark is also famous as the material used for birchbark canoes.

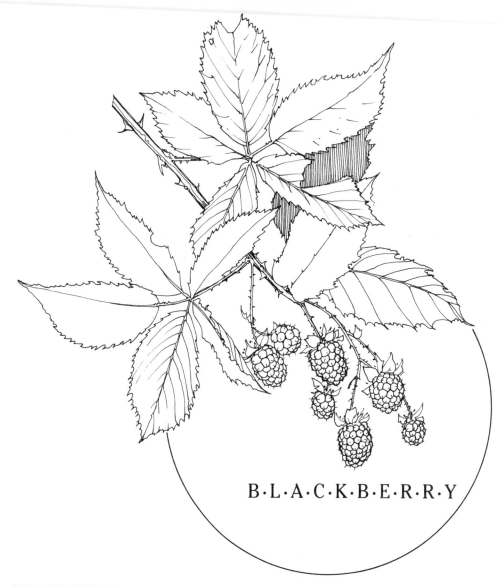

B·L·A·C·K·B·E·R·R·Y

BLACKBERRY

Botanical: *Rubus laciniatus, R. procerus,* and related species

Blackberry bushes offer a trinity of benefits to the sensitive gardener: a luscious fruit, alluring white blossoms, and a healing herb. The plant has a respected place in the traditional herbal medicine of China (where it is known as *Piao*), as well as in the European tradition. The ancient Greeks used blackberries as a remedy for gout. And in England, its leaves were applied directly to the skin to soothe burns and scalds.

Blackberry bushes grow wild throughout the United States and in many other temperate zones throughout North America and western Europe. They are especially abundant in Australia. Long, thorny stems, serrated leaves produced in a stellate pattern, loosely clustered blossoms, and shiny dark berries characterize the blackberry bush. The purplish blue berries are composed of numerous small drupelets, each containing a tiny seed. Wild blackberries, a bramble fruit, grow in meadows, coppices, forest borders, waste areas, and pastures.

The blackberry is a vigorous, expansive plant, as any gardener who has tried to thin, confine, or eradicate it knows. Once established, blackberry vines arrange themselves in dense, thorny masses. Rooting them out is difficult, since their root fragments continue to send up runners with apparent indomitability. Therefore, it is the better part of valor, and a heck of a lot less work, to make sure your blackberry patch has enough room to grow and prosper without becoming an intrusion of the rest of your garden. Blackberries can be trained to grow on supports, as raspberries do. Of course, this is most easily done with young starts. There are thornless blackberry varieties available, but these often seem to lack the full flavor of the thorny varieties.

Blackberries are propagated by layering branches, or by root cuttings. Take root cuttings about ½ inch long in autumn and store them in sand over the winter in a cool place (around 50°F). In the very early spring, when the ground has begun to loosen from the winter cold, set the cuttings into the soil. Place them vertically, 1 to 3 feet apart and cover them with 3 to 4 inches of soil. If you prefer, you can layer the branches in late summer, when their tips become slightly thickened and grow without leaves (see chapter 5 for directions for layering).

Blackberries will grow in many types of environments, but they prosper most in a loose, moist, moderately rich soil. Additions of well-rotted compost and manure to the base of the bushes in spring and autumn will ensure maximum development and health.

The berries, roots, leaves, and bark have all been used for healing purposes. The berries are said to have astringent and tightening qualities. Both the berries and the root have been used in Native American, European, and Chinese medicine to treat diarrhea and dysentery. The root is much more potent than the berries, and it is the part most often used for these purposes, as a simple decoction, or a decoction mixed with milk.

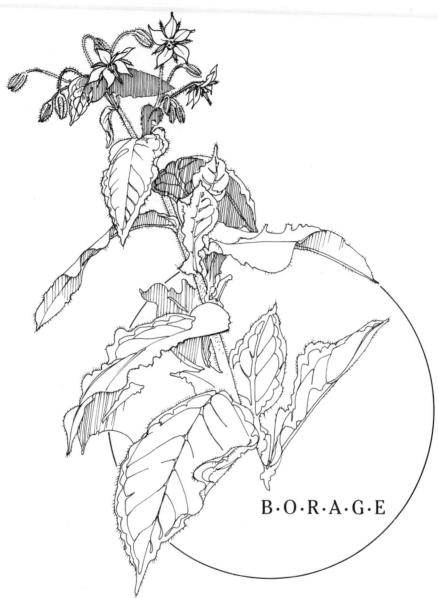

B·O·R·A·G·E

BORAGE (Talewort, Cool-Tankard)
Botanical: *Borago officinalis*

Since ancient times, borage has had a reputation for dispelling melancholy and fostering courage. Its name may come from a corruption of *corago,* "I bring courage." Or it may derive from another Latin word, *burra,* which means "a flock of wool"– perhaps reference to the plant's hairy leaves and stems. Some plant historians feel that the herb's name may have originated from the Celtic word *barrach* meaning "a man of courage." The Welsh call borage the "herb of gladness." The Romans made borage flowers into an elixir which Pliny said had the power to lighten spirits, and in Elizabethan England borage was prescribed for melancholy.

Borage, a hardy annual, is also nicknamed "bee's bread" because of the bees that pollinate it and love to hover around its flowers. The actual color of borage stems and leaves is dark blue-green, but prickly white hairs covering the whole plant give it a silvery cast. The stems are hollow and succulent; the leaves are alternate, wrinkled, and about 3 inches long. Its beautiful blue, starlike flowers are accented with black anthers. Borage is a lovely plant which usually grows to about 1½ feet high. Its branches can extend out to a width of about 3 feet, creating a wonderful rounded shape. Borage, which likes to grow with strawberries and looks attractive planted among other herbs and flowers, is thought to help discourage insects from attacking nearby plants.

The herb is believed to have originated in northwestern Syria, but now it grows in many parts of Europe and the United States, both in gardens and marginal areas. Borage can be planted from seed when the danger of frost is past. After the first seeding, it will self-sow abundantly, and the new plants can be thinned or transplanted. Transplant borage carefully when it is still quite young. A single plant will spread over a 4-foot-square area, so allow borage transplants plenty of room to expand. With enough soil undisturbed around its roots, and careful handling, borage will flourish in a new place in the garden. It prefers a loose, well-aerated soil that is moist and fairly rich, although it will grow in less favored soils, too. Composted manure should be added to the soil where borage grows. Mulching the borage bed when the young plants are a few weeks old will provide the moist environment this herb prefers.

You can gather selected leaves and flowers for fresh use throughout borage's growing season. To harvest leaves for medicinal use, gather them before the plant flowers and dry them (see Drying Herbs, chapter 6), taking care not to expose them to heat. Borage leaves discolor and lose their viable healing qualities unless they are dried in a place that is warm with plenty of circulating air. You can gather flowers at blooming time, and dry them in the same way.

Medicinally, borage has a calming and cooling effect and can help break fevers. In Europe, borage tea has been used traditionally as a strengthening tonic for convalescing patients. American herbalist William LeSassier suggests that borage is a good herb for people with high blood pressure, or those who are apprehensive or worry a lot.

Versatile borage has a gastronomical dimension to it, too. The plant was enjoyed in the Middle Ages and centuries later as a popular salad herb. Even today, savvy cooks know that the young leaves and flowers lend a refreshing flavor to salads. An infusion of borage leaves can be served cold as a beverage tea, decorated with the gorgeous, sky blue flowers. Borage flowers can also be candied and used to decorate special desserts and confections. Borage is often described as having a cucumberlike taste. This is somewhat true, but it's much the same as describing something as tasting "like chicken." It is just an approximation. You'll have to try it yourself to see if you agree.

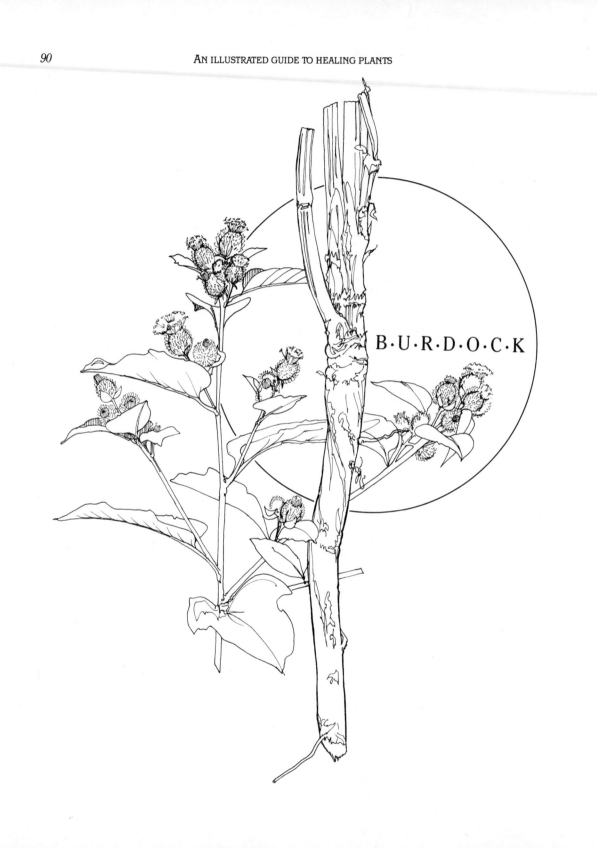

B·U·R·D·O·C·K

BURDOCK (Beggar's Buttons, Clotbur)
Botanical: *Arctium Lappa, A. minus*

Native Hawaiians credit burdock, known there by its Japanese name of *gobo,* with an ability to increase strength and endurance. Hawaiians who need stamina to perform some arduous task have been known to repeat the popular expression, "I need gobo." This sturdy plant, whose Latin name *Arctium* derives from the Greek word meaning "bear," is found in many countries of the world. As various cultures have discovered, its versatility is culinary as well as medicinal.

The burdock plant is alternately despised as a troublesome weed and sought out as a cherished healing herb. Introduced to North America by the early European settlers, it grows alongside roads, in ditches, hedgerows, and waste places throughout most of the United States and Canada. It also grows throughout Asia, and particularly Japan, where it is cultivated as a food and healing plant.

Burdock is a biennial plant with long, dull green stalks and large (up to 12 inches long), oval leaves with many veins. The leaves resemble those of rhubarb because of their size, shape, and wavy edges. Their undersides are gray and covered with fine down. The leaves and stalks usually are striped with purple patterns. In the plant's second year of growth, purple blossoms top thick seed stalks which grow up to 3 feet in height. The flowers are followed by the characteristic spherical burs covered with bristly stickers. The plant sends down a long thick taproot, which is the part used medicinally.

To grow burdock, set seeds ¼ inch deep in rows about 2 feet apart. When seedlings are established, thin them to a distance of about 6 inches apart. The plant will thrive in a deep bed of well-rotted compost, manure, sawdust, leaf mold, wood chips, and other light, loose materials. Sawdust is an especially good addition to the bed because it increases porosity and makes it easier to pull up the roots. Fine wood chips also help. If the bed is too shallow or not porous enough, the roots will be very difficult to dig up, since they grow to over 12 inches long. A thin spade or posthole digger can help to unearth stubborn roots. For medicinal use, treat burdock as an annual, harvesting its roots at the end of the growing season in the plant's first year of growth. Follow drying procedures for roots given in chapter 6. The leftover plant tops make an excellent mulch or compost ingredient.

In the cuisine of both Japan and China, burdock root is enjoyed not only for its taste but also for its strengthening and nutritive qualities. The fresh root is skinned and sliced into thin rounds and added to soups, vegetables, stir-fries, and meat dishes. Rich-tasting miso broth, fortified with sea and land vegetables, including burdock, is a classic Japanese soup. To make this simple but elegant soup, sauté peeled, sliced burdock root in a little vegetable oil for about 5 minutes. Add sliced onions (and other vegetables such as carrots and bok choy, if desired). Add about 1 cup rehydrated hiziki or wakame seaweed to the vegetables, then stir in 1½ cups of water for every serving of soup. Simmer, uncovered, until all the vegetables are tender. Combine 2 tablespoons of the soup liquid plus 1 heaping tablespoon miso for each serving in a bowl and stir until the miso dissolves. Remove the soup from the heat and stir in the dissolved miso. Serve hot. The nutritional benefits of burdock and those of the seaweeds, which contain 10 to 20 percent more minerals than land plants, make this a very healthy soup.

Europeans and Americans alike enjoy the leaves and stalks of burdock as a vegetable. You can gather the tender young leaves of first-year burdock in early spring, blanch them in water, and use them as a salad vegetable. Peeled and served in a salad or cooked like asparagus, the young leafstalks also make a savory vegetable dish. When the plants reach their second year of growth, the immature flower stalk can be peeled to yield a tasty pith. Remove all parts of the outer rind and cook this pith like the root.

In addition to its contributions in the kitchen, burdock has some long-standing medicinal applications, too. Burdock leaf poultices have been used for centuries to treat gout in Europe and China. In Chinese medicine, the seedpod is dried and used for colds, coughs, swelling in the throat, boils, and measles. Both European and Chinese herbalists have long considered burdock roots' lightly warming, moistening effect an excellent tonic for the lungs and liver, and a good blood purifier. An infusion of the leaves, or a decoction of the root, has been used traditionally as a wash for various skin problems, including acne, ringworm, measles rash, and burns. Burdock roots' nourishing and healing properties make it a very valuable plant.

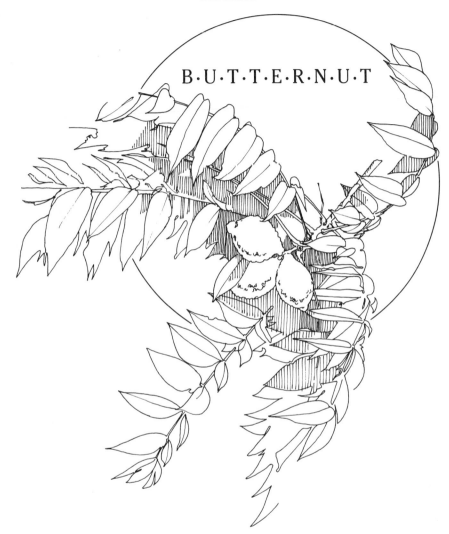

BUTTERNUT (Oil Nut, White Walnut, Lemon Walnut)
Botanical: *Juglans cinerea*

The butternut's botanical name *Juglans,* meaning "royal nut of Jupiter," suggests the highly prized status this tree has enjoyed since ancient times. Its rich, oily nuts are not the least of its treasures. The butternut tree is a native of North America and a close relative of the familiar black walnut. It grows in rich woods, along rivers and streams on well-drained soil, and also in parks, village greens, yards, and along sidewalks in many smaller communities. Its range is from Canada south to the mountainous regions of Georgia, and from the East to West Coasts across the middle to northern states. Like other members of the walnut family, the butternut prefers deep, well-drained soil and adequate moisture. Butternut trees are hardy in climates where the temperature does not drop lower than 10°F below zero.

The butternut grows to a height of 40 to 60 feet when mature. Its bark is light gray—lighter than either the black or English walnut—and it is divided into broad ridges which are somewhat furrowed. Butternut leaves greatly resemble those of the other walnuts: they are opposite and compound, with 11 to 17 leaves per stem. The fruit also looks like black or English walnuts, but it is more elliptical than the others. In fact, when unhusked, butternuts look rather like small, green-tinged lemons. The nut itself has a shell which is very tough and deeply furrowed.

Like the black walnut, butternut trees excrete a substance called juglone which is toxic to some plants. Alfalfa and lespedeza seem adversely affected, though some farmers, according to Gene Logsdon in *Organic Orcharding,* maintain that they can grow alfalfa well around walnut trees. Bluegrass, fescue, and red clover all prosper near walnuts, but many other plants and common weeds are killed by the juglone.

The medicinal part of the butternut is the inner bark, which has traditionally been used as a laxative. It should be collected according to directions in chapter 6 and dried in a warm, shady place. Butternut bark is classified as having a warming, moistening effect, so it is not appropriate to dry it in the sun. The twigs and branches, as well as the inner part of the root, have all been used for medicinal purposes, too. A healthy pruning should yield an abundant supply of bark. After the bark is dried, chop it into small pieces and powder it in an electric coffee grinder or blender.

Herbalists use the powdered bark as a mild laxative, which is reputed to not gripe or cramp the intestines. Because of its gentle action, many American herbalists consider butternut better than the stronger laxative herbs such as cascara sagrada and buckthorn, which sometimes cause intestinal cramping when used incorrectly or excessively. Butternut apparently does not encourage a dependency as some strong laxative herbs do. It is also supposed to be helpful to people who are eliminating coffee from their diet. (Because coffee is a powerful laxative, one of its withdrawal symptoms may be intestinal problems, and butternut powder has been used to help alleviate them.)

Butternut and black walnut are judged to be similar healing agents. They are sometimes used interchangeably, but the butternut is considered more efficacious. It is often used in conjunction with walnut in herbal preparations. In Appalachia, an oil expressed from the fresh butternut has been used for expelling tapeworms. Native Americans applied the bark to the skin to treat rheumatism, headache, and toothache and used a compress of strong tea made from the bark as a styptic. Early American settlers and Indians alike used a syrup made from butternut sap as a tonic. A tea made from the inner bark also served as a tonic during the early days of the United States. Another traditional use of butternut calls for rubbing the skin with the powdered leaves to stimulate and soothe sore muscles, bruises, and similar afflictions.

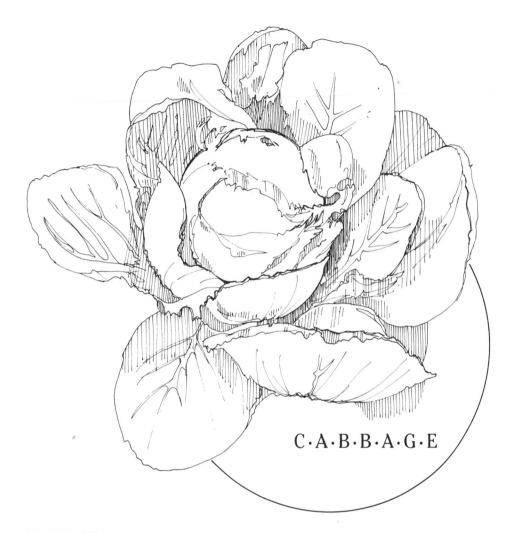

C·A·B·B·A·G·E

CABBAGE

Botanical: *Brassica oleracea*

Although cabbage enjoys a somewhat humble profile today as an unassuming vegetable, its history is rife with uses as a medicinal plant, even up to the present time. Many Greeks esteemed the cabbage as medicine, and Hippocrates recommended it for colic and dysentery. Pythagoras also praised it highly, and one Greek doctor dedicated an entire book to its healing qualities. In ancient Rome, Cato the Elder had great respect for cabbage as a healer. Cato was a well-known farmer who distrusted Greeks, and he insisted that by eating cabbage, Romans were able to avoid going to the Greek doctors.

Cabbage grows wild all over the Mediterranean region, as well as on the sea-coasts of the British Isles. In his seventeenth century *Herbal,* Nicholas Culpeper glorified cabbage and its wild ancestor the "colewort." In characteristically extravagant style, Culpeper recommended cabbage for everything from kidney stones to eye problems and short-windedness. Then, in a burst of personal commentary, he tells us:

> *This I am sure, cabbages are extremely windy whether you take them as meat*
> *or as medicine; yes, as windy meat as can be eaten, unless you eat bagpipes*
> *or bellows...*

The humble cabbage is a common garden vegetable today, available in many varieties, and as spring or late-producing winter storage types. It is an easy plant to grow and will thrive in most soils. Cabbage needs cool weather and a moist soil; it does not do well in midsummer heat and dryness, unless it is heavily mulched. You can start cabbage from seed sown in fine soil indoors or in a cold frame six weeks before the last frost in your area. Do not plant the seeds in a potting soil that is too rich, or the seedlings will be leggy. When the plants are six weeks old, transplant them into their outdoor bed. Check your seed packet instructions or a reliable book on vegetable gardening for specific guidelines on correct distances between plants. Generally, early varieties should be planted 14 inches apart, and late varieties 24 inches apart. Spacing distances in an intensively planted garden will be closer. A good mulch, and additions of well-rotted compost and leaves to the soil, will help to ensure a thriving cabbage patch. Cabbage is attacked by various insects, including the cabbage aphid, maggot, and worm. Depending on your garden's ecology, you can discourage or help to repel these insects by interplanting sage, mint, hyssop, and rosemary.

For all its well-known "windiness," cabbage has certainly enjoyed a variety of healing uses throughout the centuries. Sometimes known as "the poor man's medicine" in Europe, cabbage is high in vitamin C and sulfur. In Germany people included sauerkraut in their heavy winter diet as an effective way to add vitamin C (and helpful fermentation bacteria). Of course, much commercial sauerkraut that has been pasteurized and salted has lost both of these beneficial ingredients. In addition, cabbage and related plants containing sulfur are considered very good for cleansing the liver. Many herbalists prescribe adding cabbage to your diet as a general good practice to keep the liver healthy.

Cabbage has also been used to expel worms, soothe rheumatism and sciatica, and heal burns, wounds, and insect bites. Maurice Mességué has a rather unorthodox use for cabbage leaves. He irons them with a warm iron until they are very flexible, then he applies the leaves as a poultice to the affected parts of patients suffering from rheumatism, gout, sciatica, or lumbago. In his book *Health Secrets of Plants and Herbs,* the French herbalist also reports using fresh cabbage juice for expelling worms, and he praises cabbage as a vegetable or juice to calm those who are anxious, agitated, or depressed.

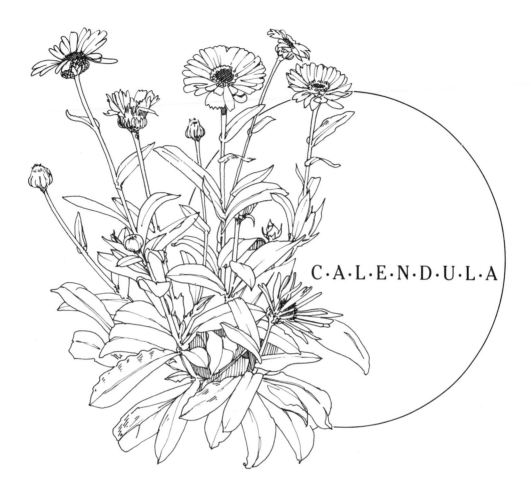

C·A·L·E·N·D·U·L·A

CALENDULA (Pot Marigold)

Botanical: *Calendula officinalis*

Calendula has been associated with the sun for centuries. Its habit of opening its flowers when the sun appears and of closing them when it sets, inspired poets of various eras and countries. In 1817, England's John Keats wrote in a poem titled "I Stood Tiptoe":

Open fresh your round of starry folds,
Ye ardent marigolds!
Dry up the moisture from your golden lids,
For great Apollo bids
That in these days your praises should be sung . . .

The calendula is a hardy annual herb whose bright green leaves and stems contain a tinge of yellow. The plant has a bushy habit, but it becomes leggy unless periodically pinched back. The leaves and stems have a slightly sticky quality; they are also rather hairy. The flowers are a rich orange-yellow color, and they open and close in rhythm with the sunlight.

Calendula is very easy to grow. Sow the seeds in late spring when the soil temperature is around 60°F. The plant prefers a moderately rich, well-drained soil, although it will proliferate in lighter soils as well. Calendula originated in southern Europe, and it will self-sow in temperate climates where winters are not severe. Temperatures below 25°F damage the plant. But given half a chance, calendula flourishes exuberantly and creates vibrant mases of bright green foliage ornamented everywhere with its sunny flowers. It looks lovely as a border. You can also allow it to fill a section of an old-fashioned flower and herb garden or sow it among vegetables, where it will deter insects.

It is the delicate petals of the calendula flower that have been used in European herbal medicine. Flowers are harvested when they are newly opened. The whole flower head is picked and set out to dry on paper, cloth, or nonmetallic screens in a warm, dark, airy place. When the flower heads are dry, the petals are picked from them and stored in airtight jars made of dark-colored glass. Care must be observed in the drying process, or the petals will lose their color and healing qualities.

Beloved by gypsies, monks, and the herbal doctors of old Europe, the calendula is a mild herb, one considered gentle enough even for children and old people. During the Civil War, calendula petals were often used to stanch wounds. Today, in Europe and in this country, herbalists use calendula petals in an ointment for dressing wounds and sores. A lotion made from the blossoms has proved soothing to bee and wasp stings. An infusion of the flower petals has been used for treating conjunctivitis and other eye inflammations. An infusion of the fresh blossoms has a traditional application in breaking fevers, by inducing perspiration. Calendula has also been used to treat toothaches and ulcers.

Powdered calendula petals mixed with arrowroot powder, cornstarch, or pure talc is a pleasant way to soothe skin rashes in both adults and children, including infants. Calendula has a place in the kitchen, too. Its petals can substitute for expensive saffron in Spanish or Indian dishes.

Be careful not to confuse the old-fashioned calendula or pot marigold with the African marigold (botanical name: *Tagetes*), which has become so popular in gardens today. The African marigold, while useful as an insect repellent in vegetable gardens, is not a medicinal herb, and should never be used when calendula or pot marigold is called for.

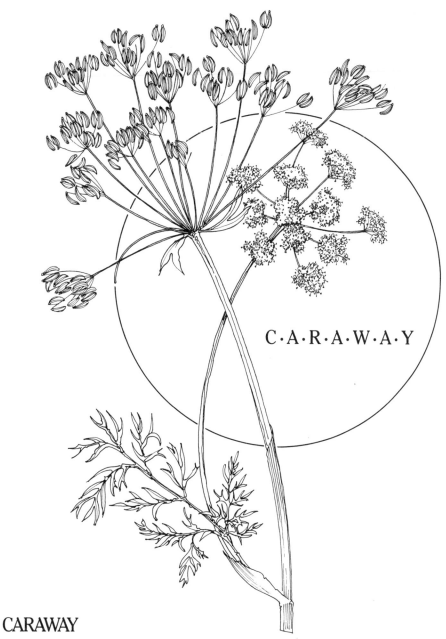

C·A·R·A·W·A·Y

CARAWAY
Botanical: *Carum carvi*

Centuries ago caraway was believed to have retentive properties, quite literally. Caraway-laced potions were used to attract and magnetize a person's love. People also mingled caraway seeds with their most prized possessions, in the hope that the seeds would protect their goods from theft, or magically hold any would-be thief in place until the owner returned.

Caraway is a biennial herb belonging to the Umbellifer family. Its feathery leaves look very much like those of its relative, fennel. Paradoxically, however, caraway is repelled by fennel and does not grow well near it. Caraway produces a small rosette of leaves and a long taproot during its first year of growth. During its second year, it sends up light green furrowed stems with the characteristic feathery leaves. Composite umbels of tiny white flowers are followed by the seeds, which are the part of the plant used for both healing and culinary purposes. Caraway requires a good deal of bright sun and warmth in order to develop its aromatic oil. It prefers a fairly heavy soil, on the dry side. The plant's long taproots can effectively break up and aerate heavy soils.

Seeds are sown directly into the plant's permanent bed. Because of its long root, caraway dislikes transplanting. Sow seeds 6 to 8 inches apart, and ½ inch deep in early spring, after the danger of frost is past. Caraway is a good companion plant for garden peas. It makes a lovely background plant in the herb garden or herbaceous border; it grows to about 2 feet tall. Harvest the seeds when they start to darken, as directed in chapter 6.

Caraway is cultivated commercially in Morocco, Holland, and England for its aromatic seeds, which enjoy many flavoring uses both in home kitchens and in the food industry. Some of its most renowned uses are as a seasoning for cabbage, onions, turnips, and meat, an addition to cheeses, rye breads, and stews, and as a pickling component.

Like other members of the Umbellifer family, caraway has properties helpful to the stomach and digestion. Caraway seeds, which are often found in substantial ethnic cuisines such as German, do in fact aid digestion and help to expel gas. Both the seeds and cooked roots of the plant are considered by herbalists to be strengthening to the intestines. Caraway is a warming, drying herb. It is slightly, and harmlessly, calmative.

One traditional European use for caraway is a colic medicine for infants. The colic medicine is made in much the same way as a simple infusion—1 ounce of the bruised seeds is combined with 1 pint of water. But instead of placing the herb in boiled water, as you usually do for an infusion, soak the seeds in cold water for 6 hours, then strain and discard them. Caraway is so pleasant and useful, it is one of the most widely used herbs throughout the world.

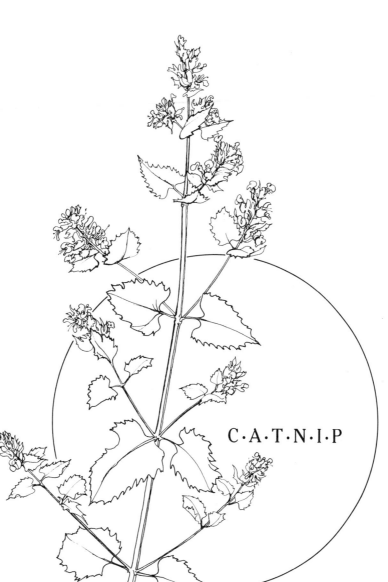

C·A·T·N·I·P

CATNIP

Botanical: *Nepeta cataria*

Catnip is a perennial that is a member of the mint family; it can be found growing wild all over Europe, temperate Asia, and North America, where it was introduced by early European settlers. The gray-green plant has a mounded shape, and displays the square stalk that characterizes members of the mint family. Its leaves are toothed and heart-shaped. It grows 2 to 3 feet high, and its stems and leaves are covered with a fine down.

The plant does not require as much moisture as do other members of the mint family. In fact, many herb growers report that catnip's most aromatic potential develops when the plant is grown in a rather sandy soil with a springtime side-dressing of well-rotted compost. Catnip can be propagated from seed, either in the fall or in the spring after the danger of frost is past. Fall-sown seeds give better results in most climates. Sow seeds in rows placed about 20 inches apart. When the seedlings sprout, thin them to about 20 inches apart as well, since the plant can grow rather large. You can also start catnip from root divisions taken from the parent plant in spring. See the instructions for making divisions in chapter 5. The plant can reach a height of 4 feet in favorable conditions and does well in full or partial sun. The flowering tops, which are the part of the plant used medicinally, are harvested when the plant is in full bloom, by cutting the plant back to 3 to 4 inches above the ground.

The attraction of cats to catnip is legendary. A great many cat owners have enjoyed watching their pet roll, jump, chew, and crash around with a bag or "mouse" stuffed with catnip. In fact, growing catnip just for cats is a worthwhile endeavor in itself. Unfortunately, though, cats don't differentiate between neat little bags of catnip and tender young shoots coming up in the garden. A word to the wise will suffice: when planning a garden, plant catnip by itself or behind some strong shrubs. Or protect it with a cat-proof fence.

Actually, catnip is not just for cats. Catnip tea was a favored beverage of the English in the days before Chinese tea arrived there. In an old English book, *The Herb Garden,* an herbal historian known simply as Miss Bardswell commented that actually catnip tea was "quite as pleasant and a good deal more wholesome" than the Chinese import which had become fashionable.

In an infusion or tisane, catnip has been used traditionally as a calmative. The root of the plant is reported to have the opposite effect, however. In her book, *A Modern Herbal,* Mrs. M. Grieve quoted one old English herbalist on the subject. Catnip root, when chewed, according to this anonymous informant, will "make the most gentle person fierce and quarrelsome." But it is the aboveground part of the plant, especially its flowering top, that is used for healing. Catnip is judged to be a good antispasmodic herb, useful for treating stomach complaints. As an ingredient in those old-fashioned household stomach tonics known as "bitters," catnip's role was to combat overacidity and overstimulation of the stomach. It also is supposed to help relax intestinal cramping, and so English and American herbalists have sometimes included it as part of an herbal laxative formula. The infusion has also been used to calm restlessness or nervousness in both adults and children. According to a contemporary American herbalist, catnip tea helps to release symptoms arising from "gut level" emotional tension such as anxiety, headache, indigestion, cramping, and the blocking of normal metabolic processes.

Adults can drink catnip tea freely, as they did in old England, but large doses of this warm beverage will act as an emetic. Catnip is also regarded as a warming herb and has been used to break fevers, but it appears to do so without raising body heat significantly. Catnip also has a moistening quality.

Never boil catnip or it will lose its volatile oils and much of its healing quality. Simply infuse the herb in water that has just been boiled and allowed to cool a few moments. Cover the container or vessel tightly as soon as you have combined the catnip and the water. See the directions for making infusions in chapter 6.

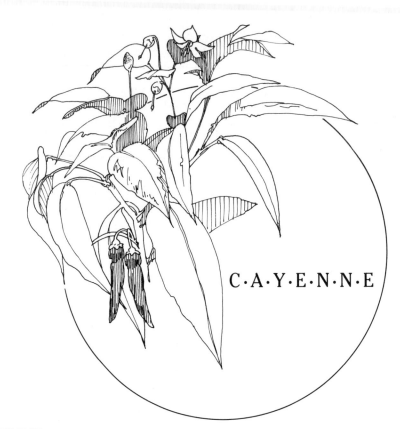

C·A·Y·E·N·N·E

CAYENNE
Botanical: *Capsicum annuum,* Longum Group

Cayenne is a shrubby perennial plant whose name, fittingly enough, is derived from the Greek word meaning "to bite." This spicy member of the pepper family is native to Africa and India, but the sixteenth century herbalist Gerard reported its cultivation in England during his time. Cayenne is grown today in most tropical and subtropical climates such as parts of Mexico and South America. Indeed, one of the cayenne pepper's most salient roles is in Latin American cuisine. It is a very conspicuous flavoring agent in many bean, rice, meat, and vegetable dishes from that part of the world. Underlying its famed enlivening ability are a number of health values.

The cayenne plant grows 2 to 6 feet high, depending on soil and climate. Its angular branches are usually slightly purple at the nodes. Its long leaves and general shape are very similar to those of sweet and hot pepper plants, and the long peppers it produces are bright red. Cayenne needs a good deal of heat and sunlight to prosper. It likes light, warm soil, too, and in this country it does well outdoors in the southern states. It can be grown indoors in a greenhouse or at a window with strong sun from a southern exposure, though its medicinal qualities may not develop as fully as those of a plant grown outdoors in its tropical habitat. Keep indoor plants moist and wash them gently every three to four weeks with a solution of Ivory soap and water, to prevent pest infestation. You can obtain cayenne seeds and young plants from some of the larger commercial herb gardens, including some of those listed in the Resource Guide at the back of this book.

The pepper pods are the part of the plant to use medicinally. Gather the pods when they are red and ripe and hang them to dry in partial sun. When they are dry, you can powder the pods in an electric coffee grinder or a blender. Do this very carefully to avoid inhaling any of the powder. Another caution whenever you are working with cayenne pods or powder is to wash your hands thoroughly before you touch any sensitive part of your body. Cayenne will cause extreme irritation of eyes, mucous membranes, or other sensitive areas with which it comes in contact.

The ground powder made from the cayenne peppers has been used for healing in a variety of ways. Cayenne opens the capillaries and soothes the stomach and mucous membranes. It has been used to tonify the stomach, intestines, and other internal organs, and to treat constipation. In the West Indies, a cayenne preparation called mandram has been used to treat weak digestion and loss of appetite. The preparation consists of thinly sliced cucumbers, shallots, chives or onion, lemon or lime juice, Madeira wine, and a few pods of the pepper mashed into the liquid.

A classic herbal formula both in the United States and England for treating constipation is equal parts of cayenne and slippery elm powder capped into gelatin capsules and taken with meals. Cayenne is taken this way in the hope that it will not act as a laxative, but will instead tone and balance intestinal function. The same remedy is sometimes used to clear mucus. Dissolved in water, the mixture also makes stimulating demulcent gargle for sore throats. If used for this purpose, one teaspoon of the mixture is made into a paste with a little water to prevent the slippery elm from forming lumps. Then more warm water is added to the paste to make the gargle.

Cayenne mixed with bran and warm water makes a wonderful comforting poultice for the treatment of chest and lung congestion. This plaster, like a ginger plaster (both of which are described in detail in chapter 6), is also good for people who tire easily, and who complain of having no energy. For treating general lack of energy, the poultice is placed over the kidney area in the lower back and covered with a warm towel. In both treatments, the person should be kept covered and warm. Another classic use of cayenne is in the form of a liniment (see All-Good Liniment, page 322).

Many healers find cayenne to be a very useful herb for treating most adults. But never give cayenne to infants, or use it internally if you have very weak kidneys.

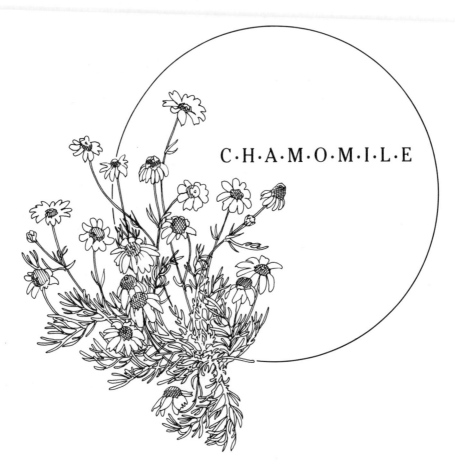

C·H·A·M·O·M·I·L·E

CHAMOMILE (Camomile)

Botanical: *Anthemis nobilis* (Roman or common chamomile); *Matricaria
chamomilla* (German or wild chamomile)

There are not many plants that enjoy being stepped on, but chamomile is one
that does. One old English saying about the plant goes:

*Like a chamomile bed
the more it is trodden
the more it will spread.*

In Great Britain, entire lawns made of the sweet-scented herb release their se-
ductive fragrance to any lucky person who walks or reclines on them. Its fresh scent
made chamomile a popular strewing herb in medieval England, at a time when the
scent of strewing herbs was the only measure used to counter the aroma of the
unwashed citizenry.

Roman or common chamomile is a compact, low-growing plant with tiny, daisylike flowers. The wild Roman (also called English) chamomile has single flowers, the cultivated variety has double flowers. The plant has a downy, grayish green appearance and a moundlike shape. German chamomile is taller and more rangy in habit, and its flowers have single petals. Roman chamomile is a perennial plant, the German is an annual. Both Roman and German chamomile share the deliciously fresh, applelike scent. (There is also a plant called corn chamomile, which looks somewhat like German chamomile, but that can be distinguished from the true chamomiles by its smell, which is rather offensive.)

Roman chamomile will grow in nearly any type of soil. The single-flowered type which grows in the wild favors rather dry, sandy soil. The cultivated type with double flowers prefers a richer soil and gives the heaviest crop of blossoms when planted in moist, slightly heavy black loam. Double flowers are considered more desirable for healing uses. Although the wild Roman chamomile is stronger pharmacologically, the medicinal alkali it contains is so concentrated that it can damage the coating of the stomach and intestines. For this reason the double-flowered form is preferred for healing uses.

Chamomile can be sown from seed. Its seed is very fine and requires a well-prepared soil to receive it, or it will disappear deep into the ill-prepared bed and never sprout. Spring sowing is recommended. It is easier and quicker to propagate Roman chamomile from the little offshoots or sets that the mother plant produces. They can be divided in the early spring and set into well-manured soil, spaced about 18 inches apart. Roman chamomile is extremely hardy, but if your winters are very severe and you don't want to risk losing the plants, mulch them heavily to protect them.

The annual German chamomile can be seeded in either fall or spring. However, the seeds have an unstable viability. Planting them in the fall helps, because viability is increased when the seeds are subjected to freezing and thawing. Once established, the German chamomile plant will reseed itself if some flower heads are allowed to remain unharvested. Both Roman and German chamomile like lots of sun. Keep the soil evenly moist for optimum growth and flower production.

Gather chamomile blossoms when they are in full bloom and dry them carefully according to the directions given in chapter 6. The flowers are quite fragile, so treat them attentively to maintain their healing properties.

In many cultures, chamomile was connected to the healing elements of the sun. Roman chamomile, often called "the plant's physician," has a reputation for reviving and maintaining the health of other plants growing near it. A classic use of chamomile tea or infusion is as a hair rinse to add "sunlight" to hair and bring out the natural blond highlights. The Egyptians used chamomile's warming quality to cure "agues," the malarial chills that plagued the ancient civilization. Dioscorides and Pliny recommended a chamomile poultice or bath to cure headaches and illnesses affecting the liver, kidneys, and bladder.

In more modern times, chamomile has been best known as a calmative. A cup of chamomile tea is a classic remedy for nervous or hysterical conditions. As a nervine, chamomile is safe and effective. Gentle to the stomach, it can also be used to relieve indigestion. Like an infusion of basswood flowers, an infusion of chamomile blossoms can be added to the bath to calm irritable or hyperactive children. The German species is especially recommended for this use, although either type of chamomile is said to work. One contemporary herbal practitioner, William LeSassier, recommends chamomile tea for pregnant women, saying that it will help produce babies who do not whine. Chamomile is one of the most ancient and gentle of herbs, still sweetly popular today.

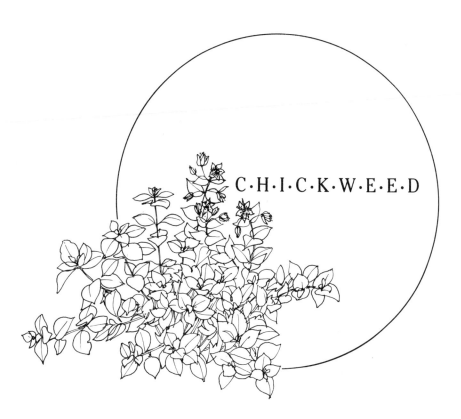

CHICKWEED

Botanical: *Stellaria media*

Chickweed is a garden weed or wild herb of temperate regions. It can be found growing under trees, especially oak trees, and in moist shady places in the woods and garden. It grows along the ground and is easily recognizable by its tangled, procumbent manner, and its small light green paired leaves and succulent stems. Its tiny flowers are star-shaped and white. Although chickweed is generally gathered from the wild, it also makes itself at home in greenhouses, gardens, and home landscapes, where there is continual moisture and at least partial shade (under a dripping faucet on the north side of the house, for instance). In such places its growth can be encouraged. Chickweed can even be transplanted from wild stands and put in a similar environment at home.

Chickweed's healing properties are designated as emollient, demulcent, and refrigerant. Culpeper's seventeenth century contemporaries in England favored this plant for cooling the liver, treating the skin problems, and checking obesity. An infusion of the whole plant has been used for bathing skin inflammations and rashes. The fresh plant, crushed in a mortar and pestle to release its healing juices, makes an effective poultice (a method described in chapter 6) for treating skin ulcers and sores.

Chickweed is probably best known as a "kidney herb" and although there is no scientific evidence to support its effectiveness, chickweed is one of the spring greens taken traditionally in this country to cleanse the kidneys and liver after a winter of heavy eating. Chickweed has a delicate taste, somewhat similar to that of spinach, and can be used in much the same way—as a fresh salad green or lightly steamed as a cooked vegetable. As a blood purifier, chickweed was one of the early European "simples." Although scientists disagree, herbalists continue to regard the humble chickweed as a safe, effective herb for generally strengthening and cleansing the system.

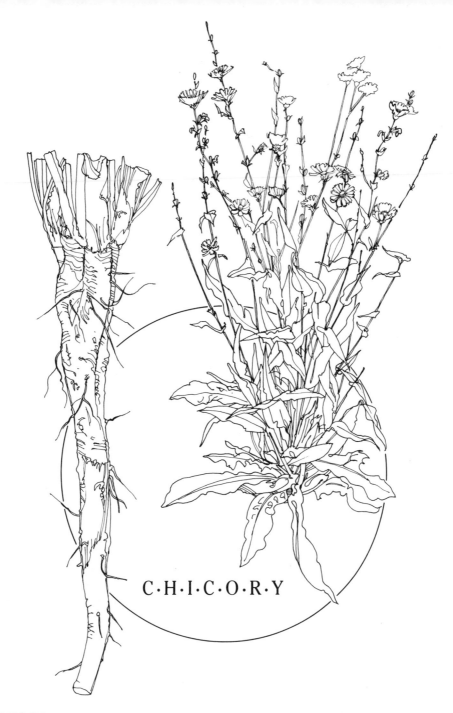

C·H·I·C·O·R·Y

CHICORY (Succory)
Botanical: *Cichorium intybus*

    The sixteenth century herbalist Parkinson described chicory as a "fine, cleansing, jovial plant," but his description would probably appall many of us today, since we tend to think of it only as a rather obnoxious weed. Chicory can be found growing wild in many countries in pastures, fields, and marginal areas. It also sometimes pops up in the midst of lawns and gardens, much to the consternation of gardeners. There are also cultivated types of chicory that are grown as vegetables, but they should not be confused with the wild form which we are discussing here.

Chicory is a perennial herb with a taproot resembling that of the dandelion. It grows between 2 and 3 feet tall, and it is easily recognized by its unkempt appearance and lovely blue flowers. Its leaves are rather sparse, and its branches are set off angularly from the main stem, which gives the plant a rather straggly look. The bases of the leaves clasp the stems. The leaves at the plant's base are large and hairy, and somewhat resemble those of the dandelion, hence its nickname of blue dandelion.

Like many strong, wild herbs, chicory is not terribly particular about what type of soil it grows in. When it is cultivated for its root, the plant does well in a deep bed in which the topsoil is mixed with amendments of sawdust and composted manure. If the bed is deep and the soil is friable, then it is easy to gather the roots in the fall of the plant's first year. You can sow the plant from seed in late spring but not much earlier or the seed will bolt. Plant seed in drills about 15 inches apart, provide the plants with moderate waterings and sun, and the crop will produce an abundance of healing roots. One caution, though: Chicory likes to spread and take over, so confine or plant it in a separate part of the garden. Harvest the roots in the autumn and follow the directions given in chapter 6 for cutting, drying, and storing them.

Europeans use the root of wild or cultivated chicory as a coffee substitute (see our recipe for herbal coffee, on page 308) or just to balance coffee's flavor. They also add the leaves to green salads. Some European cooks steam or boil the root of the plant and season it with butter, herbs, and spices.

While some people may see only chicory's dubious character in the garden, others are acquainted with its medicinal value. The roof of the plant was traditionally used to treat jaundice and other liver ailments, although no current studies bear out the efficacy of these treatments. French herbalist Maurice Mességué maintains that the reason chicory is so popular in France as a coffee addition or substitute is that it is a good "liver herb," tonifying and detoxifying the livers of those who enjoy French cuisine perhaps a bit too much. The French also believe that chicory, added to coffee, counteracts the coffee's acidic quality and its adverse effect on the stomach. A decoction of the dried root is a noted treatment for stomach acidity.

The leaves of the chicory plant also have healing properties. Bruised, softened, and soaked for a few minutes in water that has just been boiled, the leaves are a traditional treatment in Europe and in this country for skin lacerations, swellings, and inflammations. Added to salads, the young leaves, gathered before the plant flowers, are believed to have a salutary effect on the liver and kidneys, as do the bitter leaves of the dandelion. Both chicory and dandelion leaves are classified as warm and moistening, while their roots are warm and drying. In fact, chicory's traditional medicinal properties—tonic, laxative, and diuretic—are similar to those of dandelion.

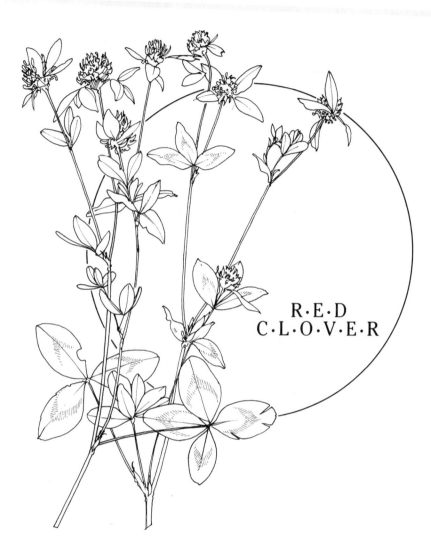

R·E·D C·L·O·V·E·R

RED CLOVER (Sweet Clover, Cow Clover, Meadow Clover, Trefoil)
Botanical: *Trifolium pratense*

Though not native to the United States, red clover has long been cultivated here as a forage crop. Children growing up in the country sometimes develop a special affinity for this wild food, especially for the naturally sweet blossoms, which they love to eat. Red clover is a leguminous plant that grows throughout the United States, Europe, and northern Asia. Considered a perennial, it usually does back after two or three years. It stands between 1 and 2 feet in height and is favored both as a forage crop and a nitrogen fixer in poor soils. Red clover makes an excellent green manure. In parts of England, the plant's rich green trifoliate leaves (clover is related to the shamrock) are considered a talisman against witches and evil. Rosy-colored clover blossoms are composed of many tiny segments that form a ball shape.

Red clover is beneficial to other plants. Its rather deep and branched roots break up compacted earth and bring up nutrients from the subsoil. Red clover thrives in a variety of soils but does not tolerate too much sand or gravel. Seed it in the spring or fall, depending on your local climate and moisture patterns.

Like alfalfa, red clover is a plant that heals the earth as well as the body. A clover ground cover is recommended to provide a living, regenerative mulch to depleted ground. Mixed with bird's-foot trefoil, vetch, and rye grass, red clover makes an excellent nitrogen-fixing cover crop. After the clover mixture has taken hold, alfalfa can also be sown. After several years of clover, alfalfa, and vetch cropping in poor soils, there will be a marked improvement in tilth, nutrient content, microorganisms, worms, and other beneficial qualities.

The blossoms are the part of the plant used for healing purposes. Red clover blossoms are one of the classics in the American and European herbal tradition. They have been used as a spring tonic for thinning and purifying the blood. The flowers are said to have a cooling and moistening effect. Harvest them when just blooming and dry them according to the directions in chapter 6. In simple infusions clover blossoms have been used to treat chest complaints such as colds, asthma, and bronchitis. The herb is also considered antispasmodic and sedative, providing a welcome relaxation for those suffering from chest constriction.

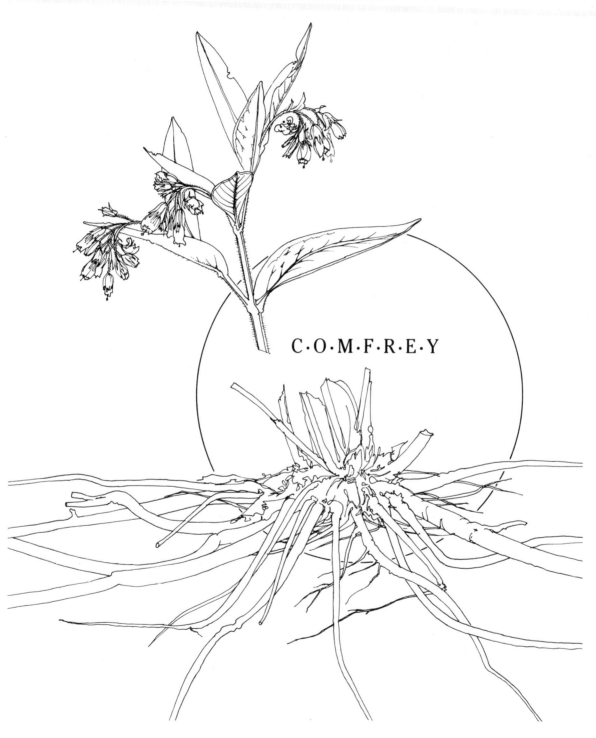

C·O·M·F·R·E·Y

COMFREY (Knitbone, Healing Herb, Boneset, Bruisewort)
Botanical: *Symphytum officinale*

Comfrey is a handsome herb from the same family as borage. The plants grow 2 to 3 feet tall, with basal leaves that are up to a foot long, elliptical, and of a deep, rich green color. They are covered with fine, rough hairs, which makes them somewhat prickly. From the clump of leaves at the plant's base rises a single stalk with smaller leaves, growing on stems that clasp the stalk. Atop this stalk grow the flower racemes. They curve over in a shape reminiscent of forget-me-nots, a close relative of comfrey. These flower stalks often contain seeds, flowers, and buds all at the same time. The flowers are either purple or cream colored and appear from May until the end of summer. Comfrey roots are about 1 inch thick and a foot or more long, with a black exterior and white interior. They grow just beneath the soil surface as spreading rhizomes and are somewhat fibrous, fleshy, juicy, and mucilaginous. Comfrey has several closely related species, including *Symphytum asperum* and *S.* ×*uplandicum.* The latter, a hybrid of *S. officinale* and another species, is popularly known as Russian comfrey. It grows to heights of 5 feet or more. But it is *S. officinale,* or common comfrey, that is most valued for its healing properties.

Comfrey is a native of Europe and Asia, but it has been introduced all over the world. It is a very hardy plant and has been known to withstand temperatures as low as 40°F below zero. Comfrey is also a prolific grower. It is often used as a food crop for goats and rabbits, and as a source of green compost. It will survive in almost any soil, but it reaches its most luxuriant growth in a loose, rich, loamy soil with a pH of 6.0 to 7.0. Applications of compost, manure, limestone, and phosphate rock will aid comfrey's growth if the soil is inadequate.

You can raise comfrey from crown cuttings with buds, from young nursery plants, and from seed, although seeds are the least reliable method. By far the easiest way to propagate this vigorous plant is from root cuttings. A piece of root of almost any size, placed in suitable soil and watered adequately, will produce comfrey plant. In fact, the main concern in growing comfrey is not how to grow it, but how to keep this perennial from spreading. It has a tendency to quickly take over an entire garden, and there is virtually no way to remove it once it has established itself on such a scale. To prevent comfrey's uncontrolled spread, plant it separately or use a containing device such as a border of sheet metal buried 1 foot deep.

Plant root cuttings 3 to 6 inches deep and 2 to 3 feet apart. Comfrey will grow well planted closer together, but the roots will be difficult to harvest. Keep weeds down with mulch. You can divide young plants in the spring as soon as the leaves begin growing. Comfrey will tolerate full sunlight but does better when it receives dappled shade at least part of the day. It prefers a moist soil and should be watered regularly, like other leafy garden vegetables or herbs.

Both the leaf and root of comfrey have been used for healing purposes. Leaves are most often used fresh, but since fresh leaves are not available all year, they may be used dried also. Gather mature leaves before the plant flowers by cutting them several inches above the crown. Spread them in single layers on screens in a shady, but warm place, as described in Drying Herbs, chapter 6. When they are dry, store the leaves either whole, lying flat in airtight boxes, or gently crumbled and stored in jars like other leafy herbs. Comfrey has an amazingly vigorous growth, and the plant will continue to send up new leaves even after three or four cuttings. For home use, though, you may find that the first cutting, taken just before the plant blooms, will suffice.

Gather comfrey roots in autumn just after the first frost. You can also harvest roots in early spring, before new leaves appear. Clean them by washing with cool running water, then cut them into thin slices and dry on screens in the sun. Comfrey root is most easily used in the form of a powder (also described in chapter 6).

In addition to containing the healing substance allantoin, the comfrey plant is rich in calcium, potassium, phosphorus, and vitamins A and C. The root is considered demulcent, mildly astringent, anti-irritant, and cooling.

Although comfrey has been used both internally and externally for over 2,000 years, recently a controversy has arisen over its potentially toxic effects when ingested. The various species of comfrey contain pyrrolidine and related alkaloids which can cause liver impairment and liver cancer. These alkaloids, mainly concentrated in the comfrey root, are moderately present in new immature leaves, and lowest in mature leaves. Health authorities do not know conclusively that the therapeutic use of comfrey tea poses a health hazard. As with even the most careful scientific research there is a certain amount of conflicting evidence and a lack of complete evidence indicating comfrey as a carcinogenic agent. However, until the issue is clarified further, we must advise against using comfrey internally. It's always better to err on the side of caution.

Fortunately, the external use of comfrey is not currently known to pose a carcinogenic risk. Herbalists throughout the ages placed comfrey high on their list of popular and effective external remedies. Comfrey's principle use, as some of its common names indicate, has been for mending wounds and broken bones. The name comfrey itself derives from its uses in medieval times when it was known as *confirmare* meaning "to make firm or strengthen." The genus name, *Symphytum,* derived from the Greek *sympho* meaning "to unite," also refers to comfrey's healing uses.

This highly acclaimed herb elicited one of Culpeper's more exaggerated statements:

The roots being outwardly applied cure fresh wounds or cuts immediately, being bruised and laid thereto; and is specially good for ruptures and broken bones, so powerful to consolidate and knit together that if they be boiled with dissevered pieces of flesh in a pot, it will join them together again.

Although comfrey might not work as well as Culpeper claims, it has been seen to have an effect on cuts, burns, skin ulcers, boils, hemorrhoids, sprains, and fractures. (To make a comfrey poultice, follow the directions under Compresses, Poultices, and Plasters in chapter 6.) Powdered comfrey root, sprinkled on minor cuts, bruises, and mild burns, seems to promote their healing.

All parts of the comfrey plant contain allantoin, a substance used in some pharmaceutical preparations to increase cell growth. The roots contain the highest amounts of this healing substance. It is the allantoin in comfrey that makes the herb a good external remedy. In fact, comfrey may work so well to heal open wounds and cuts that it must be administered carefully. If the wound is not disinfected first, it is possible that comfrey would cause the surface skin to cover an infection. If that happens, the wound would have to be reopened, disinfected and allowed to heal again. Herbalists often combine goldenseal root powder with comfrey root powder in order to include some antiseptic properties. Of course, you should always consult a qualified health practitioner for treatment of any serious or deep cuts.

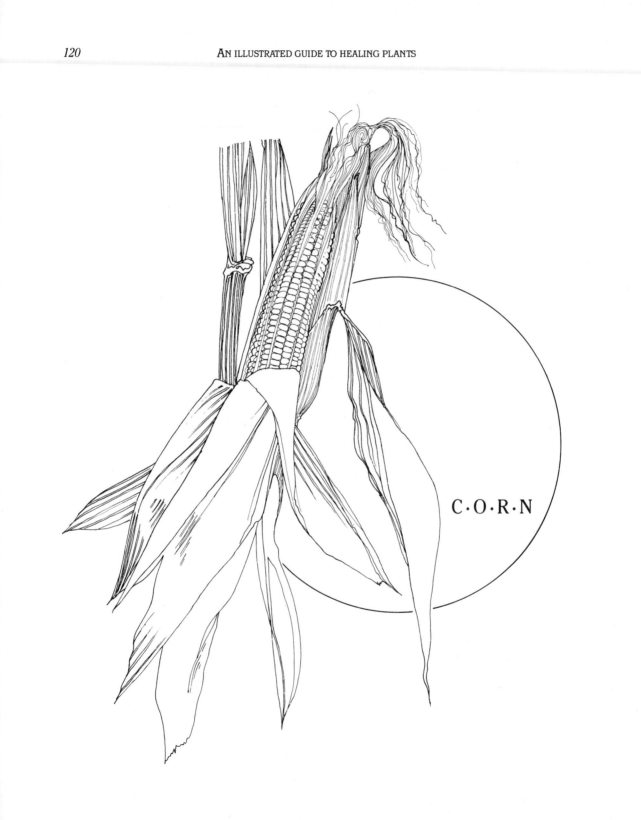

C·O·R·N

CORN (Maize)
Botanical: *Zea mays*

The tall, stately corn plant is America's greatest contribution to the world's food supply. A staple of Indian diets in both North and South America, various other cultures also have high regard for corn's medicinal uses. Spanish explorers in South America were impressed with:

> the remarkable curative properties of corn, which is not only the principal article of food in America, but is also of great benefit in the treatment of affections of the kidney and bladder, among which are calculus and retention of urine. . . .

So wrote Garcilaso de la Vega in the late 1500s. European settlers learned of corn's healing uses from Native American peoples and transmitted this knowledge back to Europe. Eventually, corn even made its way to China (where it is called *Yu-Shu-Shu*) and earned an esteemed place in the Chinese pharmacopoeia.

The corn plant grows between 6 and 8 feet in height, depending upon soil and moisture. It has shiny, bright green leaves, and a thick, fibrous stalk. The ears are covered by husks, with a layer of corn silk between the ear of corn and the green husk. Corn, an easy crop to raise, requires a growing season of approximately 70 to 80 days and plenty of warm sun. It will grow in many types of garden soil but prospers best with additions of well-rotted compost. It is a very heavy feeder. Early varieties are planted in drills after the danger of frost is past. Later varieties are usually planted in hills. Heavy mulching with hay and other organic materials is suggested to hold moisture in and to control weed populations. But some weeds that grow with corn actually seem to increase its health and yield. Biodynamic gardeners recommend inclusion of deep-rooting purslane, pigweed, and lamb's-quarters in corn rows to provide moisture-holding ground cover and to bring up nourishment from the subsoil for the heavy-feeding corn plants.

Both the corn itself and the corn silk between the ear and the husk have been used for healing purposes. To dry the silk, lay it in very thin layers on muslin, or on a nonmetallic screen in a warm, airy room such as an attic or drying shed. It will take between one and two weeks to dry. After drying, corn silk should be stored in an airtight container made of dark glass. Be sure to use it within one year.

Cornmeal and soft corn porridges, both easy to digest, have been traditional sources of nourishment for invalids. Pioneer American settlers and Indians used cornmeal poultices extensively. The early settlers boiled cornmeal with milk and applied it to burns, inflammations, and hard swellings. In Appalachia, salted cornmeal is still a traditional poultice for treating inflammations.

The Native Americans taught the early settlers of this country to make tea from corn silk. The early Americans drank the tea by itself or added its soothing, demulcent qualities to formulas for infections of the bladder, kidneys, and urinary tract. Corn silk tea is also considered diuretic, and is used for this purpose in Europe and in China.

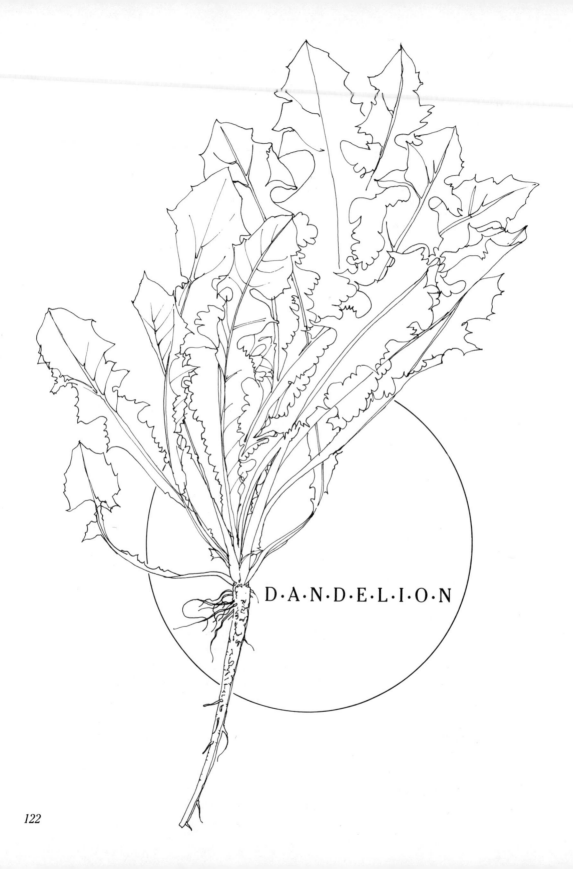

D·A·N·D·E·L·I·O·N

DANDELION (Lion's Tooth, Wild Endive)
Botanical: *Taraxacum officinale*

Winner of a rogue's reputation wherever it grows in lawns, pastures, fields, and gardens, dandelion is perhaps the world's most famous weed. It is also one of the oldest and most versatile of the healing herbs. Dandelion's botanical name means "the official remedy for disorders," and since ancient times, the plant has lived up to that title. To medieval European herbalists who worked with the Doctrine of Signatures, the bright yellow flower of the dandelion was a sign that it was good for the liver. One ounce of the fresh leaves contains large amounts of vitamin A and calcium, as well as substantial amounts of vitamin B_1, vitamin C, sodium, potassium, and trace elements.

Dandelion roots are thick and dark brown on the outside, with a white milky interior. The crown of the plant, where stem and root meet, can be several inches long when dandelion is grown in a deep mulch. The leaves of dandelion plants grow in a rosette form against the ground. They are shiny, hairless, and toothed—which accounts for the origin of the plant's name—a corruption of the French *dent de lion* or lion's tooth. The plant sends up its bright yellow, round shaggy flowers on succulent stems. Most children know that when broken, these hollow stems ooze a milky liquid. Before the flowers rise on these stalks, they are formed as compact buds deep within the rosette of leaves.

All parts of the dandelion are edible and considered useful for healing. Traditionally in Europe and America, bitter-tasting fresh dandelion greens were a favorite spring tonic. Even before the greens emerge, the "blanched" rosette of leaf stems, often found buried under mulch or dirt, makes an excellent salad ingredient. Later, as the leaves get larger, tight flower buds remain buried in the rosette base. These are also quite a good vegetable. Once the flower stalks have reached their full height, dandelion greens are generally too bitter to eat. But the fresh flowers can still be enjoyed as a colorful addition to salads or cooked dishes. Then in the fall, after a hard frost, the bitterness of dandelion leaves is dispersed and you can enjoy them once again.

You can usually easily locate a source of wild dandelion, but digging out the roots can be a problem. They are deep and tenacious and can seem almost impossible to unearth from some soils. In addition, in many places that dandelion grows—such as lawns—it's not practical to dig down deep to extract the entire root. If you're fortunate enough to find an organic field that has just been plowed, you can usually find dandelion roots that are already turned up or easily pulled out of a trench or crest.

If you decide to grow your own dandelion plants, a good trick is to plant them atop a narrow raised bed of loose soil with additions of sawdust or fine wood chips to help make it porous. When harvesting time comes during the second year, you can easily pull the roots out sideways. You can collect dandelion seed from wild plants if you wish to cultivate the plant. Sow the seeds about 12 inches apart in shallow drills. Harvest dandelion flowers from cultivated beds before they go to seed to avoid an unwanted proliferation of the plant.

The root of the plant is the part most often used for healing purposes. It has been used in European herbal medicine for centuries to treat diabetes. In the spring, the root contains levulose, a sugar easily assimilated by diabetics. By autumn, this sugar has changed to inulin, a starch also easily assimilated by diabetics. Collected either in the spring or fall, fresh dandelion roots can be peeled, parboiled, and sautéed to be served as a tasty vegetable. Stronger in flavor than the highly cultivated vegetables many of us are accustomed to, the dandelion root has a marked taste which is both slightly sweet and bitter.

Dandelion root is a classic European remedy for liver diseases, particularly those involving deep congestion of the liver. Some herbalists also cite its digestion-aiding and laxative abilities. Dandelion root, which is considered diuretic, is categorized as having warming and drying properties, whereas the leaves are warming and moistening. Many European herbalists regard dandelion as one of the best herbs for building the blood and curing anemic conditions.

For year-round medicinal use, chop the roots into small pieces and dry them in a warm, airy place, or in a slow dryer at a temperature not over 100°F. People with generally sensitive stomachs may benefit from the roasted fresh root. Chop and roast it in the oven until it turns a rich brown color and feels very brittle. Roasted dandelion root is sometimes used as a coffee substitute or as an addition to coffee. Like chicory root, which is used in the same way, dandelion root is believed to strengthen the liver, as well as the spleen, pancreas, and kidneys. In fact, it acts as an antidote to many of coffee's detrimental effects on the body. You will find in chapter 6, a recipe for an herbal coffee substitute made with dandelion roots.

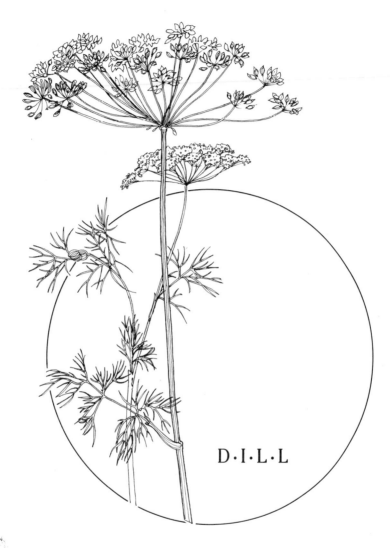

D·I·L·L

DILL

Botanical: *Anethum graveolens*

Dill boasts a well-established tie to the ancient but sophisticated civilization of Egypt. Records found in Egyptian tombs suggest that doctors considered the herb a powerful digestive aid even in those long-ago times.

Dill is a native of the Mediterranean region and southern Russia, where its use in the local cuisine is well known. Dill also grows wild among the corn plants in Spain, although it is not found in cornfields in other European countries. It makes a beautiful background plant in the herb garden, and aside from its medicinal uses, both the leaves (called dillweed) and seed can be used to advantage in breads, soups, pickles, meats, and salads.

Dill is a hardy annual member of the Umbellifer family, and it greatly resembles its relative, fennel. It is smaller than fennel, however, attaining a height of 2 to 2½ feet at maturity. The plant seldom develops more than one smooth, shiny, hollow stalk, which displays feathery, fernlike leaves. Dill produces yellow flowers in the umbrellalike clusters characteristic of all umbellifers. After flowering, the plant develops the crescent-shaped seed for which it is famous.

Dill is easy to cultivate in loose, fairly rich soil and full sun. You may want to start seedlings in a cold frame or greenhouse and transfer them outdoors after danger of frost is past. If seed is sown directly into the plant's permanent bed, drills should be spaced 10 inches apart. Dill seed ripens during a hot summer in about 6 weeks; in cooler weather, it can take up to 12 weeks. Drill will often reseed itself if you let some of the flowers go to seed in the garden.

Do not gather dill leaves until the plant has established itself well. Then you can pick leaves in small amounts from each plant throughout the growing season until the plant begins to flower. The fresh leaves can be used immediately in cooking, but for year-round use and storage they must be dried. To do this, place the leaves on nonmetallic screens, in a warm, dark place. For the best results, dill leaves should dry within two days. More drying time than that may ruin their color and flavor. Harvest dill seeds when they re light brown, following the directions in chapter 6.

European and American herbalists regularly use dill leaves and seeds to dispel flatulence, increase mother's milk, and treat breast congestion which may come with nursing. Dill is also considered to be stimulating to the appetite and gently beneficial to the stomach. A simple tea of dill seed or weed may be taken several times daily to treat any of these conditions. A mild infusion of dill seeds is used by some herbalists to relieve colic in babies.

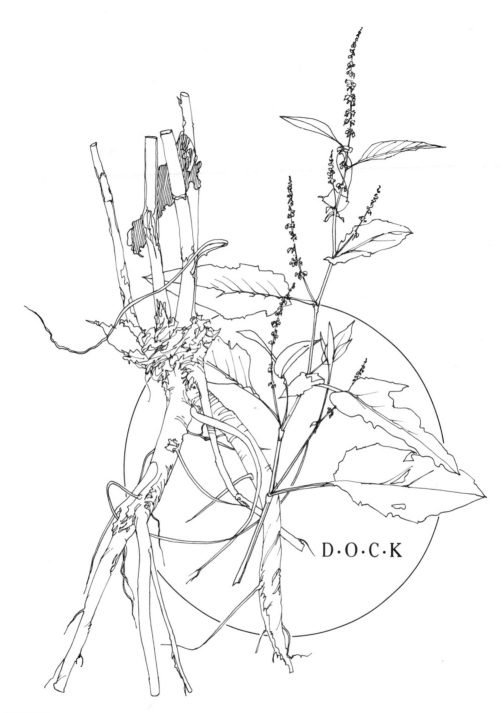

D·O·C·K

DOCK (Curled Dock, Yellow Dock)
Botanical: *Rumex crispus*

Dock is a perennial plant related to rhubarb and buckwheat. There are many varieties of the plant, but the one most often recommended for medicinal purposes in both European and Chinese medicine is the wild yellow or curly dock. Yellow dock grows in pastures, wooded areas, and marginal areas in many countries with a temperate climate. The plant reaches up to 5 feet in height in favorable conditions. It prefers a loose, loamy soil with adequate moisture, but it can be found growing in thin, dry, gravelly soils as well. The yellowish green leaves of dock have curly or wavy edges, grow between 6 and 10 inches in length, and emanate from a central crown. The stem of the plant rises from 1 to 3 feet high, and in the autumn it is easy to spot yellow dock because of the rust-colored sheaf of seeds it develops. They resemble somewhat the seed sheaths of the buckwheat plant, but are much smaller. The root of the plant, the part most often used for healing purposes, is 8 to 12 inches long. It is fleshy and usually not forked, with a reddish brown exterior and white interior.

Gather dock roots in the fall after the seeds mature, but before the first frost. You may need to use a narrow spade to unearth the deep roots, or you can harvest roots from plants growing on loose banks or hillsides to simplify the task. Clean and dry harvested roots either in slices or whole, according to the directions given in chapter 6.

It is possible to cultivate dock of deep, porous garden beds, as you do burdock, dandelion, and other root crops. If dock isn't abundant in the fields and waysides where you live, then it is definitely worthwhile to plant some in your garden. You may have to gather your own seeds from wild plants, but dock is usually quite prolific in its uncultivated form, so that's a simple task. It may be more difficult to unearth the root, but the wild root is bound to have more healing qualities. Remember, in general there is a significant difference in potency between wild and cultivated plants used as medicine.

When gathering dock (or any wild plant), you should always check locally to make sure that the area has not been sprayed with herbicides or pesticides, and never forage on private land without the owner's permission, of course. In the early spring, you can exploit the tonic properties of the dock plant's new leaves, adding them to fresh salads. Their unique lemony flavor makes them pleasant as a steamed green, seasoned with a little garlic and olive oil. Dock leaves are rich in both vitamins A and C; in fact, the late Euell Gibbons claimed that they contain nearly four times more carotene (a substance that is changed to vitamin A inside the human body) than carrots. Like dandelion greens, dock leaves are tasty only when young and tender and again after autumn frost has removed the leaves' bitterness.

Dock root has a reputation among Western herbalists as an effective tonic and cleanser for the whole system. They use it to strengthen the circulatory system, the blood, liver, kidneys, and bladder. Dock has been identified as a laxative for many years, and its effectiveness for this purpose has been substantiated by scientific research. A tea made from the root of the plant is famous in Chinese medicine as a treatment for chronic constipation. In his book, *Secrets of the Chinese Herbalists,* Richard Lucas describes the traditional Chinese use of the same species of dock root (which they call *Ch'in-Ch'ao-Mai*) for this purpose. Dock root is not allowed to boil as most roots are. Instead, the Chinese herbalist places a teaspoonful of the chopped roots in a cup, pours boiling water over them to the cup's rim, covers the cup, and allows the tea to steep for 30 minutes. Then the root is strained off, and the tea reheated and drunk. According to Lucas:

> *The Chinese point out that the problem of constipation varies with different people, so that the amount of yellow dock tea taken daily depends on individual needs. For example, some people may find that less than the average three or four cups daily is sufficient, while others may need more.*[2]

Dock root is also said to have a cooling and drying effect. It has been used externally in the form of an ointment or herbal bath treatment for skin conditions such as eczema, itches, sores, hives, and ringworm. Herbalists who treat these conditions with dock also recommend that the person drink dock root tea several times daily, until their condition improves.

In Tibet, dock leaves are used in moxibustion, a healing technique employed with acupuncture (this technique is described in chapter 3). The leaves are dried, rolled together, pounded, and sifted into a medium coarse powder. Then this powder is rolled between the palms and formed into cones. The yellow dock is also used in Tibet for treating arthritis. In this treatment, a poultice is made of the leaves, and the root is also made into a beverage tea.

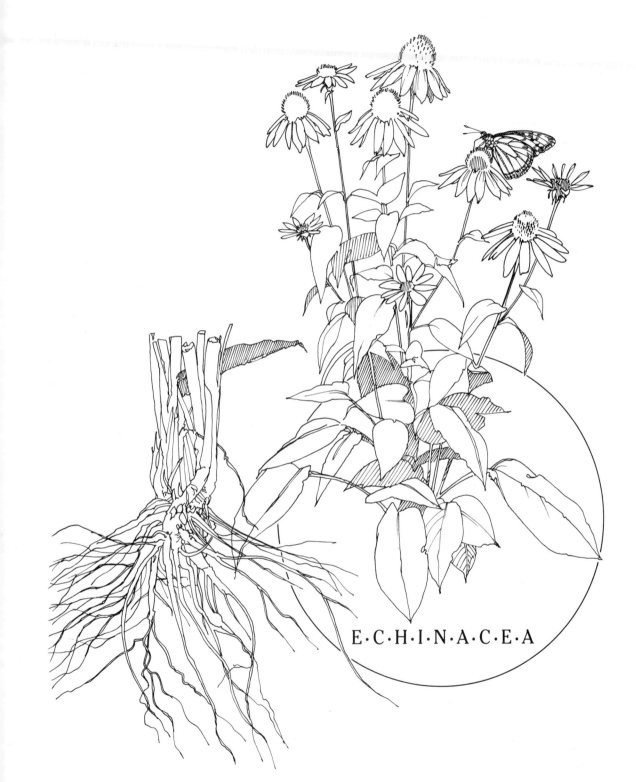

E·C·H·I·N·A·C·E·A

ECHINACEA (Purple Coneflower, Black Sampson)
Botanical: *Echinacea purpurea, E. angustifolia, E. pallida*

Echinacea is a native American plant from the Composite family. It is indigenous to the central plains states from the northern to southern boundaries of the country, where it grows on road banks, prairies, fields, and in dry, open woods. The plant is perennial and grows from 1 to 5 feet in height. It has alternate, lance-shaped leaves with toothed margins. The top leaves lack defined stems. Echinacea's flowers resemble those of the black-eyed Susan in form. Their color ranges from purple to white, and their bold symmetry is strikingly beautiful.

The root, which is the part used for healing purposes, is collected in the late fall of the third or fourth year of the plant's growth, but not after the fourth year. Echinacea is one of the last plants to go dormant in most herb gardens. After several hard frosts it will die back, and that is the time to harvest the root. It should be cleaned and dried according to directions in chapter 6. The crown of the plant can be replanted after the root is harvested, but the resulting plant will not be as medicinally potent.

Echinacea is easy to start from seed. You can achieve a good germination rate if you wait until the air temperature is 70°F to sow the seed. The plant does well in raised beds, with additions of kelp, compost, and rock phosphate. It likes alkaline soil and trace minerals, full sun, and moderate moisture.

According to Melvin Gilmore, an anthropologist who studied Native American medicine in the early part of this century, echinacea was used "as a remedy for more ailments than any other plant in the plains states."[3] In its growing range, all the Indian tribes used the plant to treat snakebite and the bites of poisonous insects. Native Americans also used the juice of the plant to bathe burns and added the juice to the water sprinkled on coals during traditional "sweats," taken for purification purposes. Some Indians used echinacea juice to make their hands, feet, or mouths insensitive to heat, in order to hold, walk on, or "swallow" hot coals and fire during ceremonies.

Many American herbalists still regard echinacea as one of the very best blood purifiers, as well as an effective antibiotic. It is one of the main ingredients in an antibiotic herbal medicine created by Dr. Ed Alstat, a pharmacist and naturopath in Oregon (who is interviewed in chapter 2). Naturopathic doctor Michael Tierra calls *Echinacea angustifolia* "the best herb for blood and lymph purification." According to Tierra, echinacea neutralizes acid conditions in the blood associated with lymphatic stagnation. Dr. Paul Lee, founder of the Platonic Academy of Herbal Studies, describes echinacea as "our leading herb on the list of immuno-stimulants." Dr. Lee is referring to what he believes is echinacea's ability to confer "nonspecific immunity to disease." Medical researchers in Germany, Russia, and China have shown interest in echinacea and are investigating its properties.

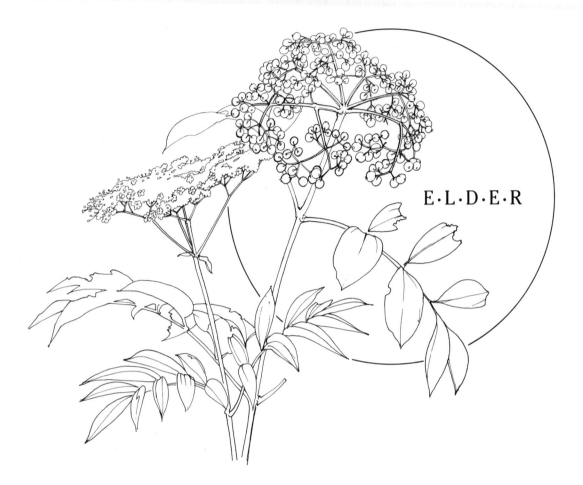

E·L·D·E·R

ELDER

Botanical: *Sambucus nigra*

The elder was a favorite remedy of European gypsies, and in fact, the plant was so widely used in Europe that it earned the epithet "the medicine chest of the country people."

Myth and superstition have always surrounded elder in European countries. Its wood has been used in Russia, Bohemia, and Sicily to drive off evil spirits and harmful creatures. In England, the tree was cultivated as a protection against witches. Perhaps the assignment of such mystical powers to the elder has its basis in an ancient belief that Christ was crucified on a cross of elder wood.

Roman healers, and ancient English and Welsh "leeches" (as physicians were called) all used elder for healing, as did students at the famous Salerno School in eleventh century Italy. In the seventeenth century, John Evelyn spoke its praises in his *Herbal*, saying:

> *If the medicinal properties of its leaves, bark and berries were fully known, I cannot tell what our countryman could ail for which he might not fetch a remedy from every hedge, either for sickness, or wounds.*

In *Cymbeline*, Shakespeare calls it "the stinking elder." The plant does have a strong odor, which repels insects, and also some people. As Mrs. M. Grieve notes in *A Modern Herbal:*

> *The whole tree has a narcotic smell, and it is not considered wise to sleep under its shade. . . . No plant will grow under the shadow of it, being affected by its exhalations.*

While such descriptions may sound rather unpleasant there are plenty of folks who are not put off by the smell of elder, and who really enjoy being around the plant.

Elder can be found growing both as a wild and cultivated plant throughout Europe and North America. It is considered a shrub but can resemble a tree as well. It grows 6 to 10 feet in height. The plant has pale gray, deeply fissured bark. Its leaves are serrated, divided opposite and in arrangements which usually contain five leaves. They are dark green above and lighter green underneath. The core of both the trunk and branches of elder has a white pith, which in the small branches can be blown out easily. These small branches have been hollowed out to make country flutes, whistles, children's popguns, and straws to blow on fires. The roots of elder are very branched, and will penetrate walls if planted near them. Elder flowers are creamy white and carried in clusters. They are followed by the berries, which are dark purplish blue. An elder shrub covered with its creamy umbels, or drooping under the weight of its shiny berry clusters, is a familiar sight in the countryside.

The plant is propagated from cuttings or seed, or sometimes from suckers. Since it is a rather slow process to grow the plant from seed, most people prefer either of these two methods. Take cuttings in the fall according to the instructions in chapter 6. Elder grows best in rich, moist soil and partial shade. It makes a lovely ornamental shrub and can be planted in a hedgerow or as a roadside plant.

The elder has boasted an extensive list of healing uses throughout history. Its leaves, flowers, bark, and berries have all been used. You can collect and dry the leaves of the plant in midsummer, according to the directions in chapter 6. Elder leaves are considered purgative, expectorant, diuretic, and diaphoretic. Boiled with linseed oil, elder leaves are a traditional English remedy for hemorrhoids. The leaves are strained off after the oil has absorbed their green color, and the affected part is treated with the oil. A few leaves can be applied afterward and covered with cotton cloth. Elder leaf ointment (see the recipe for Green Elder Ointment, in chapter 6) is another traditional English remedy, used to treat wounds and bruises.

A cosmetic water made with elder flowers is an old-fasioned cosmetic lotion for the skin. A tisane or infusion made from dried elder flowers has also been used to soothe irritated skin. Herbal baths made with flower infusion were traditionally used to calm nervous or anxious people. You can prepare an elder bath, following the general instructions for herbal baths in chapter 6. Elder flower tea has also been used for inducing perspiration in cases of influenza and for treating sore throats and colds. Cooled elder tea is a traditional and soothing medicine for eye irritations. Gather elder flowers when they are in early bloom and dry them in a warm, airy place, but not in an oven or dryer unless it has a thermostat that can be set at no higher than 80°F. The flowers of the elder are delicate, so watch them carefully as they dry to make sure they do not discolor.

Elderberries have been a traditional remedy for constipation, colic, diarrhea, colds, and rheumatism. The viburnic acid in the berries apparently promotes perspiration, which seems to hasten the conclusion of these disorders. Elderberries make a famous traditional wine that is drunk warm in tiny doses for colds, and they also make a delicious syrup (see Making Herbal Syrups, chapter 6). Homemade elderberry jelly and jam are special treats from the kitchen.

The inner bark of the elder tree is considered a strong purgative and has been used by herbalists in this manner since the time of Hippocrates. For external use you can prepare an emollient ointment with elder bark, by following the same method described in Making Herbal Salves and Ointments, chapter 6. Gather the bark in autumn from young trees according to the General Guidelines for Harvesting in chapter 6.

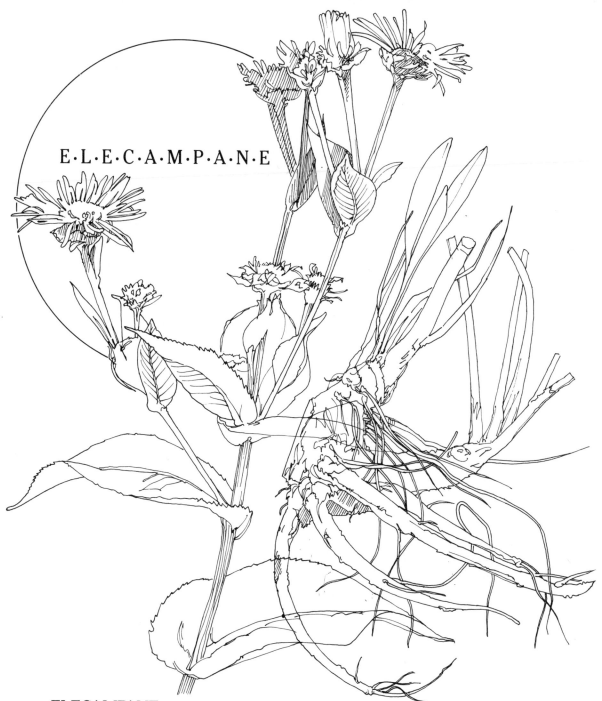

E·L·E·C·A·M·P·A·N·E

ELECAMPANE (Elfdock, Horseheal, Scabwort)
Botanical: *Inula helenium*

Elecampane inherits two of its common names from its early medical applications. "Horseheal" was derived from its use by veterinarians in treating pulmonary disorders in horses. "Scabwort" came from the herb's reputed effectiveness in healing scabs on sheep.

Elecampane is a beautiful herb whose leaves resemble those of the mullein plant, and whose flowers look like sunflowers. The plant can be found growing wild throughout Europe and the temperate zones of Asia, as far as southern Siberia and northwestern India. In North America, it grows from Nova Scotia to North Carolina, and then westward to Missouri. Elecampane is a tall plant—it reaches heights of 4 to 6 feet. It has a stout, deeply furrowed stem which is branched at the top. At its base, the down-covered plant displays a rosette of large, oval leaves that are 1 to 1½ feet long and up to 4 inches across. These leaves are downy and have toothed margins. The leaves that grow on the stem itself are shorter and broader and clasp the stem. Elecampane flowers are bright yellow and are produced in large terminal heads 3 to 4 inches across. The perennial rootstock is large, succulent, branching, and aromatic.

The best way to propagate elecampane is from offshoots or root cuttings taken in autumn from a mature plant. The root pieces should be about 2 inches long. Cover them with slightly moist, sandy soil and store them over the winter in a room with a constant temperature between 50° and 60°F. The roots will develop into new plants by spring, and you can set these out after the danger of frost is past. Place them in rows 3 feet apart, with about 18 inches between plants. Elecampane can also be grown easily from seed started in flats indoors or in a cold frame in early spring. Set out the transplants after the danger of frost is past. Elecampane prefers a clay loam that is moist and well drained in a damp, somewhat shaded environment.

The root is the part of the plant used for healing purposes. It is harvested in the autumn of the plant's second year, after two hard frosts. For medicinal purposes, elecampane root is considered good only in the second year of its growth. In ancient Rome, elecampane was regarded as a good aid in overcoming postbanquet indigestion.

"Let no day pass without eating some of the roots of elecampane condited [preserved] to help digestion, to expel melancholy and sorrow and to cause mirth," wrote Pliny, many centuries ago. And if it is as good at expelling melancholy and causing mirth as Pliny suggests, we modern people should consider eating it more often! The venerable physician Galen brought the mysterious medicine of Rome into brief focus when he wrote that elecampane root is "good for the passions of the hucklebone." Perhaps this is what prompted Pliny to extol it for causing mirth.

Both European and Chinese herbalists have used elecampane root to treat complaints of the lungs and throat and other pulmonary disorders. In China, the native species of the plant is known as Hsuan-Fu-Hua. In the form of syrup, lozenges, or candy, elecampane is considered a soothing treatment for asthma and bronchitis.

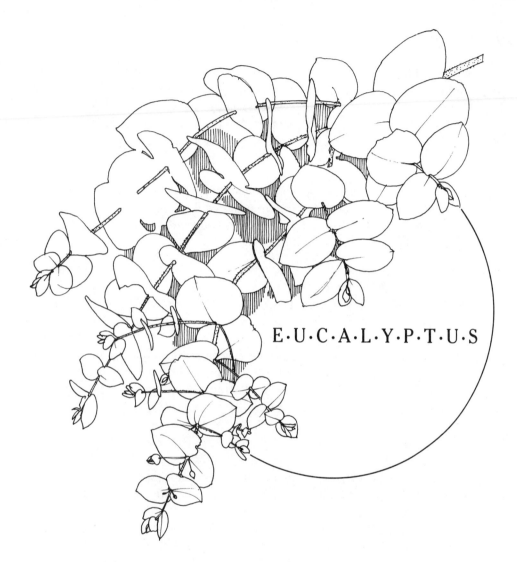

EUCALYPTUS (Blue Gum, Fever Tree)
Botanical: *Eucalyptus globulus,* and other species

The eucalyptus is one of the tallest trees in the world. In its native Australia, specimens that reach 480 feet in height have been found. This beautiful tree, with its long, narrow blue-green leaves, has become naturalized in many parts of the world. It is now found in southern Europe, South Africa, Tahiti, India, and Central America. In the United States, its outdoor habitat is limited to the southwestern states and California.

It has the potential to grow in the southeastern states as well, but it has not yet been established there.

In much of its introduced range, the tree has been planted in swamps in order to dry them and thus reduce the breeding sites for malarial mosquitoes. It may be that the strong, purifying aroma of eucalyptus also helps to repel insects and disperse stagnant air. The tree has smooth, pale gray bark that peels off in thin strips from time to time, exposing the greenish underlayer of the trunk. As Gene Logsdon notes in *Organic Orcharding:*

> *Most [eucalyptus trees] bloom beautiful fragrant blossoms and are first-rate bee trees. What's more, the trees of many species adapt well to alkaline soils, windy conditions, and considerable drought, although they do better with a good supply of moisture.*

In Arizona, eucalyptus are planted as windbreaks to protect citrus groves. In the process, they attract bees to the orchards, too.

This fast-growing tree is not cold hardy; it cannot tolerate temperatures below 27°F. In England, where climate does not allow the permanent planting of eucalyptus, it is cultivated like the bay tree, in large containers that are moved into the greenhouse in the winter. The tree does have some drawbacks. It is dangerous planted near buildings, playgrounds, sidewalks, and similar frequented areas because its large, gangly limbs tend to snap off in windstorms. Eucalyptus roots are troublesome in clogging water lines and sewage lines, as the plant seeks moisture.

Of the many species of eucalyptus, it is the "blue gum" or *Eucalyptus globulus,* that has been most valued for its medicinal properties. The aromatic oil, which develops in the leaves of the mature eucalyptus tree, is considered a very useful healing substance. It is an ingredient in many commerical preparations designed to clear mucus from the nose and lungs. In traditional herbal practice eucalyptus oil is judged antiseptic, astringent, and stimulant, with a warming effect.

The leaves of the mature evergreen tree can be identified by their shape: they are longer, narrower, darker, and droopier than the leaves of the immature tree. In fact, the leaves are often described as swordlike. The leaves of the immature tree are rounder, lighter colored, and stiff. The tree develops the longer, oil-rich leaves after about five years of growth. You can gather leaves at any time and use them either fresh or dried. To dry them, place them on nonmetallic screens in a warm room. Spread the leaves thinly to keep them from fermenting before they dry; eucalyptus leaves are thick and resist dehydration.

You can make a simple eucalyptus infusion by steeping a handful of fresh or dried leaves for 20 minutes in a quart of water that has just been boiled. This tea makes a stimulating astringent addition to the herbal bath and can also be combined with rubbing alcohol and used as a refreshing after-shave. Probably the most popular use of eucalyptus is as a cleanser for the lungs and lymph systems. A classic remedy to clear the nose and help dry mucous conditions is to inhale the vapors of hot eucalyptus leaf tea. The steaming tea is placed in an open pot on a table or on the floor, and the ailing person sits or lies near the pot and breathes in the trailing vapors of the eucalyptus infusion.

You can also use the oil distilled from the leaves for this purpose, either in an electric vaporizer or in the old-fashioned style described above. The oil is considered safe to use in this way, but like all distilled herb oils, it is very potent, so exercise caution when using it. Never apply eucalyptus oil directly to the skin, but dilute it first with water, vegetable oil, or rubbing alcohol. Always keep eucalyptus oil away from your eyes. For internal use, never administer more than a few drops of eucalyptus oil at a time, and be sure to dilute it with water to make a tea. These same precautions apply to oils distilled from rosemary, peppermint, pennyroyal, and other herbs.

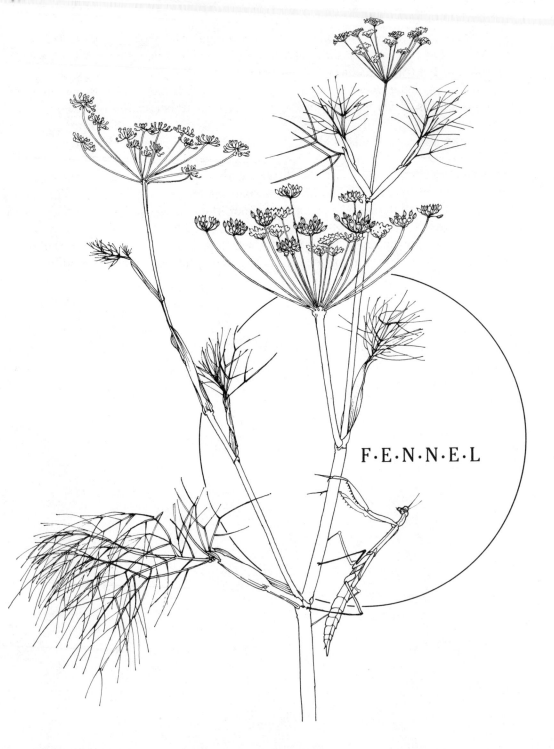

F·E·N·N·E·L

FENNEL

Botanical: *Foeniculum vulgare*

The ancient Greeks consumed fennel to obtain courage and a long life, the ancient Romans to keep their waistlines trim. Fennel's herbal uses of yore also include a digestive aid, eyewash, and insect repellent. It is one of those herbs with a dual history of medicinal and culinary uses.

Fennel is a beautiful perennial plant, a relative of dill, anise, and caraway. It is native to the Mediterranean region, where its stalk and leaves are eaten as a delicacy. The plant grows 4 to 5 feet tall, and has bright green, shiny, smooth stems and feathery fernlike leaves. Its bright yellow flowers are produced in umbels and are followed by the aromatic seeds, which are used medicinally.

Fennel thrives in moderately rich soil and likes plenty of sun. You can sow it outside as early in spring as you can work the soil. Sow the seed lightly in drills 6 inches apart and keep the area moist for two weeks, at which time the first leaves should appear. Thin the plants to stand 6 inches apart as they mature. Gardeners who favor companion planting say that fennel has an adverse effect on bush beans, caraway, tomatoes, and kohlrabi. In turn, coriander and wormwood have an adverse effect on fennel, so all of these plants should be kept away from each other in the garden.

As the plant matures, you can pick moderate quantities of the leaves from time to time for kitchen use. Harvest the seeds when they turn brown according to the guidelines provided in chapter 6. To winter over the plant in cold climates, dig up the taproot with about 3 inches of stem at the end of the plant's first growing season. Bury the root in a cold frame or trench, or in a bucket of sand in the cellar until spring, when you can replant it. Keep fennel plants being wintered over in this way cool, but not damp.

As a healing herb, fennel has been used to soothe the stomach and intestines, to relieve flatulence, to expel worms, to sweeten the breath, as a gargle, an eyewash, and to increase milk in nursing mothers. For all of these purposes the seeds are made into a tea that is drunk two to three times daily. In poultice form, fennel has been used to relieve swelling in the breasts of nursing mothers. The herb is considered mildly and gently calmative.

In Italy, the tender young stalks are harvested by cutting them at the crown. Italians serve them fresh in salads or steamed and sautéed with a little garlic and olive oil. Cooked this way, fennel is a favorite accompaniment to pasta dishes in southern Italy. There is a bulbing variety that produces large, succulent overlapping stems and is prepared in a similar fashion. The French pair the delicate, licoricelike taste of fennel with fish—in soups, stews, and sauces. One favorite treatment in French Provençal cooking is to grill fish over burning stalks of dried fennel. Americans, too, are now learning to appreciate this sweet, pungent, aromatic herb.

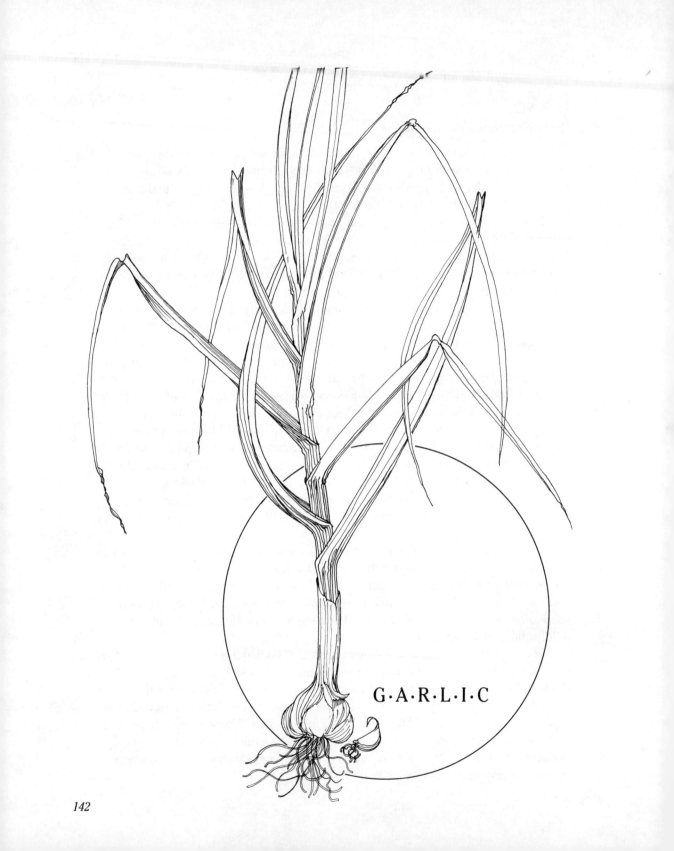

G·A·R·L·I·C

142

GARLIC
Botanical: *Allium sativum*

Garlic, the "stinking rose" of the herb world, is one of the most ancient healing plants. It is thought to be native to China, and it has been esteemed in the medical tradition of that country for thousands of years. No doubt the early Egyptians were aware of garlic's antibiotic properties, too. Hieroglyphic records show that laborers consumed large amounts of garlic while constructing the pyramids. In China and in Europe, garlic has been used to guard against plagues and infectious diseases. In Greece and Rome, it was eaten extensively; the famous Roman physician Galen praised it as the common man's heal-all. Throughout Europe, garlic has traditionally been both a food and a prominent herb in botanical medicine. In North America, Native Americans ate garlic regularly and used it for a variety of healing purposes. The traditional medicines of both Europe and China have employed garlic for respiratory problems.

The bulb of the garlic plant, which is the part used medicinally, is compound and composed of individual cloves, or sections. From this bulb the leaves rise up flat and straight, looking somewhat like the leaves of the onion, to which garlic is related. The flower stalk rises directly from the bulb, displaying a globe-shaped white flower head.

Garlic is an excellent herb for the garden. Planted around fruit and nut trees, it helps to repel moles. Placed near roses, it helps to keep aphids at bay. In fact, companion planting lore has it that garlic will keep a large variety of insects away from the more delicate garden vegetables and herbs. It is easy to cultivate, too. It likes light soil with good drainage. Plant the individual cloves 2 inches deep and about 6 inches apart in early spring, at the same time you plant onion sets in your region. If you garden intensively in a raised bed, the plants can be less than 6 inches apart. Additions of well-rotted compost will ensure a good crop. Harvest garlic when the top growth of the plant begins to die down. Once harvested, allow the bulbs to cure outdoors in the shade for several days before you store them.

Garlic tea, made by infusing several chopped cloves of garlic in 1 quart of water, has been used as a gargle, or taken internally for colds and flu (see the recipe in chapter 6 for an expectorant garlic syrup). Placed externally on a cut, on a wound, or simply on the hands, or the soles of the feet, garlic's antibiotic qualities are said to be quickly absorbed into the bloodstream. A fresh clove of garlic placed on the gums may soothe an abscessed tooth or other inflammation in the mouth. A cotton ball soaked in garlic oil is an old-time European remedy for treating ear infections. (Never place a clove of garlic in your ear, however! It can lodge there and complicate the ear problem.)

Chinese herbalists traditionally used garlic to treat certain forms of high blood pressure. A number of Western physicians and researchers in Germany, France, and Switzerland have also reported success in treating high blood pressure with garlic.

Garlic has an age-old reputation as a plant that stirs sexual appetite and rambunctious thoughts. In many Eastern religious traditions, yogis, monks, and nuns eliminate garlic from their diets for these reasons. Congruent with this belief, Culpeper reported his view of garlic:

> *Its heat is very vehement; and all vehement hot things send up but ill-savored vapors to the brain . . . it will . . . send up strong fancies, and as many strange visions to the head; therefore, let it be taken inwardly with great moderation.*

The smell of garlic on a person is accepted as an endearing quality in countries such as Korea and Italy. In this country, however, it is not. If you like the healing properties of garlic but not its smell, try soaking in a hot bath for 15 to 20 minutes after using it. You'll find that most of the garlic aroma dissipates in the bath.

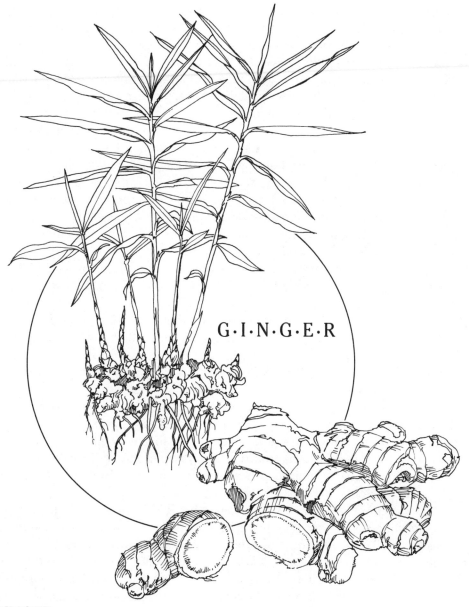

G·I·N·G·E·R

GINGER

Botanical: *Zingiber officinale*

Ginger, an exotic tropical plant with highly aromatic flowers, originated in China and later spread to Spain, where it was grown as early as the sixteenth century. The conquistadores brought ginger from Spain to the New World, and it was eventually established as a major commercial crop in Jamaica. Today ginger, with some well established culinary roles, is widely grown in the West Indies, Africa, India, and southeast Asia. Ginger is an important ingredient in Chinese and Japanese cuisine, and it has even come to be one of the spices used in making all-American pumpkin pies. Ginger not only spices food with its warming pungent taste, but it assists in the digestion of rich, fatty foods and helps to relieve flatulence.

In Hawaii, ginger plants bear pinkish white flowers on stalks that reach heights of 8 to 10 feet. The species found in China *(Zingiber officinale)* has yellowish green flowers and grows about 2½ feet tall. The leaves of the plant are swordlike, and the stalk is a cane, similar to a cornstalk. The rhizome, which is the part used for medicinal purposes (it is commonly called gingerroot, although it is not a true root), is fleshy, aromatic, and covered with a thin greenish skin. In tropical climates, ginger is planted outdoors in autumn, and the ginger "root" is ready for harvest by midsummer of the following year, after the leaves die down.

In the United States, ginger can be grown outdoors in Florida, Hawaii, and the southernmost parts of California, Arizona, New Mexico, and Texas. It thrives in raised beds with additions of well-composted manure and kelp. The plant is propagated from pieces of the rhizome, which contain "eyes," as do potatoes. For best results each root piece planted should contain two eyes. Set the root cuttings 3 inches deep and at least 12 inches apart.

Ginger can be successfully grown in greenhouses or indoors in bright light if the climate is not warm enough for outdoor cultivation. For best results, be sure the rhizomes you plant are young, fresh roots. You will recognize them by their light green color. In this country about the only place to get young ginger is in Oriental grocery stores in large cities. (The Chinese often prepare fresh, tender ginger as a spicy vegetable.) Most of the ginger roots sold in supermarkets and other food stores are older roots, identifiable by their tough, light tan skin. You can plant these too, but the success rate will not be as high as for young rhizomes.

Plant each piece of rhizome in a container that is 12 inches in diameter and at least 10 inches deep. The soil mix should be loose and rich (compost, leaf mold, and peat moss are all good additions), and the container must have good drainage. Line the container with a layer of gravel before adding any soil. Keep the soil evenly moist (not soggy) and the temperature a constant 70°F or more during the first several weeks after planting. In fact, your ginger plant will need warm temperatures and ample humidity throughout its life in order to thrive. The cuttings will take about a month to sprout. Keep the plant in direct sunlight as long as it doesn't dry out.

If you do not wish to plant the tuberous rhizomes right away, you can keep them fresh for months in the refrigerator, or by storing them buried in a box of dry sand in a cool room. To dry the root, remove the thin layer of skin and slice the root into thin disks. Dry the slices in the sun or in a well-ventilated room according to the directions given in chapter 6.

The Chinese call ginger *Chiang* and use it extensively as a botanic medicine. Ginger's acrid, pungent, sharp taste has heating and drying properties, and Chinese healers prescribe its use especially in autumn and winter. A classic Chinese remedy for colds, flu, and coughs is an invigorating tea made from fresh gingerroot. It is found to be very helpful in eliminating mucus. Chinese medicine also specifies ginger for nausea, hangover, and general debility. Ginger is slightly diuretic and is said to strengthen the kidneys, bladder, and uterus by "warming" them and thus increasing their vital energy. In China, women with delayed menstruation or menstrual cramps commonly drink gingerroot tea.

You can vary the strength of ginger tea according to your needs. Usually, three or four thin slices of the fresh root are simmered in a pint of water for anywhere from 10 to 30 minutes. Ginger is an effective and safe herb. A cup of hot ginger tea is a heart-warming antidote to a cold winter day, especially after the chilling effects of frigid air and blistering winds. Chinese healers say that even moderate amounts of ginger tea have the power to strengthen the lungs and kidneys.

Ginger has some useful external applications for healing, too. In his book *Healing Ourselves,* Japanese herbalist Naboru Muramoto recommends ginger compresses, baths, and oils for general debility, gout, arthritis, headaches, and spinal pain. Most of these treatments require the freshly expressed juice of a ginger root. You can extract the juice by finely grating the ginger into a bowl and then gathering the grated ginger into a cheesecloth or jelly bag. Then squeeze out as much of the juice as you can into a bowl. You can even squeeze out the juice with your fingers, if nothing else is available. (See the recipe for Ginger Compress in chapter 6 for complete directions.)

Ginger compresses are highly regarded in Oriental medicine. They are used on the forehead to relieve sinus congestion. They are placed on the chest to break up congestion from colds, flu, bronchitis, and other pulmonary complaints. They have a history of use in treating kidney problems, arthritis, and rheumatism. Chinese women apply ginger compresses to the lower back and abdomen to relieve menstrual cramps.

You can turn leftover compress water (which should not be kept more than one day) into an invigorating footbath that promotes circulation throughout the whole body. To make an extra-strength bath use about 2 pounds of gingerroot and 1 gallon of water. Follow the same method you use to make a ginger compress. Add this mixture to a hot bath to revitalize your whole body when it is sore from hard work, multiple bruises, or arthritis or bursitis.

Ginger oil made by combining equal parts of ginger juice and cold-pressed sesame seed oil has medicinal value, too. This oil can be massaged into the skin in place of a ginger compress. Japanese herbalist Naboru Muramoto describes the traditional Japanese treatment of spinal and joint problems with a ginger oil massage in his book

Healing Ourselves. Muramoto also recommends placing a piece of cotton soaked in ginger oil in the ear to provide relief from earache.

In the Tibetan system of medicine, ginger plays a role in many preparations used to treat ailments emanating from an imbalance of the phlegm humor (the humors of Tibetan medicine are described in chapter 3). Like garlic, onions, and cayenne pepper, ginger is regarded as promoting overall circulation of energy in the body and acting as a stimulant for those who are debilitated, lethargic, or convalescing from an illness.

A recent discovery, reported in the *New England Journal of Medicine* in 1983, is that ginger is useful in treating vertigo. A study showed that powdered ginger taken in capsule form was as helpful as dramamine in treating motion sickness.

Its long list of uses both for healing and cooking make ginger a most worthwhile herb to include in your medicine chest and spice rack.

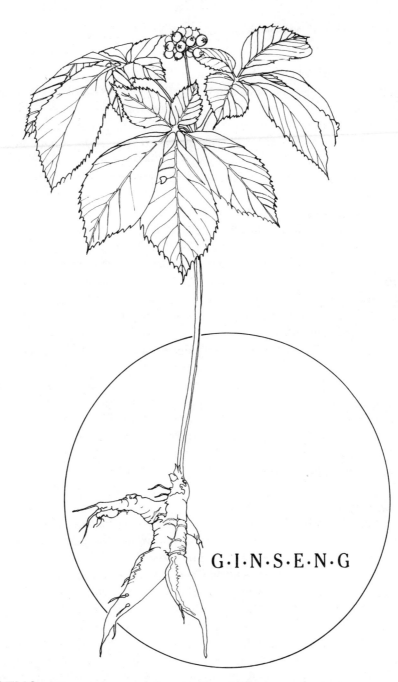

G·I·N·S·E·N·G

GINSENG (Man Root, Root of Life, Root of Immortality)
Botanical: *Panax* species

Steeped in colorful lore, ginseng ranks among the most fabled of ancient healing plants. Its legendary medicinal uses, persisting since ancient times, range from nerve calmative and expeller of evil to heart tonic and aphrodisiac. Most of the outrageous cure-all claims have taken their place in fascinating volumes of folklore, but ginseng is still quite a respected herb among natural healers. Until recent times, there existed no scientific research to make or break ginseng's fantastic image.

Ginseng is native to North America, as well as to China. Wild American ginseng (*Panax quinquefolius*) is protected by law in many states because populations have declined from years of radical overharvesting. The growing range of wild ginseng runs from Pennsylvania north into Canada and south to Georgia along the Appalachian Mountains, then west to Minnesota. Centuries of high demand have sparked an overharvesting of ginseng in the Orient, too. *P. shinseng*, the Oriental species, still grows wild only in very remote regions of China, Japan, and Korea.

Wild ginseng grows in a solitary fashion, although at times several plants can be found growing near each other. In the wild, American ginseng cohabits with other shade- and moisture-loving plants such as wild ginger, may apples, goldenseal, rattlesnake fern, and jack-in-the-pulpit. It can be found under ash, basswood, oak, elm, hickory, maple and other deciduous trees, and to some extent under pines, cedars, and firs. American ginseng has a particular affinity for shady north slopes, where there is loose, rich soil and leaf mold from the forest cover.

In its first year the plant sends up but one leaf. The second year it produces two leaves, each divided in turn into five leaflets. In its third year, it produces a third leaf and some greenish yellow flowers, followed by clusters of red berries. The mature ginseng plant is from 10 to 20 inches high. The root is cylindrical, long and tapered with prominent wrinkles, sometimes called "threads," marking its growth. It is often forked at both the bottom and sides, creating a shape somewhat reminiscent of the human body, and inspiring one of ginseng's common names, man root.

Today, many herbalists grow their own ginseng in semiwild or cultivated settings. If you own or have access to land whose ecology includes a north slope with a good stand of hardwood trees or mixed hardwoods and conifers that produces a shade canopy of 70 percent or more, you have the right kind of wild environment for the cultivation of ginseng. Ginseng needs a rich, light, well-drained soil, too. You can grow the plant from seed or young "starts," which you can purchase from a number of the growers listed in the Appendix at the back of the book.

Ginseng seeds have a hard covering that must be softened for efficient germination. Some recent research has shown that ginseng seeds are softened by birds, who eat the ripe ginseng berries. As the seeds pass through the bird's digestive system, hydrochloric acid in the bird's stomach prepares them for germination. To simulate this natural process, gardeners can soak the seeds in a mixture of 1 part liquid household bleach and 9 parts water for 5 to 10 minutes. Then rinse the seeds thoroughly. Sow ginseng seeds in the fall by pressing them into soil to a depth of ½ inch. They take anywhere from eight months to two years to germinate. If you would prefer to get a head start on growing a crop of ginseng, it would be expedient for you to start with young plants.

It is best to leave plenty of space between ginseng plants, as that is their natural preference. Five feet between each plant is a minimum. Ample spacing between plants seems to decrease ginseng's susceptibility to certain diseases. Check the plants for root and leaf diseases regularly, or the entire planting may be destroyed. To lessen the possibility of plant disease, gardeners in the Orient allow ground from which ginseng has recently been harvested to lie fallow or at least to be planted to a different crop for several years before any more ginseng is replanted there.

Some growers of semiwild gardens cover their ginseng plants with wire mesh to keep away deer, mice, rabbits, and other hungry wildlife. Some gardeners drive sheet metal barriers into the ground surrounding the roots to ward off moles. According to Chinese tradition, however, metal should not be placed near the growing plants. James A. Duke, chief of the Economic Botany Laboratory of the USDA, noted in a report "Chinese Anti-Cancer Plants" that when he planted ginseng in collars made of tin cans, despite Chinese advice to the contrary, 75 percent of his plants died.[4]

Ginseng can also be cultivated in a more civilized garden setting, as long as you can provide a well-shaded bed. Some growers construct arbors of lath strips or lattice to cover the top and both sides of the ginseng beds. These arbors should provide a 70 percent shade cover. Cultivated ginseng should be grown in a soil with plenty of leaf mold and well-rotted compost and manure added to it. The soil should be slightly damp, as it would be in a woodsy setting. A mulch layer of decaying leaves at least 2 inches thick is a healthy addition to a cultivated ginseng bed. It provides nutrients as the leaves decay and also helps hold in soil moisture.

Ginseng is a challenging plant to grow, and it is not a plant for the impatient gardener. At the very least, ginseng must grow for six or seven years before its root is ready to harvest. Nine years of growth produces a far superior root. The root is said to get better with age, and ginseng can grow to be very old indeed. In recent years, potent, valuable specimens have been found with growth rings indicating their age to be 400 years.

Cleaned, fresh ginseng root is sometimes eaten raw immediately after harvesting. The fresh root is supposed to contain much more of the active principles, called ginsenosides, which have been found to possess adaptogenic (antistress) properties than does the dried root. However, ginseng can be processed for storage in a number of ways. The Chinese and Koreans have developed a method of processing ginseng, which they believe retains the active principles and preserves the root very well, too. They clean the fresh roots and put them in a basket, which is in turn placed in a closed earthenware steamer. The steamer is set on top of an iron pot of boiling water. This water often contains the Chinese herbal bark known as *sa woo,* and its medicinal essence penetrates the roots as they steam. The steaming continues for one to four hours. Then the roots (which must never be smoked) are carefully dried over a slow-burning wood fire or in a drying house. After a week to ten days the dried roots are dark red or maroon, and translucent, hard, and brittle—yielding what is known as Red Ginseng in the herb trade. You can also dry ginseng roots in the sun after washing them thoroughly. Spread on a screen or cloth, they will take one to two weeks to dry thoroughly. When dry, store them in a glass jar.

Harvesting ginseng roots was the very stuff of which legends were made in ancient China, where a special guild of ginseng hunters called *va-pang-suis* searched for the plant at night with tiny bows and arrows. The plant, it was said, emitted a light of its own, and moved around at night. It was only with the tiny arrows with string attached to them that the hunters were able to catch the roots. James Duke, a researcher at the USDA Economic Botany Laboratory, challenged the Chinese belief that ginseng moved around at night. Doubting such a claim, he planted 100 ginseng plants in an experimental garden. When he found that the next morning nearly half of the roots had moved (or been moved) out of the hole, but were uneaten, he replanted them. Again half the plants were disturbed during the night. Dr. Duke now professes some credence in "Chinese sayings that are difficult to believe."[5]

In modern times, Russia, China, and Korea have engaged in a good deal of scientific research in an attempt to document the medicinal claims for ginseng. The noted Russian scientist I. I. Brekhman has conducted extensive research on ginseng's ability to increase the body's resistance to illness. In his research, Brekhman has found that ginseng was able to relieve signs of stress and help subjects cope with tension-creating situations. Apparently, ginseng positively affects the adrenal cortex, relieving its need to produce stress-combating hormones in large amounts.

Other scientists have been investigating ginseng's medicinal uses in various specific diseases. At the Third International Ginseng Conference held in Korea in 1981, Japanese scientist Dr. M. Kimura reported positive treatment of diabetic patients with ginseng.[6] At the same conference, another Japanese scientist, Dr. Morio Yonezawa, reported research using ginseng extract to prevent radiation-induced bone marrow damage. According to Yonezawa, one injection of the extract produced a restorative effect after a patient's exposure to radiation. In a related study, Dr. Yoon Seok Chang of the Seoul National University Hospital in Korea reported that in two comparative studies on 50 patients with cervical cancer, oral doses of red panax ginseng restored bone marrow functions that had been damaged by radiation.[7]

There has been much controversy in the United States over the efficacy of this unusual plant. Some people praise it while others deride it as a mere placebo. Oriental herbalists offer an explanation for ginseng's mixed reviews, based on their medical tradition. Chinese medicine considers ginseng, one of the most yang herbs, to be suited for health problems related to deficiency. For someone with a very strong yang condition, the effects of ginseng will hardly be noticeable. Ginseng is actually contraindicated for those whose yang condition is causing high blood pressure. On the other hand, for those whose condition is yin (more frail), ginseng is considered beneficial.

The Chinese and Native American tribes both use ginseng to treat impotence. Tibetan doctor Shenphen Dawa Rinpoche recommends ginseng to men over 45, for whom he calls it the "king of medicines." The Chinese also use ginseng in treating senility, debility, diabetes, hypoglycemia, uterine disorders, mental illness caused by nervous exhaustion, anemia, dyspepsia, and arteriosclerosis. Various Native American tribes have used ginseng for sexual ailments, to increase fertility, as a panacea and a reviving tonic, as well as for stomach disorders, headaches, fevers, and coughs.

Perhaps more research will shed some light on the mysteries of a plant that is supposed to shine by itself at night.

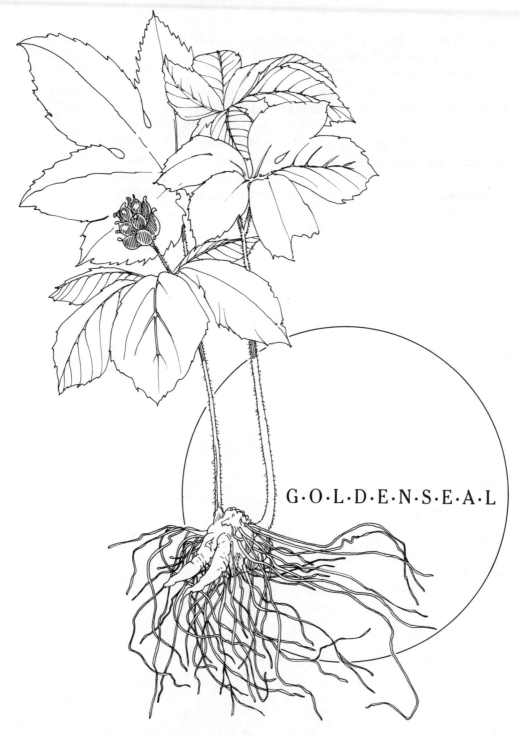

G·O·L·D·E·N·S·E·A·L

GOLDENSEAL (Yellow Root, Orange Root, Yellow Puccoon)
Botanical: *Hydrastis canadensis*

Goldenseal, sometimes called "poor man's ginseng" because of its reputed tonic effect on the entire body, does bear a certain resemblance to its more famous relative. Both plants grow in the same range and habitats, are about the same size, and look somewhat similar. Both have been overharvested due to ever-increasing popularity and demand.

Goldenseal, an herb native to North America, was first discovered and used by the Cherokee Indians. The plant grows on shady, northern hillsides and in the rich soil of river deltas. It is most plentiful in the Ozarks, the Appalachians, and the Mississippi and Ohio River valleys. But it also grows in the province of Ontario, Canada. From southern Ontario and New York State, the plant can be found in the wild westward to Minnesota and south to Georgia and Kentucky. It was cultivated at the turn of the twentieth century in Washington and Oregon, where modest stands of it can still be found.

Goldenseal is a perennial with a yellow rootstock, marked by annual growth rings, just as ginseng root is. Goldenseal's purplish stems grow about 1 foot tall and bear two large, five-part leaves that are slightly hairy. The plant develops one flower head, which is either greenish white or rose colored. This singular flower turns into a fruit that resembles a large raspberry. The root, which is seldom more than 2 inches in length, is the part of the plant used for healing purposes. The plant is easily identified when its berry is fruiting, but it is best to harvest the root in the late fall, after the topgrowth has died back. People searching for wild goldenseal usually make one trip to find and identify the plant's habitat and location, and a second trip to harvest the root.

Wild goldenseal is not very easy to find these days. Like wild American ginseng, it has been harvested to near extinction ever since herbalists first took note of its healing properties in the 1800s. For this reason it is better to grow the herb at home in a semiwild garden environment. Goldenseal can also be grown from pieces of the rootstock or from seed. (See the Resource Guide at the back of the book for sources of goldenseal plants, rootstock, or seed.)

Like ginseng, goldenseal grows best on north slopes with a 70 percent shade canopy. It can also be cultivated in beds shaded on top and the side, receiving the most sun by simple arbors made of lattice or lath strips. You can try growing grapes on top of the arbors and accomplish two gardening feats at once.

Set the goldenseal plants or rootstocks in the ground ½ inch deep and at least 8 inches apart. The soil should be rich in leaf mold or compost. From rootstock or seedlings, it takes two to three years for the plant to develop a harvestable root. From seed, it takes five years. Harvest the root in the late fall of the plant's third to fifth year, depending upon whether you have grown it from seed or rootstock. Wait until the topgrowth dies back, and several hard frosts have occurred before harvesting. Dry and store the root according to the guidelines in chapter 6.

Indian tribes who lived within goldenseal's growing range used this native plant extensively. As the European settlers came to know the plant, they adopted many of the healing uses known to the Indians. Fresh goldenseal root soaked in water was used as an eyewash. A tea of the root cleansed skin conditions such as acne and eczema. The same tea was also used by early American settlers as a douche to treat vaginal infections.

Goldenseal has been found to contain alkaloids known as berberine and hydrastine, which are astringent and also have mild antibiotic properties. Many modern American herbalists consider goldenseal one of the best herbs available in North America. Goldenseal's influence is warming and drying, properties which are considered useful in correcting problems of the mucous membranes. The herb is also employed as an antiseptic. As early as 1650, a Jesuit priest reported using the bruised leaf to close and disinfect cuts and wounds.[8] The powdered root is also sprinkled directly onto cuts or wounds to disinfect them and promote rapid healing.

A solution of goldenseal and myrrh gum powder in warm water is sometimes used as a douche for treating vaginal infections. The herb is also regarded as a good stomach tonic. And like ginseng, goldenseal has often been used for treating symptoms associated with exhaustion of the adrenal glands: stress, anxiety, nervousness, asthma, and allergic reactions. Goldenseal is also an emmenagogue, or substance which brings on menses. It should not be used by pregnant women.

Herbalists always practice great discretion when using goldenseal to treat any internal condition. The herb has cumulative effects on the system, so it is employed in very small doses for no longer than one week at a time. The alkaloids contained in this herb are known to be toxic in large doses. Used correctly, however, goldenseal is considered a very effective herb for correcting a variety of conditions.

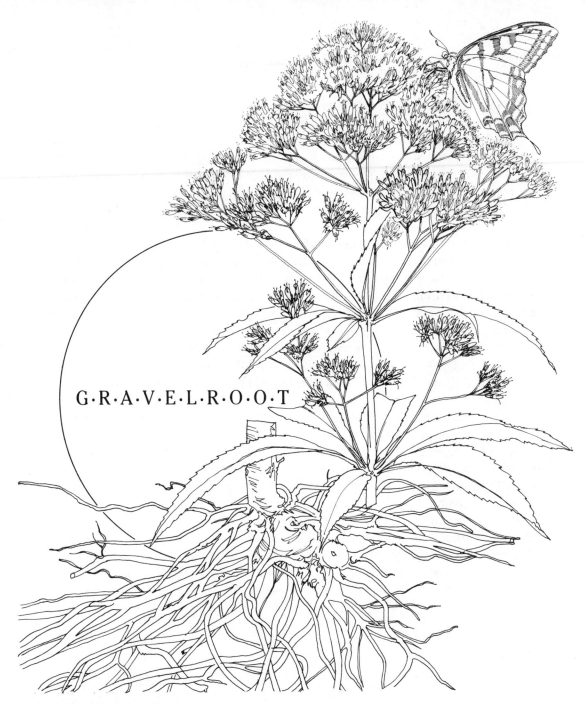

G·R·A·V·E·L·R·O·O·T

GRAVELROOT (Joe-Pye Weed, Purple Boneset, Queen-of-the-Meadow)
Botanical: *Eupatorium purpureum*

Gravelroot is a large perennial plant that grows from 3 feet to as much as 10 feet high. Its stem is rigid and hollow, or partially hollow, with purple tinges above the leaf joints. Its leaves are rough and crinkly above, but downy underneath. They circle the stem in whorls of four or five every couple of inches. The flowers are usually pinkish or purple and form a dense umbrella at the top of the plant. Gravelroot often grows in impenetrably thick masses. It grows wild in North America from Canada all the way to Florida, and west to Texas and the Dakotas. It prefers rich lowlands, stream banks, moist woods, and swamps or marshes.

Gravelroot likes full sun or partial shade and rich, well-drained soil. Springtime applications of well-rotted manure or compost are beneficial. Start seed indoors in flats and move the seedlings outside when the danger of frost is past. The seed is fine and is sown much as lettuce seed is sown, about ¼ inch deep in well-prepared soil. You can also propagate the plant from rootstock divisions made in the fall when the root is harvested. Winter over the divisions in a bucket or box of sand in a cool room or cellar. Harvest the root in the late autumn of the plant's second or third year and dry it according to directions in chapter 6. The crown of the plant can also be replanted and will produce another harvestable root in two to three years.

The gravelroot plant has a long history of healing use. Its botanical name comes from a king in ancient Roman times, Mithridates Eupator, who used the plant medicinally. The common name of gravelroot comes from its use in eliminating gravel or stones from the kidneys and bladder. Native Americans use the root for this purpose, and so do Chinese herbalists. Gravelroot has also traditionally been used by European and American herbalists to treat lower back pains, lumbago, gout, and rheumatism. Native Americans and early settlers used the leaves and root of the plant to produce the profuse sweating needed to break fevers. One of the plant's vernacular names is Joe-Pye Weed, after an Indian healer who became famous for his successful treatment of typhus fever with gravelroot.

Gravelroot is most commonly used as an ingredient in herb formulas or by itself as a decoction of the dried root. You should be aware though, that in large doses gravelroot is an emetic, and although it has been used in many different ways over the years, it can be toxic if used in a casual way.

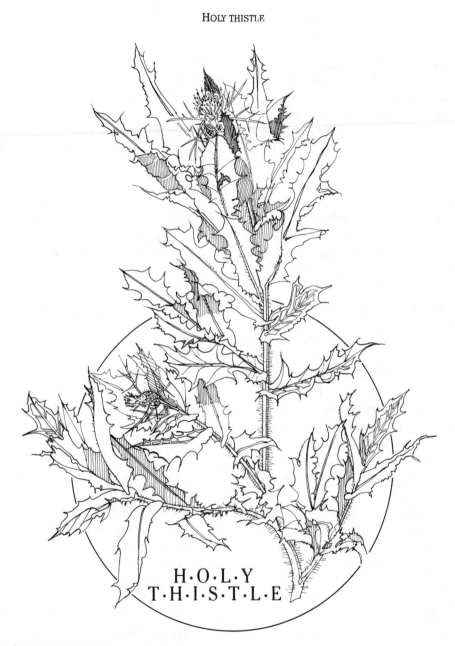

H·O·L·Y
T·H·I·S·T·L·E

HOLY THISTLE (Blessed Thistle, Spotted Thistle)

Botanical: *Cnicus benedictus*

In the Middle Ages, holy thistle and angelica were the two most common medicinal herbs in Europe. Holy thistle grows wild in stony areas of southern Europe, where it is thought to have originated. It is also a common wayside plant in the eastern United States and in parts of the Southwest. The plant, which is rather downy, reaches about 2 feet in height, has many branches, and toothed, spiny lobed leaves. The flowers are pale yellow and appear in green, prickly heads. The holy thistle's leafy parts are used for healing purposes.

Holy thistle is a hardy plant. You can sow it directly into its permanent bed in early spring. Plant the seed about 6 inches apart and ¼ inch deep. It thrives in good garden soil, with spring additions of well-rotted compost. The plant is ready for gathering in early summer. One-third of its growth can be cut back at that time. Often, three or four such cuttings can be taken during the growing season, so a small patch of holy thistle will produce enough of the foliage to last all year. Harvest the plant before it flowers each time, so that it does not have the opportunity to self-sow and become a garden pest. Dry the leafy parts according to the general directions in chapter 6.

The holy thistle, as its name implies, has been highly respected as a healing herb in Europe for many centuries. Although most of its traditional uses have not been substantiated by modern research, this is an herb with a rich history. By the mid-1500s, it had become popular in medieval "physick" gardens as far north as England.

Holy thistle's properties are tonic, diaphoretic, emetic, stimulant, and emmenagogic. Considered a tonic for the heart, holy thistle has been used traditionally to increase circulation. It also is used to promote perspiration and break fevers, and to increase production of milk in nursing mothers. A simple infusion of the herb, either fresh or dried, has been used to purify the blood and act as a general tonic. A cup of the tea is taken twice a day. In large amounts, the tea was used to induce vomiting. In normal doses, though, holy thistle is considered a gentle stomach tonic.

In medieval times, the plant had a reputation as an herb for the nervous system, and it was used in treating melancholy, mental agitation, and other nervous disorders, often in combination with valerian, wood betony, and sage. The name "holy thistle" probably was derived at least in part from the herb's ability to make people more relaxed, calm, and peaceful. This gentle herb is still popular as a mild calmative.

All of the thistles (including artichoke) are considered tonics for the liver. Holy thistle, which has a warming, drying effect, is especially popular among contemporary herbalists for liver problems, particularly those associated with alcoholism.

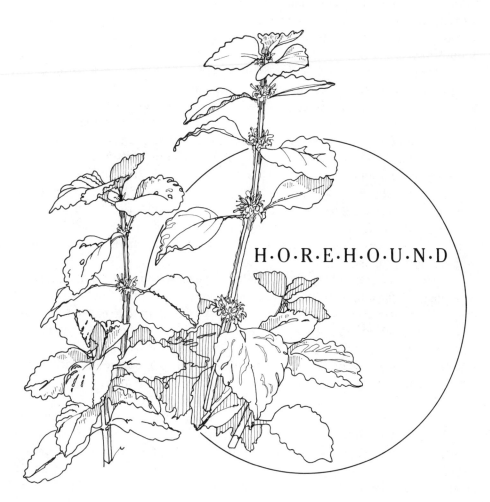

H·O·R·E·H·O·U·N·D

HOREHOUND

Botanical: *Marrubium vulgare*

The history of the horehound goes back at least to ancient Egypt, where it was known by several prestigious names—Eye of the Star, Seed of Horus, and Bull's Blood. Horehound is a perennial member of the mint family. It is a bushy plant with woolly silver-white leaves that are wrinkled and opposite and carried on quadrangular hairy stems. Its flowers are white and displayed in whorls that circle the tips of the stalks that bear them. A common wayside plant in both Europe and the United States, horehound is usually found growing in poor, dry soil. It is most easily propagated from cuttings or root divisions taken in either spring or fall. You can also propagate it from seeds, sowing them ⅛ inch deep and 1 inch apart in the spring after the danger of frost is past. When the seedlings begin to develop, thin them to stand about 9 inches apart.

In the garden, as in the wild, horehound thrives in sandy soil in a warm, sunny location, an environment that encourages a maximum concentration of the valuable herbal qualities in the plant's leaves. Horehound has a characteristic musky odor, which some people find disagreeable, but the smell dissipates as the herb dries.

The plant does not bloom until its second year, but you can harvest horehound in its first year by cutting back the plant by about one-third of its total topgrowth. In subsequent years you can harvest the plant more fully by cutting back foliage to about 4 inches above the ground, just before it flowers. Two or three cuttings a year can be made, depending on your climate and growing conditions. Harvest and dry the leaves according to the directions in chapter 6. If the horehound plant is allowed to flower, its seeds will self-sow widely in the garden, transforming it from a valuable herb to a garden nuisance.

Horehound has enjoyed a number of healing uses throughout the histories. It was thought to be one of the bitter herbs that formed part of the first Passover rite of the Jewish people. Powdered horehound leaves have been used to expel worms, and an ointment made with the leaves has been used to soothe itches and wounds. In large doses, the herb was used as a laxative. Greeks, Romans, and medieval Europeans used horehound for snakebites, dog bites, and to counteract vegetable poisons. Culpeper reported its use in bringing on menses and in helping to expel afterbirth.

But horehound is definitely best known as a remedy for coughs and pulmonary complaints and in the treatment of colds. A strong infusion of horehound is used by herbalists to promote perspiration and has been used for breaking fevers. Many people in both Europe and America brew horehound tea as soon as they feel a cold coming on. If a cold has already set in, horehound tea taken three times daily is considered a valuable aid in expelling mucus.

Horehound syrup and cough drops are famous old-fashioned cold remedies from the 1800s, but the use of horehound leaves in cough syrup goes back at least to the 1600s. See page 317 for a recipe that re-creates the soothing properties of this time-honored remedy.

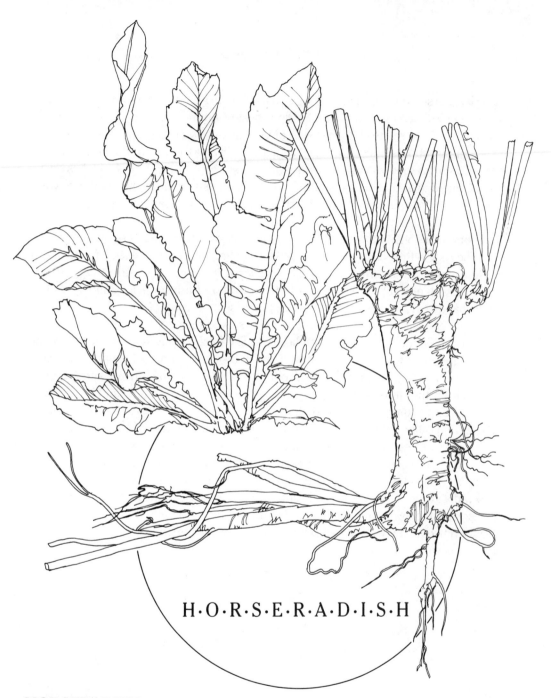

H·O·R·S·E·R·A·D·I·S·H

HORSERADISH

Botanical: *Armoracia rusticana*

Horseradish is a vigorous herb believed native to Hungary or Russia. A perennial plant that is now well established throughout the temperate regions of Europe and

America, horseradish produces elongated toothed leaves that grow about 2 feet high. Although it's a perennial, horseradish does best when treated as an annual. The plant does not develop seeds in its first year of growth, but you can propagate it from root cuttings about 6 inches long, taken from a straight root. Plant the cuttings in early spring, as soon as you can work the soil. Set the cuttings 12 to 15 inches deep and about 18 inches apart. The plants do best in full sun in a deeply tilled bed with substantial additions of well-rotted manure and compost. They like frequent watering, too. Horseradish spreads rapidly, so you may want to contain it by planting it in bottomless 5-gallon containers or by using some other kind of barrier.

The root is the part most often used for healing purposes. Dig it up in late fall. If you do not harvest the roots regularly you should replant with fresh cuttings every three years to prevent deterioration of the crop. Store fresh roots for culinary and medicinal use in dry sand in a cool, dark place, such as a cellar.

From earliest times, horseradish root has served the people of many cultures as a stimulant, diuretic, antiseptic, and laxative. The fresh, grated root and leaves of the plant, a source of vitamin C, have been used in the past to prevent scurvy. If you've ever eaten freshly grated horseradish root as a condiment, you already know how well it clears the sinuses. Its major active principle is known as allylisothiocyanate, or mustard oil. European herbalists have used an infusion of the root to treat asthma, coughs, and other pulmonary complaints. The same infusion has also been used to treat kidney stones, edema, and albuminuria. The grated root, in poultice form, is a well-known European treatment for easing chest congestion and muscle aches and pains. According to the early twentieth century English herbalist Mrs. M. Grieve, horseradish root contains "so much sulfur that it is serviceable used externally as a rubefacient in chronic rheumatism and in paralytic complaints." Horseradish has also been used to expel worms in children, to promote perspiration, and to relieve facial neuralgia.

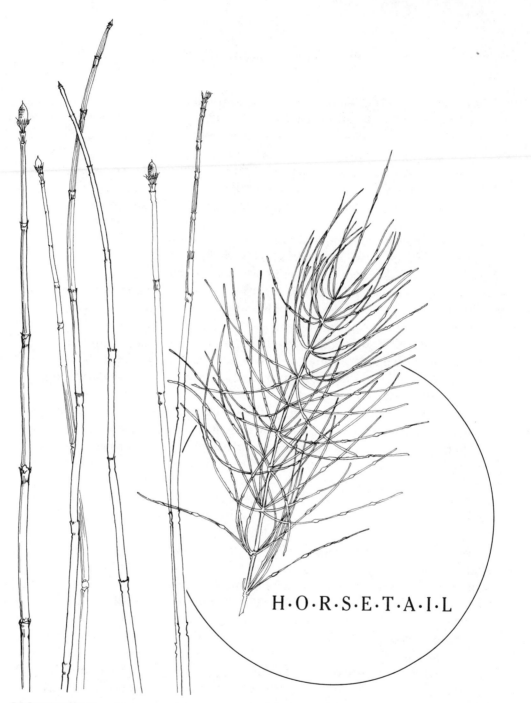

H·O·R·S·E·T·A·I·L

HORSETAIL (Scouring Rush, Shavegrass)
Botanical: *Equisetum* species

In the Carboniferous era when dinosaurs reigned supreme on Earth, gigantic plants resembling horsetail probably formed a large percentage of the vegetation.

They reached heights of 50 feet, and their remains survive today in our planet's vast coal reserves. Today's horsetail plants grow to heights of 3 to 6 feet. Like contemporary lizards, they are but tiny reminders of their larger ancestors. They still thrive in shaded, water-soaked environments such as creek and river banks, flood plains, pond and lake edges, and marshes. Various species of this genus grow in virtually all parts of the temperate and tropical world.

There is no other plant quite like horsetail. Even without knowing its botanical history, you can sense its primitive vigor and mystery when you stand in the midst of a horsetail "grove." The plant, which has really changed very little from prehistoric times, is an evergreen that reproduces both sexually through the production of spores (like ferns do), and asexually through the production of tubers and stolons. These rhizomes run laterally underwater or in wet claylike soils, often forming dense mats which help prevent erosion. In early spring the plant sends up a short, fertile stalk that's about 1 foot tall and resembles a miniature Christmas tree with successive whorls of scaly bright green branches. Spore-bearing catkins are produced at the top of the central stalk. Soon after they are produced, these spores literally spring away from the parent plant and are distributed by wind and water.

The catkin-bearing stalk then dies down, and the second stage of the plant shoots up—a barren hollow stem with bamboolike nodes or joints. These joints have a black ring that marks their presence and sets off the stem's lovely light green color. As the season progresses the stem's color darkens, until by late summer it is a deep olive green. The entire stem is scored by 16 to 27 very fine vertical grooves.

Horsetail makes a beautiful addition to a water garden. Considered a hardy plant, its perennial root is protected in winter by both the mud and water that cover its bed. Horsetail will also grow near walls or in other moist, shady places. You can purchase small plants from some of the herb nurseries listed in the Resource Guide. Or, you can propagate the plant from root sections collected from wild horsetail stands in the spring when the plant begins to send up its spearlike stems. Set these root divisions just under the surface of soft soil at the edges of the water garden. The roots take hold best when they are planted so that the water just slightly covers them.

Horsetail is extremely high in silica (an oxide of silicon), which makes up as much as 40 percent of the total herb.[9] You can get a sense of how this affects plant tissue by picking a stem and rubbing it between your fingers. There is a brittle, squeaky quality due to the deposits of silica beneath the stem's fine ridges. This abrasive characteristic has been utilized all over the world for cleaning dishes, sanding wood, and polishing metal. It has given rise to some of horsetail's nicknames, such as scouring rush, Dutch rush, pewterwort, and shavegrass (which comes from "shaving" or sanding wood). The silica content of horsetail sets it apart from virtually all other herbs. Oatstraw is another herb also high in organic silica compounds and is sometimes used instead of horsetail.

Although it contains only trace amounts of calcium, horsetail tea has been a traditional herbal treatment for mending broken bones. According to a theory developed by French scientist Louis Kervran, it seems to be the herb's high silica content that prompts such healing, through a process he calls "biological transmutation."

In keeping with its unusual appearance and growth pattern, horsetail also has two other medicinal uses that are related but slightly different. The barren canelike stems are picked in spring and used fresh in an infusion that is thought to help build the kidney's strength. Gathered in autumn, the mature barren stalks are assigned diuretic and cooling properties and are believed to be eliminating to the kidneys. Because of this, herbalists most often add fall-gathered horsetail to formulas calling for a soothing diuretic. When needed for its silica content, horsetail should be gathered in autumn, also. In fact, it is believed to be partly because of its higher silica content that fall-gathered horsetail acts as a diuretic. In Europe horsetail herb tea was also used to stop bleeding, both internally and externally.

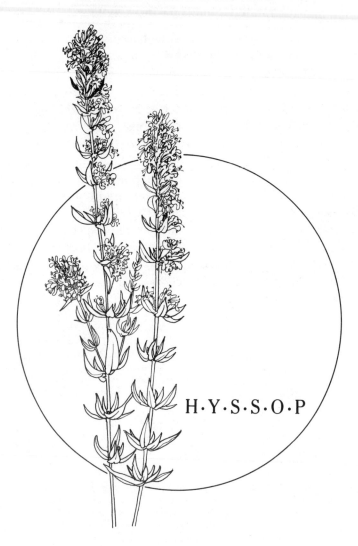

HYSSOP

Botanical: *Hyssopus officinalis*

    Hyssop's name comes from the Greek *azob* meaning "holy herb." In ancient times, hyssop was used to cleanse and purify both people and sacred places. In the Bible, in Psalm 51, David says, "Purge me with hyssop and I shall be clean." The plant has a pungent, bitter taste. Today, the volatile oil of the plant is used in both the perfume industry and in the making of liqueurs, especially Chartreuse.

    Hyssop is an evergreen herb that grows from 1 to 2 feet high. A member of the mint family, the plant has square stems and small, opposite leaves that are lance-shaped and stemless. Its flowers are either red, white, or bluish and are displayed in whorls. Hyssop, especially the blue-flowered variety, is often used as a border plant, backed by rosemary and lavender. The plant prefers a dry, sunny location and a chalky soil.

You can start hyssop from seed in the spring, after the danger of frost is past. If you plan to start the seed indoors, plant it four weeks before the date of the last projected frost in your area. Sow the seed in drills ¼ inch deep. You can also propagate hyssop from spring cuttings. The cuttings can be rooted either indoors or out, but they need a cool, shady place as a rooting environment. When the cuttings have taken root, place them in their permanent bed, spaced about 1 foot apart. A side-dressing of composted manure can be given in the spring. You can also propagate hyssop from divisions made in either the spring or fall. The young plants need frequent watering (every few days) at first, but after they are established they prefer a dry environment.

If you have some grapevines, you might consider planting hyssop around them. The herb is said to increase the grape yields and enhance the flavor of the fruit. Or, try planting hyssop near your cabbages. Many gardeners claim it makes a good companion for cabbage and helps keep destructive insects away. Hyssop is also well known for its ability to attract bees to the garden.

Once the plant gets to be about 18 inches high it is fairly mature, and you can begin to cut back the tops frequently to keep the leaves tender. Use the hyssop tops you cut throughout the summer to add zest to salads or soups, or in teas. Or you can dry and use the tops for health purposes. After making several small cuttings, cut back the entire plant to about 4 inches above the ground just before it flowers and dry the leaves and stems according to the directions in chapter 6.

Traditionally, hyssop has been used in treating pulmonary complaints. It has a reputation as an expectorant, stimulant, and diaphoretic. A warm infusion of the plant, or a blend of hyssop and horehound, can be used for colds, fevers, coughs, and sore throats. To make an infusion of hyssop alone, use 1 ounce of the dried herb to 1 pint water; to make an infusion with hyssop and horehound use ½ ounce hyssop, ½ ounce horehound, and 1 pint water. Follow the directions for making infusions in chapter 6.

Hyssop has also been used in compress form to relieve muscular aches and pains and rheumatism. An infusion of the fresh green leaves is considered an antirheumatic tea. The prescribed dosage for this ailment is 1 cupful 3 times daily. Bruised, fresh hyssop leaves have also been used for healing minor cuts and bruises. They are applied directly to the affected areas and held in place lightly with some cotton cloth and adhesive tape. Hyssop contains volatile oils which modern pharmacologists believe may be mildly antiseptic and useful for such topical applications. No other pharmacologically active principles have so far been identified in this herb, but it retains its place in herbal tradition nonetheless.

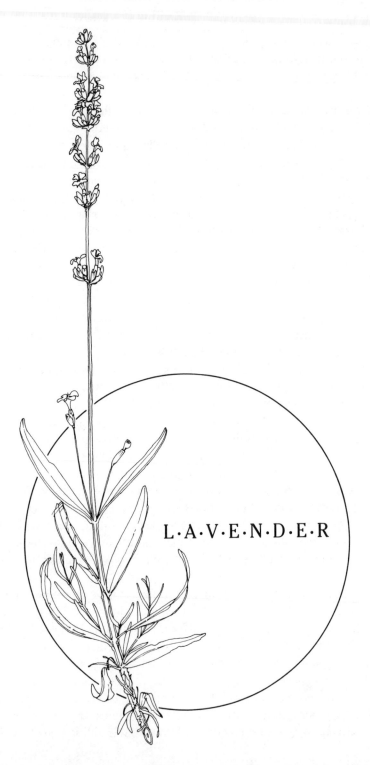

LAVENDER
Botanical: *Lavandula* species

Lavender, derived from the Latin *lavare,* meaning to wash, was esteemed in ancient Rome as a sensual fragrance for the bath. Lavender became popular in medieval Europe for a variety of healing purposes, and it's been with us ever since. "It is the wonder and joy of the south in its blue dress, and its scent is God's gift to earth. No scent could be sweeter," says French herbalist Maurice Méssegué.[10] In many parts of Europe, stalks of lavender leaves and flowers were set in linen closets to impart their fragrance to sheets, pillowcases, blankets, and comforters. Though used in a more limited manner today, lavender still scents sachets, perfumes and colognes, soaps, and other aromatic infusions.

Lavender is a bushy perennial with woody stems and small, opposite, gray-green leaves. The highly aromatic flowers, which appear in midsummer, grow on long spikes and range in color from pale lavender to deep bluish purple. Lavender plants are from 1 to 4 feet tall, depending on their age. If left to grow undisturbed for many years, mature plants spread in both height and girth and develop a dense tangle of thick woody stems.

There are three main species of lavender. English lavender, also known as "true lavender" is *Lavandula vera.* This species, and also the spike lavender, *L. spica,* are known for the delightfully aromatic fragrance that we associate with lavender. The French lavender, *L. stoechas,* has a scent more reminiscent of rosemary than lavender.

The English variety is most commonly grown because it is the most aromatic. Both the English and French lavenders prefer a sandy, coarse, rather dry soil. Lavender needs good drainage and does very well planted on slopes facing south or southwest. Planting either the English or French lavenders in this way helps develop the plant's essential oils in the flowering tops. Planted in a richer soil instead, without a southern exposure, the flowers will not be as finely scented or medicinally potent. Unlike the English and French lavenders, the spike lavender, *L. spica,* prefers a rich soil.

Lavender can be propagated from seed. It takes about 1 month to germinate and about 2½ months more before the seedling is ready for transplanting. Because of its slow-growing habit, many gardeners perfer to propagate lavender from cuttings, layerings, or division of roots. Cuttings are perhaps the most common method, and they are taken in early spring or late summer. Cuttings are actually not cut but are pulled from the plant by grasping a strong, healthy shoot and pulling it downward so that a small heel comes along with the stem. Root your cuttings in sandy soil in a pot. Keep them in shade, and when the weather grows colder, place them in a cool room for the winter. Set them out in spring in their permanent bed. As the young lavender plants grow, cut them back a little to encourage bushiness.

A native of southern Europe, lavender does not fare well in harsh winters. The plants suffer from wind, both in summer and winter, and should be situated in a protected area. Damp, low-lying places and areas prone to frost pockets are not ideal places to plant lavender. Cutting it back and mulching it heavily with straw will help the plant to winter over. In climates where winter temperatures frequently drop below freezing, it is best to cultivate lavender in pots and bring it into the greenhouse during the winter.

Harvest lavender flowers by snipping the stems about 6 inches below the flowering spike. Then dry them in a cool, airy room, either in bunches hanging down from rafters or lines, or laid flat in thin layers on nonmetallic screens.

Although the wonderfully refreshing and delightful scent of lavender is reason enough to grow and use it, the plant has a long history of medicinal aspects, too, although no modern research has been done to verify them. Lavender has always been attributed calmative properties and has been used to relieve nervous headaches and depression. As a nervine it has an uplifting, purifying influence, unlike some nervines that are somewhat stupefying. Just inhaling its heady aroma brings promise enough to anyone of lavender's therapeutic uses. The flowers can be prepared in a simple infusion and used in several ways to calm jittery nerves. Taken several times a day in teacupful doses, an infusion of the flowers can help relieve nervous conditions, as can a lavender bath. An infusion of the flowers can also be used as a gargle for sore throats and colds. Warm lavender tea applied in a compress to the head can relieve a headache. Or place the compress on the chest to relieve congestion and cold symptoms.

Lavender also has apparent stomachic properties, and an infusion drunk as tea or placed in the bath is used by European herbalists to stimulate the appetite, relieve stomach or intestinal flatulence, and soothe colic. Because of its calmative and antiseptic qualities, children in rural villages in France are regularly given lavender baths to keep them in good health. Lavender tea is considered an excellent vermifuge, too. Many households also keep a bottle of lavender essence as a remedy against insect bites, cuts, bruises, and aches, both internal and external. In France, country dwellers hang small bunches of lavender in the corners of rooms to keep flies and mosquitoes at bay. Fresh lavender flowers can also be rubbed over your skin to deter obnoxious insects.

You can make a lavender oil extract at home (see directions in Herbal Oils, chapter 6) and enjoy its many worthwhile uses. Lavender oil can be added to a porcelain pot full of just-boiled water, and the resulting steam can be inhaled for relief of colds, bronchitis, or flu. In Europe, veterinarians have used lavender oil to rid animals of lice and other pests. It is also one of the principal ingredients in a famous Chinese medicinal oil, called "White Flower Oil," which is used for headaches, dizziness, nervous tension, dyspepsia, and as an insect repellent, applied sparingly to exposed skin surfaces.

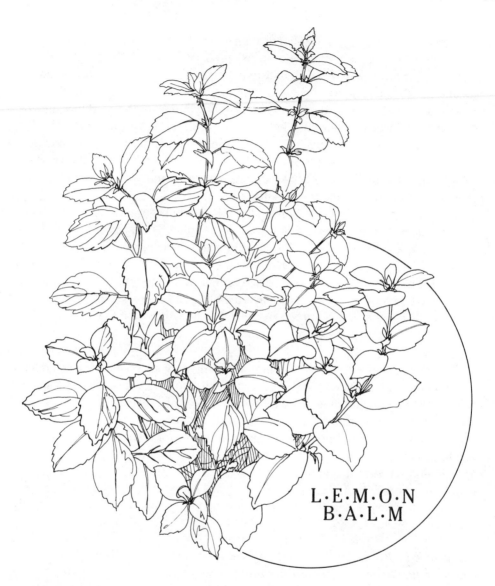

L·E·M·O·N
B·A·L·M

LEMON BALM

Botanical: *Melissa officinalis*

Lemon balm is among the most fragrant of herbs. A member of the mint family with a habit of growing in beautiful mounded shapes, lemon balm leaves release a lemony fragrance when crushed. Sniffing the bruised leaves is invigorating and therapeutic in itself. In olden times the herb was strewn about the house to provide a clean and festive atmosphere. Today lemon balm fills out potpourris and similar scented herb blends.

Lemon balm, which has the square stem that characterizes the mint family, grows from 1 to 2 feet high and has ovate, toothed leaves. Its white or yellowish flowers appear in small bunches in midsummer. The plant likes shady places and rich, moist soil. You can propagate lemon balm from seed, which will germinate in three to four weeks. Sow seed indoors in late spring and plant the seedlings outside when they are about 4 inches tall. Lemon balm is easy to propagate from root divisions taken in the early spring. In the autumn, the topgrowth dies back and the plant can be mulched with compost or leaf mold at that time to enrich the growing environment and provide some winter protection. The plant will spread, but much more slowly than most of the other mints.

The leaves of the lemon balm are used for healing purposes. Pinch or cut back the plant once before it flowers, so it will bush out again. Then, just before it prepares to bloom again, cut back the plant to within 3 inches of the ground. Dry the fragrant leaves still on their stems, in a dark, warm, airy place. An airy attic makes a good drying room for balm. Light will discolor its leaves, and too long a drying time will cause it to lose its aroma and healing qualities. Take care also not to use too much heat. Because lemon balm is a rather fragile herb, it is best to try to dry the leaves within a two-day period and to monitor their progress carefully during this time.

Lemon balm has a history of use in treating the nervous system. Arabian doctors of the ninth and tenth century were perhaps the first to notice its ability to dispel anxiety and heart palpitations. They described it as a "gladdening" herb, and that description was one that remained with the plant for centuries. In the seventeenth century, balm was often mentioned as a good medicine for disordered nerves. A favorite remedy for headaches and nervous conditions used in Europe in the sixteenth and seventeenth centuries was Carmelite water, made of lemon balm, lemon peel, angelica root, and nutmeg.

Herbalist Maurice Mességué today uses balm in the same way. In *Health Secrets of Plants and Herbs* he says:

> ... *people in despair, people who feel defeated by life: for all of these I recommend this wonderful herb, because it brings comfort and restores the joy of life to even the most melancholy.*[11]

According to Mességué, an infusion of lemon balm is also useful for stomachache and irregular menstruation. The fresh plant, either crushed or in a lotion, can be used to ease pains of neuralgia, rheumatism, or bruises, according to this French herbalist.

Lemon balm has also been used to dress and heal wounds since ancient times. Pliny and Dioscorides both mention its usefulness as a vulnerary. And in *A Modern Herbal,* Mrs. M. Grieve explains:

It is now recognized as a scientific fact that the balsamic oils of aromatic plants make excellent surgical dressings; they give off ozone and thus exercise anti-putrescent effects.

Lemon balm also makes a cooling tea for the feverish. A simple infusion is thought to be helpful in bringing down fevers.

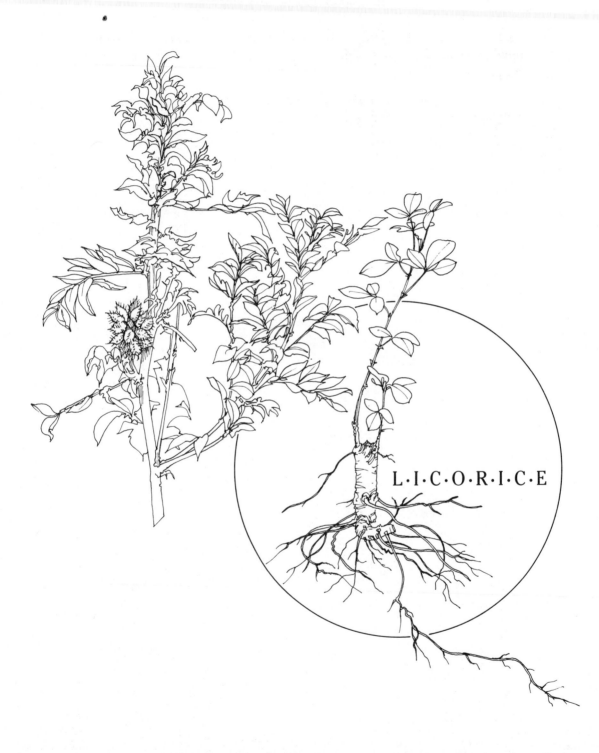

L·I·C·O·R·I·C·E

LICORICE
Botanical: *Glycyrrhiza glabra,* and other species

The Blackfoot Indians of the Dakotas steeped the leaves of wild licorice plants in hot water and used the tea to wash the inside of the ear to treat earache. Many Native American tribes ate the root both fresh and roasted. Even today in Appalachia and other parts of rural America, children enjoy chewing on licorice root as a pleasant treat.

The taste of licorice has universal appeal. It finds its way into syrups, lozenges, candies, medicines, and even fancy liqueurs. The licorice plant has almost worldwide distribution, with fifteen or more varieties found in different locations. In southern Europe and in the Near East as far as Pakistan, two licorice species are found both wild and cultivated. These two species supply most of the licorice used in Western countries for medicine and flavorings. They grow in sandy soil, often near streams or where there is an ample supply of water, and they thrive in hot climates where there is no danger of freezing. The wild licorice native to North America, *G. lepidota,* grows on prairies, near lake shores, along the edges of roads, and in fields in the northwestern, midwestern, and some eastern states.

The kind of licorice used in Chinese medicine is found in the cooler climates of Mongolia, Siberia, and the Ural and Caucasus Mountains in central Asia. It seems to have a more intense flavor than the other licorice species we've discussed.

Licorice is a graceful shrub with woody stems and spreading pinnate foliage. Surprisingly, it belongs to the Legume family, which also includes peas and snap beans. Licorice grows from 3 to 6 feet tall; its foliage and flowers are very much like those of vetch. The sweet-flavored roots of the plant often grow to depths of 4 feet, with many branching rootlets spreading from them. It is these roots, collected from the plant in its fourth year of growth only, that are used for healing purposes.

Licorice is most commonly propagated from root sections, which may be saved from parts of the harvested root. You can also propagate it from crown divisions or from suckers. Licorice thrives in rich, fine soil, like the sandy loam found in bottom lands, or in creek and river beds. It will not grow well in clay soil. When cultivating the plant, add plenty of well-rotted compost to its bed. Space plants about 18 inches apart. The best roots are formed in climates with plenty of moisture in the early part of the growing season, and a dry, hot midsummer where the plant can bake in the hot, rich soil.

In order to cultivate licorice in a greenhouse, you must provide a deep, roomy pot–36 inches deep and 36 inches around is a good size–and a sandy loam soil with good drainage and fertility. The plant requires lots of strong sunlight or full spectrum artificial light in order to flourish in a greenhouse culture.

Harvest the plants' roots in the autumn of their fourth year of growth; by the fifth year, they will be too woody to be used.The best way to harvest them is to dig a trench or hole to the side of the plant and pull the plant sideways toward the trench. Wash the roots carefully, cut them into rounds, and dry them on screens according to directions in Drying Herbs, chapter 6.

In European herbal medicine, licorice has primarily been used to relieve sore throats, bronchitis, laryngitis, coughs, and other chest complaints. The dried root of the plant is made into a simple decoction, or into a syrup, to treat these conditions (see the recipe for Licorice Syrup on page 317). In Chinese medicine, licorice is also used to soothe the throat, coughs, and difficult breathing. In addition, it is used extensively as a neutral or harmonizing herb in many herbal formulas. Chinese, Japanese, and Tibetan herbal doctors believe licorice acts mainly on the liver. As the traditional Japanese physician, Naboru Muramoto, says in his book *Healing Ourselves:*

> *By aiding the liver in discharging the poisons it filters from food, the licorice allows the kidneys to filter in turn and to eject these poisons from the blood once they have been released from the liver.*[12]

About two-thirds of all Chinese herbal formulas incorporate pleasant-tasting licorice for this reason.

Because of its perceived positive influence on the hormonal system, the Chinese have also used licorice to strengthen and balance the female reproductive system. Licorice contains compounds similar to those found in ginseng and sarsaparilla, which are thought to help the adrenal glands function more smoothly in conditions of stress and exhaustion. Because of this quality naturopaths have used licorice in treating hypoglycemia, diabetes, and Addison's disease.

Licorice is considered a building herb for the kidneys that helps the body tissues to retain water. Because of this property, herbalists deem it to be good for those who are dehydrated or thin, but not good for people with edema, pregnant women in the last trimester (when edema tends to develop), or people who are overweight because of water retention. These restrictions should always be kept in mind when licorice is used. Also, to be safe, if you have high blood pressure or heart trouble, do avoid large amounts of licorice. The overconsumption of candies containing licorice extract has caused some people to develop symptoms of edema and related problems. Accordingly, the Food and Drug Administration (FDA) is now investigating the use of licorice extract in candy making, with a view toward setting industry standards. For someone with knowledge of licorice's properties, the herb should pose no problem, if used cautiously. The Chinese, who have been using licorice for thousands of years, consider it one of the safest herbs.

In addition, a substance called carbenoxolone has been isolated from licorice in recent years. It has been used in England for a number of years in the treatment of gastric ulcers.

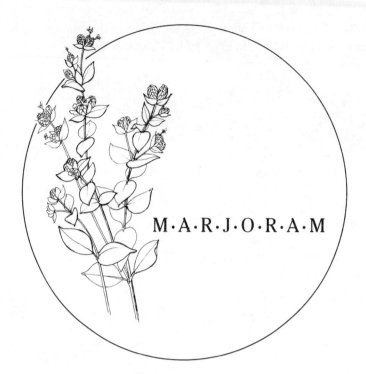

M·A·R·J·O·R·A·M

MARJORAM (Sweet Marjoram, Knotted Marjoram)
Botanical: *Origanum majorana*

A native of Portugal, marjoram is a tender perennial that is usually treated as an annual because it cannot winter over in many areas. Its name comes from the Greek and means "joy of the mountains." It has a bushy habit that you can increase by pinching back the tips of the plant during the growing season. Its leaves are small and ovate, and its white flowers form tiny knotlike shapes before opening, prompting one of its common names, knotted marjoram. There are many species of marjoram, but the one best known today as a culinary herb is *Origanum majorana,* or sweet marjoram. It is related to oregano and shares many of the same culinary properties.

Marjoram seeds are small and slow to germinate. You can sow the seeds indoors in flats and cover them with a fine layer of soil. Cover the flat with glass to increase humidity, but keep the flat out of direct sunlight. Transplant the seedlings outdoors after all danger of frost is past. The herb enjoys a sunny location and a well-drained soil to which well-rotted compost has been added. Space plants 6 to 8 inches apart in their beds. Pinch back each plant right before it begins to bloom. Later in the season, when the plant is ready to flower again, cut back the entire plant to 1 inch above the ground and dry the leaves according to the directions given in chapter 6.

If you want to save your marjoram from one year to the next, you can pot up the plants in a loose, fairly rich potting soil and bring them indoors during the winter. When you're ready to set out the plants the following spring, divide them when you unpot them and you will increase the number of plants in your marjoram patch. In warm climates, root division is the most common method of propagation.

In European countries marjoram has traditionally symbolized youth, beauty, and happiness. The French put sprigs of this herb into hope chests and linen closets. Marjoram has been used as a calmative since the days of the Roman empire. Herbalists in ancient Rome also used the plant to alleviate painful menstruation, to promote urination, to relieve injuries and bruises, and to treat conjunctivitis and other eye diseases.

Marjoram is still used by European herbalists as a nervine and calmative. Maurice Mességué says of marjoram:

> *It is indeed one of the most sedative herbs I know, soothing for people who cannot sleep owing to the pace of life today, soothing for those suffering from the pangs of love, for jagged nerves, for feverish excitement...*[13]

The steam from a hot infusion of marjoram can be inhaled to clear the respiratory passages during a bout with a cold or flu. Cooked to a comfortable temperature, the same infusion makes a fine gargle for sore throats or mild mouth infections.

Most of us know marjoram best as a kitchen herb. Pinches of marjoram enliven French and Italian cuisines and add zest to soups and stews. Use this herb in small pinches for healing purposes, too. Despite its ostensible mildness, marjoram is actually a strong herb, and it should be taken carefully. A simple infusion consists of eight pinches of the dried herb (a pinch is what you can pinch between your thumb and first finger) combined with 1 pint of water that has just been boiled.

Marjoram gargles can be strong, since they are not intended for internal consumption. For a gargle, make an infusion using ⅛ cup of the dried herb to 1 pint of water. Be very careful not to swallow any when you gargle. A strong infusion can be used as an inhalant for respiratory problems as well. A pad soaked in marjoram infusion can be placed atop the nose and sinus areas to relieve sinus problems and hay fever.

Marjoram should not be used during menstruation or by pregnant women, as it tends to irritate the uterus.

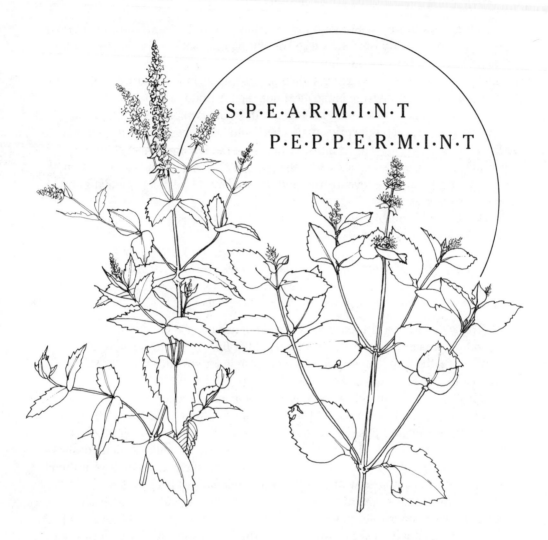

S·P·E·A·R·M·I·N·T
P·E·P·P·E·R·M·I·N·T

MINT

Botanical: *Mentha piperita, M. spicata*

Mints have cool, stimulating, and refreshing properties. The clean, uplifting scent and taste of these herbs have been valued in all parts of the world since antiquity in cooking and in healing. There are countless varieties of mints, which are themselves only a part of the vast family, Labiatae. Other family members include sage, hyssop, thyme, horehound, marjoram, pennyroyal, savory, catnip, and balm. There are many species and varieties of mints. Medicinally they are all generally diaphoretic, carminative, and stimulating. Mints interbreed very easily, so once a seed type or rootstock has been selected, it is propagated by root division and cuttings.

Three species of mint—peppermint, spearmint, and pennyroyal—are especially prominent in herbal medicine. Pennyroyal is discussed on page 207. Peppermint and spearmint both like to grow in rich, moist, well-drained soil, as do many mints. They will grow in partial shade as well as direct sunlight, but their roots must be kept cool and moist wherever they are grown. Like most mints, peppermint and spearmint spread quickly, and you will find it helpful to keep them under control by growing them in bottomless 5-gallon containers or confining them with barriers of buried sheet metal or sunken railroad ties. Although both these mints are perennials, their vitality may diminish after four or five years, and beds should be dug up and the plants divided and replanted in new situations.

PEPPERMINT

The square, purplish stems of the peppermint (*Mentha piperita*) grow from 2 to 4 feet high. The plant has a spike of small violet flowers that grow in whorls. Peppermint leaves are a deeper, richer color than the bright, vivid green of spearmint. Peppermint is easy to grow. Individual leaves can be picked as needed throughout the growing season, and the entire plant can be cut back to within 3 inches of the ground right before it flowers. Dry the leaves for storage as directed in chapter 6.

Peppermint is more stimulating to the circulation than spearmint and a stronger remedy for alleviating flatulence, dyspepsia, and indigestion. The Chinese treat peppermint as a great summer simple. While most Americans cool off with cold beverages, the Chinese refresh themselves with hot peppermint tea. In addition to aiding digestion, drinking a mild infusion of peppermint leaves you feeling comfortably cooler. This is because it brings more blood to the skin, where evaporation then wicks away body heat. A strong infusion of the herb will produce copious perspiration, and one of peppermint's traditional uses has been in breaking fevers.

Peppermint contains menthol, thymol, and other volatile oils that give the herb a variety of therapeutic properties. Any herb that contains significant amounts of menthol, as peppermint does, has a slight antiseptic quality. Peppermint tea has been used as a gargle for sore throats and to wash wounds. A simple infusion of this wonderfully aromatic herb is a classic headache remedy, and it has also been used to relieve tension, insomnia, nervousness, and trembling. A strong cup of peppermint tea, taken at the first sign of a cold or flu, may help ward it off. If the bug does bite, peppermint tea is a soothing treatment for dry cough, fever, and other cold-related symptoms.

Peppermint has been, and still is, one of the most widely used herbs in the world. Commercially, peppermint is among the most important world herb crops. It is grown on a large scale in many European countries, as well as in the United States. Tons of peppermint, distilled into oil, finds its way into toothpaste, soap, bath oil, candies, syrups, gums, and many medicinal preparations. For the home herbalist and gardener, peppermint is one of the most reliable and rewarding plants in the garden. It is simple, vigorously beautiful, easy to grow, and gently safe for healing purposes.

SPEARMINT

Spearmint (*Mentha spicata*) grows about 2 feet high and has wrinkled, lance-shaped leaves with toothed edges. Its small pinkish or lilac flowers are arranged on a spike in whorls or rings. Like peppermint, the plant can be cut back to within 3 inches of the ground just before it flowers and then dried, according to the directions in chapter 6. Spearmint is usually propagated by division in either spring or fall.

Although we are well acquainted with the refreshing menthol flavor of spearmint in candy, gum, and toothpaste, not too many of us seem to practice many of the plant's medicinal uses. In former times, spearmint was one of the most commonly and widely used herbs. From ancient Rome right up through the seventeenth century, its branches were strewn on floors at banquets and feasts to liven the air as partygoers crushed the leaves underfoot. Branches hung around the house disinfected the air. Cooks added the herb to many meat and vegetable dishes and salads and welcomed their guests with a cup of refreshing spearmint tea. Herbal healers exploited the plant no less.

Spearmint is not as strong as peppermint and has often been given to children, and to aged or convalescing people. It exerts a mild tonic, antispasmodic, stimulating, and diaphoretic influence. Traditionally, it has been used for mild cases of flatulence, indigestion, nausea, motion sickness, and heartburn. Spearmint is one of the most famous and popular simples, taken in the form of a simple infusion.

When steeped in white vinegar the herb has had some traditional use in washing head sores. A strong decoction of the leaves and stems has also been used to alleviate severe chapping of the hands. Mice are said to have an aversion to spearmint, and some people have reported that strewing some of the dried herb in areas where mice were a problem has sent them to other locales.

Still, spearmint is best known for its role in calming the stomach.

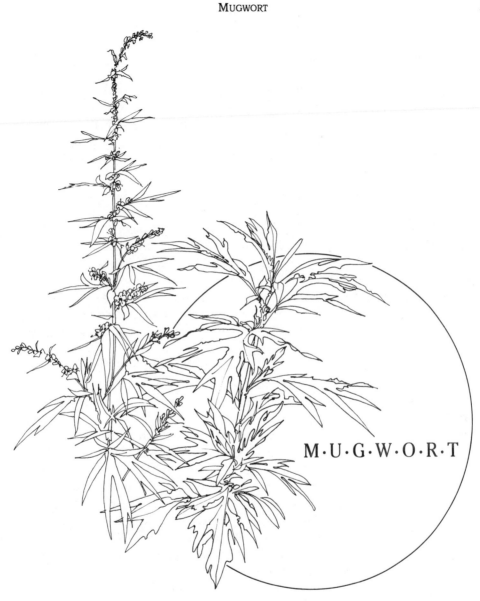

M·U·G·W·O·R·T

MUGWORT

Botanical: *Artemisia vulgaris*

This relative of the well-known wormwood or absinthia plant is popular in both Eastern and European herbal medicine. Its name is thought to have originated when mugwort was used in making beer, before hops became the traditional bitter. Or, mugwort's name may be derived from the Old English word *moughte,* which means moth, because the herb has traditionally been used to repel moths from woolen garments.

A perennial plant that spreads wherever it is planted, mugwort grows from 2 to 5 feet tall. Mugwort has leaves that are lobed either once or twice, with rounded to lance-shaped segments. The leaves are bright green on top, or sometimes purple, and whitish underneath, with a fibrous, downy texture. The plant generally resembles other plants in the mint family, and its distinctive fragrance is rather reminiscent of sage. Mugwort can always be identified by its strong, slightly heady aroma. It can be found growing wild along roadsides, hedgerows, stream banks, and waysides throughout Europe, Asia, and North America.

You can grow mugwort from seed or from divisions made in the spring or fall. Seeds are easily started indoors in flats. The plants germinate quickly, even at a temperature as low as 55°F. Plants are also available from some herb nurseries (see the Resource Guide at the back of the book for mail-order sources). Mugwort grows best in moist, rich, well-drained soil. Dig some compost into its bed before you set out the young plants and fertilize the bed regularly in the spring and fall. A thick layer of loose straw or leaf mulch will add to the organic material available to the plants and will help hold in soil moisture, too.

Mugwort is usually gathered just as it begins to flower. Cut the plant back to 4 inches above the ground and dry the stems and leaves according to the directions in chapter 6. You can remove the leaves from the stems after they are dry and store them in airtight jars.

Mugwort is considered an emmenagogue, and both Chinese and European herbalists have used it to regulate and bring on menses. The plant has also been used as a remedy for nervous disorders including hysteria, shaking, and epilepsy. In a compress, mugwort tea has been used to relieve muscle spasms. The Chinese also use mugwort tea to cure sleepwalking, a treatment which brings to mind mugwort's related European use as a stuffing in little "dream pillows," which were said to induce vivid, clear dreams when placed under the head.

The species of mugwort found in Japan is milder in taste than the species found in this country and in Europe. The Japanese, who consider mugwort a healing food and herb, often eat it as a cooked vegetable or salad green. They also incorporate mugwort into preparations for convalescents.

Mugwort is used in conjunction with acupuncture therapy in Oriental medicine. The downy fibers on mugwort leaves are separated and dried in the sun. They are then rolled into sticks or cones called moxa. Tibetan physician Shenphen Dawa Rinpoche says that "moxa" was originally a Tibetan word that was later adopted by the Chinese and Japanese, along with the Tibetan technique of moxibustion. This use of mugwort is called moxabustion (see page 50), or simply moxa, and it involves skillfully burning the cones or sticks above appropriate acupuncture points on the body. The mugwort adds its warming properties to the heat of combustion, resulting in a very stimulating therapy. Of course, this treatment should only be attempted by someone with the proper intensive training it requires.

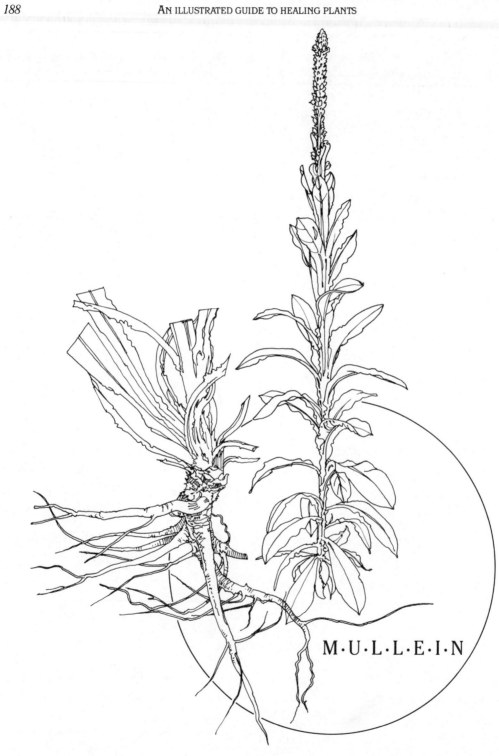

M·U·L·L·E·I·N

MULLEIN (Torches, Candlewick Plant)
Botanical: *Verbascum thapsus*

Mullein is the plant Ulysses took with him on his legendary sea voyage to protect himself against the wiles of the enchantress Circe. In India, mullein is considered a safeguard against evil spirits. Medieval Europeans dipped the plant in suet and used it as a torch, or they ignited the furry down of its leaves as tinder.

Mullein is a stately and hardy biennial herb with long, furry leaves and tall yellow flower stalks. During its first season, it produces only a leaf rosette at ground level. The leaves are from 6 to 15 inches long and somewhat resemble those of the foxglove. The soft, dense mass of white hairs that covers the leaves makes them feel thick. During the second year, the plant sends up a stout, fibrous stem with a white pith. The furry leaves, arranged neatly to ensure efficient flow of rainwater to the plant's roots, grow smaller as they ascend the stalk. Yellow flowers are produced at the top of the stalk.

The mullein plant is propagated from seed, which is available from some herb nurseries. Or you can collect seed from wild mullein. You can find mullein growing wild all over the United States (it grows in temperate Europe and Asia, too). It springs up in dry, marginal areas where the spartan conditions allow it to maximize the development of its beneficial oils. In the garden, too, mullein does best in a light, sandy soil that is not rich. Sow seed directly into the permanent bed after all danger of frost is past.

The flowers, leaves, and roots are all used for healing purposes. Mullein flowers bloom individually on the towering flower stalks and should be handpicked as they open. Dry them quickly in a warm place in the shade and store them in a dark place in an airtight container. Harvest the leaves before the flowers bloom, taking no more than one-third of the leaves from any plant. Collect the roots in the autumn. Many herb gardeners recommend cutting off the entire flower head before the seeds ripen, because mullein is a prolific self-sower that could get out of control in the garden.

Mullein flowers have bactericidal properties, and are well known among herbalists for their ability to relieve respiratory problems and earaches. The flowers are considered stronger than the leaves, and are assigned antispasmodic, demulcent, emollient, astringent, and sedative qualities in addition to the bactericidal ones.

For respiratory problems, a simple infusion of ¼ cup dried mullein flowers to 1 pint water is a classic treatment. The mixture should be carefully strained to remove petals and stamens, which will otherwise irritate the mucous membranes.

An oil produced by macerating the fresh flowers and allowing them to infuse in olive oil has been used to treat earaches or discharges from the ear, frostbite, and bruises, as well as for piles and other inflammations of the mucous membranes. To make the oil, place several handfuls of mullein flowers in a glass container and cover them with olive oil. Let the mixture steep for seven to ten days, then strain off the flowers and bottle the oil.

Although the whole mullein plant is considered sedative, the root is stronger in this quality than the leaves or flowers. (Note that mullein *seeds* are toxic and should never be used for any reason.) A decoction of the root, leaves, or flowers can be taken for calmative purposes.

Euell Gibbons once reported that the young women in Amish communities, who are not permitted to use makeup, sometimes use mullein instead. The fresh leaf, when rubbed vigorously against the cheek for a few moments, produces a noticeable rosy hue.

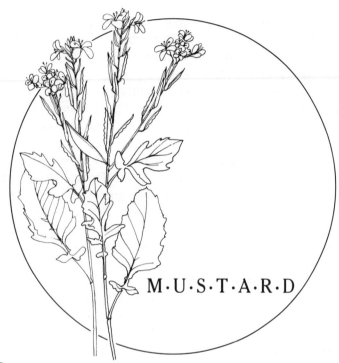

MUSTARD

Botanical: *Brassica hirta* and *B. nigra*

Mustard is a member of the genus Brassica, which also contains cabbage, kohlrabi, and broccoli. Both white and black mustard have been cultivated for centuries as a salad green and a medicine. White mustard is an erect annual plant with a delicate appearance; it grows about 18 inches high. It has pinnate leaves and large yellow cruciferous flowers. The seed pod in white mustard is carried on the plant horizontally. It is hairy, roundish, and has a flattened, sword-shaped beak. The seeds are white in color. Black mustard grows to about 3 feet in height and resembles white mustard in general conformation, except for its seedpods, which are carried erect on the plant. The pods are smooth and flattened and hold black seeds about half the size of white mustard seeds. It is the seeds of both plants that are most commonly used for healing purposes.

Because mustard plants take most of the summer to produce seeds, some gardeners prefer to sow mustard seed in late summer, so the plants will winter over and produce their seeds by around May of the following year. Sow mustard seed ⅛ inch deep in rich, well-drained, moist, well-prepared soil. Thin the plants to about 9 inches apart. Mustard is a heavy feeder and should be fertilized regularly with compost and manure. It needs a soil with a pH of no less than 6.0. Harvest the seeds just after the pods change color, from green to brown. Spread the seeds in thin layers in screens or pieces of cheesecloth and air-dry them in a warm place for two weeks. Be sure you harvest right after the color change, because otherwise the pods will burst open and scatter their seeds all over the ground.

Both white and black mustard seeds have been used to treat cases of chronic constipation. French herbalist Maurice Mességué recommends 1 teaspoon of macerated mustard seeds mixed with a little water to be taken on an empty stomach each morning for two days.[14]

White and black mustard seeds are often ground to a powder for healing purposes. They can be powdered in a blender or an electric coffee or spice grinder, or with a mortar and pestle. The active principles contained in mustard seeds are mustard oils which contain an irritating substance called allyl-isothiocyanate.

A plaster made of black mustard seed powder mixed with linseed meal is a classic remedy for relief of congestion from colds and flu, asthma, backache, and sciatica. The plaster is heated to a temperature between 104° and 110°F for best results. (See Poultices and Plasters, in chapter 6.)

Black mustard seed powder in a footbath is a European treatment for headaches and a preventive measure taken when a cold seems to be coming on. To make this footbath, dissolve ¼ cup black mustard seed powder in 1 pint of water that has just been boiled. Then add this to about 3 cups of very warm water in a porcelain basin, and soak your feet for five to eight minutes.

A decoction of whole mustard seeds can be used to aid digestion or stimulate the appetite. Put 15 pinches of seed in 1 pint of water that has been boiled. Let the mixture stand for 20 minutes, then strain off the seeds. Three cups a day of this tea may be taken for two weeks. In larger amounts (1 teaspoon of mustard powder to a glass of tepid water) mustard seed is an emetic.

Mustard is a good healing herb, but a strong one, and it must be used with care. Anemic people should never use mustard, nor should those with acid stomach, ulcers, or flatulence accompanied by distension of the abdomen.

The young leaves of both species of mustard plants are tasty additions to salads and are believed to have a salutary effect on the liver. There are vegetable varieties of mustard, too, which are cultivated for their leaves. Mustard greens are an important part of Chinese and Japanese cuisine, and of course their robust taste is a classic ingredient in Southern cooking. Mustard greens may be steamed or stir-fried or added to vegetable or meat soups and stews.

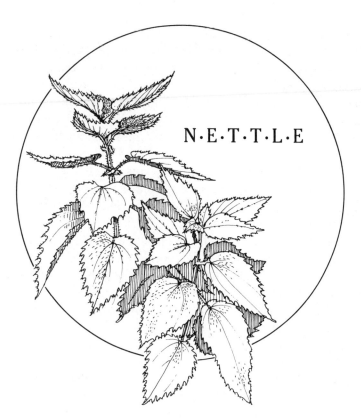

NETTLE

Botanical: *Urtica dioica*

A Scotch poet named Campbell, of an earlier century, once wrote of nettle's amazing versatility:

> *I have eaten nettles, I have slept in nettle sheets, and I have dined off a nettle tablecloth. The young and tender nettle is an excellent potherb. The stalks of the old nettle are as good as flax for making cloth. I have heard my mother say that she thought nettle cloth more durable than any other species of linen.*[15]

Nettle is a thorny perennial plant that grows between 2 and 3 feet tall. It is often found in the wild in moist, nitrogen-rich soils. The plant has toothed, heart-shaped leaves and in its general configuration it resembles some of the mints. Nettle produces both male and female flowers that are greenish in color. The male flowers appear in racemes, and the female in clusters. Mature nettle plants are covered with stinging hairs that can cause severe dermatitis if you touch them.

Nettle is easily propagated from runners taken up in either the fall or spring from an established stand of the plant. Nettle plants especially like the semishady, moist environment of creek beds, with their fertile, fine soil. Garden conditions that resemble these will produce a fine bed of nettles. Because nettle spreads so rapidly, you should plant it within barriers, or in bottomless containers.

You can pick nettles in the spring to use fresh or just before they flower if you intend to dry them for future use. Be sure to wear heavy protective gloves when you harvest nettles. Spring harvesting should be moderate—about one-third of the plants' growth. Just before the nettles flower, cut the plants back to about 4 inches above the ground with shears or a knife. Hold each plant at the bottom while you cut it. Dry according to the directions in chapter 6, then carefully strip the dry leaves from the stems and store them in airtight jars.

The nettle plant can be found in the temperate regions of Europe and Asia, as well as in South Africa, Australia, and the Andes. Although the "stinging nettle," as it is also called, has a rogue's reputation, it is one of the most versatile healing plants. It contains an array of vitamins and minerals, and the young leaves are delicious steamed or added to salads. In Scotland, Ireland, and other countries, nettles are made into soup. In fact, the most famous yogi of Tibet, Milarepa, was supposed to have lived solely on wild nettles for several years. He made them into soup. It is said that his skin turned green from eating so many nettles, and that his soup pot had a green crust from cooking nettles so often in it! A little cooking removes the sting but not the good taste from young nettle leaves.

Nettle's iron content has made it a traditional treatment for anemia. Herbalists in many countries consider it a generally strengthening herb and recommend it for pregnant women and nursing mothers. Nettles are credited with increasing the milk supply in lactating women, too and are considered a good nutritive builder for the liver.

Nettles have diuretic properties, too. Combined with an equal amount of gravelroot in a simple infusion, they are given to treat some cases of edema. Some European herbalists suggest drinking nutrient-rich nettle tea regularly for several months, in conjunction with proper diet and exercise, for those who want to lose weight.

Footbaths of nettle tea are an old treatment for rheumatism. Steep 1 cup of the fresh nettle leaves in 1 pint of just-boiled water for ten minutes. Then strain off the leaves and add the infusion to about 3 cups of hot water in a porcelain basin. Bathe the feet in the evening for eight to ten minutes.

Pregnant women of many Native American tribes used nettle regularly during pregnancy, not only because of its building and diuretic qualities but because it was thought to produce small, healthy babies, making delivery easier.

Nettles can also be used as an expectorant. To remove mucus from the lungs, herbalists sometimes recommend eating steamed nettles dressed with a little apple cider vinegar. People suffering from a calcium deficiency, though, should avoid this treatment because the vinegar may leach calcium from the body.

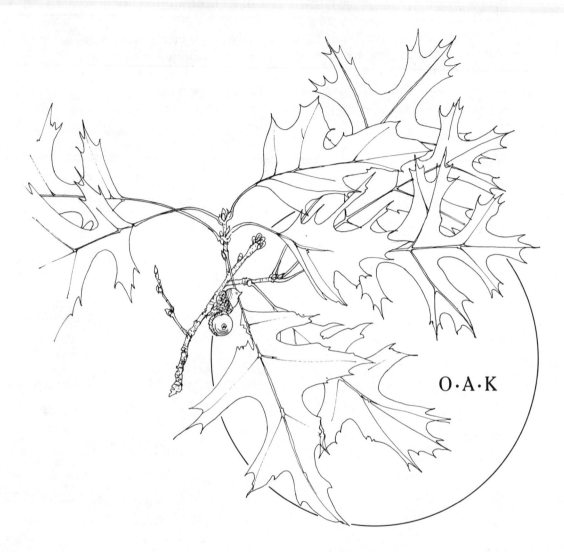

O·A·K

OAK (White Oak, Red Oak, Black Oak, Live Oak, Scrub Oak)
Botanical: *Quercus* species

In ancient mythologies the oak was the adjoining door connecting the two parts of the year. The old Celtic word for oak derives from the Sanskrit word for door. Poet Robert Graves fittingly points out the oak in *The White Goddess* as a bastion of strength: "Midsummer is the flowering season of the oak, which is the tree of endurance and triumph."[16]

There are over 200 species of oak, ranging from the scrub oak, which stands less than 6 feet high, to the black oak, which reaches heights of over 100 feet. Oaks are among the slowest growing of all trees. It takes the trunk of an oak tree about 80 years to reach 20 inches in diameter, and as the tree gets older its growth proceeds even more slowly. In England, there are oak trees that are over 1,000 years old. The largest of these, the Courthorpe Oak in Yorkshire, measures 70 feet in circumference. Because oak grows so slowly, it is one of the strongest and most durable woods. Oak furniture, beams, tools, and pegs survive longer than items made of most other hardwoods.

Oak trees prefer a fairly heavy, rich clay soil as a growing medium. They like adequate moisture and lots of sunlight. Patient gardeners can plant the acorns of many species of oak as soon as they ripen in late summer. Bury the acorns about 1 inch deep in soil which has some leaf mold and compost added to it. Small oak trees of many species can also be purchased from nurseries.

For the Native Americans, oaks were one of the most important plants. Acorns formed a staple part of the diet of many tribes, in addition to providing mast for animals like deer, squirrels, bear, and turkeys. Before acorns can be eaten the astringent tannic acid they contain must be removed, and the Indians had several ways to do this. In one method, the nuts were cut open and shelled, then ground and placed in a finely woven basket. The acorn meat was then leached in a stream for a day or two and dried or eaten fresh. A simpler method consisted of burying a basket of shelled acorns in a sandy stream bank for a few months. When the basket was retrieved, the greenish blue mold growing on the acorns was saved and used to treat infections. It is the leaves and bark of the oak tree that are used for healing today. Most oak species have gray fissured bark and smooth lobed leaves. The various species differ slightly in form, but the medicinal qualities of all oaks are the same. You can collect oak leaves and dry them during the summer. Collect the bark from young branches in the spring or from the tree trunk in the fall. (See directions for collecting and drying bark in chapter 6.)

Oak leaves and bark, rich in tannin, are very astringent and antiseptic. The tannin apparently can help stop bleeding and heal distended tissue. French herbal healer Maurice Mességué has a high regard for oak leaves and bark:

> *I prescribe them internally in small doses, and externally in larger doses, for all cases of hemorrhage such as nosebleeds, cuts and so on. I also prescribe them for ulcers, spitting of blood, blood in the urine, vaginal discharge, heavy periods, piles, incontinence of urine, diarrhea, varicose veins, eczema and bleeding gums. In fact I would advise you to put your trust in the oak tree, in its remarkable powers of healing . . . Just a few leaves of the oak tree can make a whole host of troubles disappear.*[17]

In *A Modern Herbal* Mrs. Grieve tells how medical researchers in the nineteenth century noted that British tanners who inhaled the finely powdered bark of the oak while curing hides rarely suffered from tuberculosis, because of the tightening and drying effects of the bark on their lungs.

A simple decoction of oak bark has been used to treat diarrhea or dysentery. This same decoction has also been used as a douche to treat leukorrhea, as a gargle for mouth and throat inflammations or infections, or applied locally, for bleeding gums and piles. Oak bark decoction, made into a footbath by placing the decoction in a porcelain basin with about 3 cups of hot water, is considered by herbalists to be strengthening and purifying, especially when there are sores, ulcers, or infections present. Footbaths are taken for about eight minutes, preferably in the morning. See chapter 6 for instructions on making a decoction.

A poultice for wounds can be made by bruising fresh oak leaves and placing them directly on the affected area, then covering them with a very warm cloth. The leaves can be used for footbaths or as a gargle, too. Place seven leaves in 1 pint of water that has just been boiled. Let the mixture steep for ten minutes, then strain and discard the leaves.

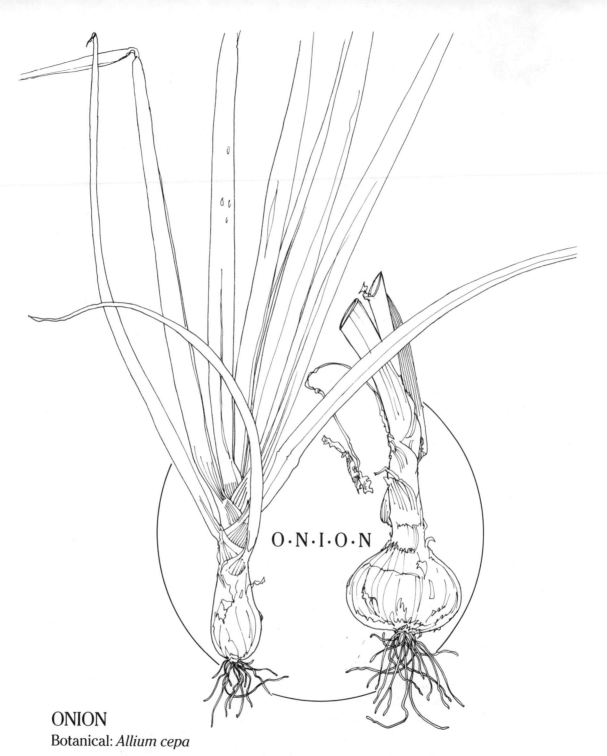

O·N·I·O·N

ONION
Botanical: *Allium cepa*

Onions are familiar plants to most people, because of their popularity as a
vegetable. Many gardeners grow onions, but not so many realize how well traveled

the humble vegetable has been throughout its history. The onion is believed to have originated in Afghanistan or Persia. In China, it is still called the "Mohammedan onion." It was cultivated thousands of years before the Christian era by the Egyptians and Chaldeans, and later on won favor with the Greeks and Romans.

Onions need rich, well-drained soil and a long daylength for best growth. The plants do not like clay, sand, or gravel soils. You can prepare the onion bed in the autumn for planting the following spring by working in liberal amounts of well-rotted compost. Wood ashes or kelp are good additions for the onion bed, whose pH should be around 6.0. If the pH is too low, add some lime. Onions prefer cool weather while their leaves are growing and hot weather for bulb formation.

Onions are easy to grow from seeds or sets. The soil should be dry when either seeds or sets are planted. There are many onion varieties available to gardeners today, including short-day varieties for southern gardens. Most varieties take about 100 days to mature. If you are planting from seed, start the seeds indoors in flats. Cover with ½ inch of well-rotted compost and keep moist until germination occurs.

Planting onion sets is a faster way to get to harvesttime. When planting sets, leave 6 inches of space between plants and make sure to press the little bulbs into the ground firmly. Some gardeners suggest covering the entire plant, so that birds cannot find them. If necessary, after the plant has taken hold and is growing, cut off its flower stem while it is young to prevent bolting, which will stop bulb formation. Onions are harvested when the leaves fall over and turn yellow-brown. Harvesting is a two-step process. First loosen the bulbs with a spading fork. A few days later, pull them gently out of the ground and let them cure for several days in the sun. A good way to store onions is to braid their stems and hang them in strings. Keep stored onions in a cool room.

The humble onion, so beloved in cuisine by both the simplest cook and the most sophisticated chef, is also among the most versatile and ancient herbal medicines known to man. The onion has been used in poultices, teas, and syrups. It has been juiced, boiled, sliced, chopped, and fried to treat illnesses ranging from earache to high blood pressure.

Onions stimulate digestion and cleanse the intestines. (They should not be eaten by those with sensitive stomachs, however.) They stimulate sweating. Onions have been used to expel worms, to calm jittery nerves, to soothe coughs and colds, and to induce urination. In Chinese medicine, the onion is used to relieve high blood pressure. According to herbalist Richard Lucas, it is also employed in Europe as a diuretic to help eliminate fluid in heart and lung sacs.

According to an article in the *West London Observer*, English scientists are investigating the possible effect of onion on blood clotting. They take their cue in this research from the French, who treat blood clots in the legs of horses with garlic and onion. Their pilot investigations showed that boiled or fried onion, given to people with fatty diets, apparently increased the body's ability to dissolve blood clots.

One old-fashioned remedy for asthma and bronchitis calls for eating slices of raw onion, or inhaling onion fumes. Onion juice, expressed in a juicer and mixed with honey, is another old asthma remedy. The mixture, which should be made fresh daily, is taken in teaspoon doses three to four times a day. Another treatment for this ailment consists of placing fresh, thin onion slices on a plate, covering them with honey, and allowing them to remain covered overnight. In the morning, the honey is scraped off and used in the same dosage as described above.

Other old-fashioned onion remedies include taking a piece of onion with some salt on it and applying it to burns to draw out the heat. Severe headache was often treated by pounding two onions into pulp and mixing them with salt and olive oil. This mixture was made into a poultice and placed on the head. Onions pounded into a pulp and made into a poultice have been used for boils and abscesses, too.

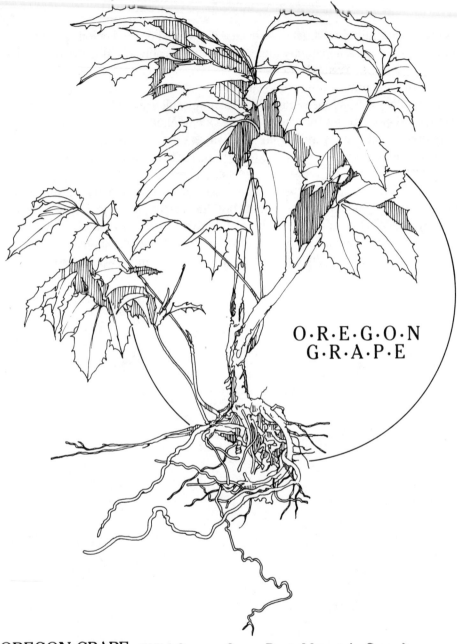

O·R·E·G·O·N
G·R·A·P·E

OREGON GRAPE (Wild Oregon Grape Root, Mountain Grape)
Botanical: *Mahonia aquifolium*

Oregon's state flower blooms on this attractive, fast-growing shrub, which is popular in ornamental landscaping. Oregon grape has shiny dark green leaves, resembling holly leaves in their shape, color, and spininess. The plant's flowers are small and yellow-green. They are followed by the berries, which turn dark purple-blue when they are ripe. The clusters of berries resemble small bunches of grapes, and they are edible.

The shrub can reach 6 feet in height, but it usually grows about 3 to 4 feet tall. It prefers a shady location and a fairly rich, well-drained soil (although we have seen it do well when cultivated in full sun and rather heavy soil). Its natural range is from Colorado west to northern California, then north to Canada. You can propagate Oregon grape from cuttings taken in midsummer. The new plants will be ready to set out the following spring. Oregon grape can be grown from seed, too. Collect seeds from the berries in the fall, and plant them outdoors so that stratification (exposure to cold temperatures) occurs. Plants can also be obtained at many landscaping nurseries.

The root is the part of the Oregon grape that is most often used for healing purposes. Do not gather it before the second year of the plant's growth, in late autumn, or in climates where the ground does not freeze during the winter. After harvesting the roots, you can replant the root crowns, and they will sometimes produce new plants. Some herbalists suggest digging up the earth around the roots, and making the harvest by pruning away one-fourth to one-third of the roots with shears, leaving enough of the root system for the plant to survive. Clean and process the roots according to directions in chapter 6.

Oregon grape is ranked by some herbalists among the most outstanding native American herbs. Its bright yellow root is high in the alkaloid berberine, which is a constituent of other powerfully healing plants such as goldenseal. Many American herbalists believe that Oregon grape stimulates liver activity and the secretion of bile. It is said to strengthen weak livers, and in the process, alleviate liver-induced symptoms such as headache, toxic blood, poor digestion, and lack of warmth. It is also regarded as an excellent blood purifier, although these claims have not been verified by scientific research. To the root is assigned a warm, drying influence. Modern herbalists use it to cleanse the spleen, as well as the liver and blood. The herb should not be used by anyone with an overactive liver, a condition created by overeating or eating too much rich food. Oregon grape is commonly prepared in a simple infusion, using ½ ounce of dried root to 1 quart of water (follow the directions under Infusions in chapter 6). It is usually taken 1 cup at a time three times daily until relief is obtained. Oregon grape is often used in herbal formulas, too.

The berries of this striking plant are considered cooling and have been used in an infusion to break fevers. Gather them in late summer when they are fully ripe and preserve them in a syrup, or dry them. They make a tasty jam, too.

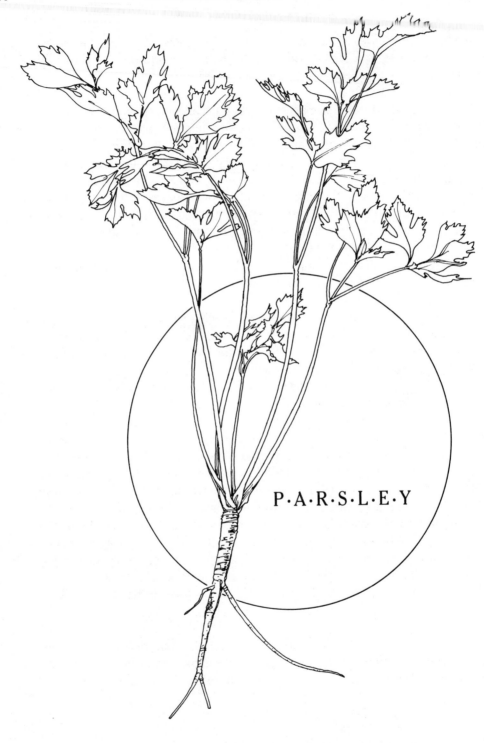

P·A·R·S·L·E·Y

PARSLEY

Botanical: *Petroselinum crispum*

Merry parsley, as it was known in the Middle Ages, is best known today for its versatility in the kitchen, but it is also valuable for medicinal purposes. Parsley is thought to have originated in Turkey, Sardinia, Algeria, and Lebanon, where it still grows wild today. The ancient Greeks had a high opinion of parsley, and associated it with Hercules, the mythological symbol of strength. They fed parsley to their racehorses to give them stamina and awarded crowns of parsley to the victors of athletic contests. And they wore chaplets of parsley at banquets in the belief that the herb would help keep them sober. It may be that our modern custom of using parsley as a decorative garnish derives from this ancient Greek practice. But if parsley can't keep people sober, at least it has the power to freshen the breath and neutralize indigestion. These properties are due to parsley's high content of chlorophyll. Ironically, today many people ignore their parsley at the end of a meal and eat a breath mint instead.

Parsley is a small, bright green herb which sends up numerous juicy stems ornamented with sprightly, curly or flat leaves, depending on the variety being grown. Curly-leaved parsley grows about 6 inches tall and has a rather mounded shape, especially when pinched back to encourage bushiness. The flat-leaved variety is taller—about 12 inches in height. Although it is really a biennial, parsley is commonly treated as an annual and harvested in its first year. That's because the leaves are the part used in cooking; the second year parsley blooms and goes to seed, producing far fewer usable leaves. The plant requires a very rich soil that is kept moist. It does not like to be transplanted, but can be, if seedlings have well-developed root systems and are carefully handled.

Parsley seeds are notoriously slow to germinate. Some gardeners suggest stratifying the seeds to speed germination. Place seeds between layers of wet white blotting paper and place them in the refrigerator for about two weeks. Sow seed in the spring, in drills ½ inch deep. The bed should be well tilled and enriched with humus-rich compost. Thin seedlings to 3-inch spacing as they mature further, to 6-inch spacing. Parsley can be pinched back throughout the growing season to supply leaves as needed for cooking. Harvest the whole plant in late summer for use in healing preparations. Both the leafy parts of the plant and its roots can be used medicinally.

Parsley is a powerhouse of vitamins and minerals. It contains vitamins A and C, calcium, thiamin, riboflavin, and niacin, making it a good addition to the diets of anemic people. During the Middle Ages, and on into the eighteenth century in Europe, parsley was a favorite "simple." It was used as a diuretic and as a liver tonic to break up kidney stones, to bring on late menses, and to soothe coughs.

In France and other European countries, a poultice of chopped, fresh parsley is used to prevent painful swollen breasts in nursing mothers. The same poultice has been applied to relieve insect bites, too. A simple infusion of parsley leaves and stems (about ½ cup of the fresh herb to 1¾ pints of water) makes a soothing skin lotion or shampoo. This same infusion, in a footbath, is considered by some to be useful for treating menopausal symptoms, asthma, and painful periods.

Parsley root is one of the five major laxative roots used by European herbalists, who often use a decoction of the roots and leaves to treat skin diseases, vaginal discharge, and circulatory troubles.

Keep in mind that too much fresh parsley can irritate the kidneys, although it is unlikely that you will eat more than two handfuls in one day, anyway. Like other strong diuretics, parsley is not recommended for medicinal use during pregnancy.

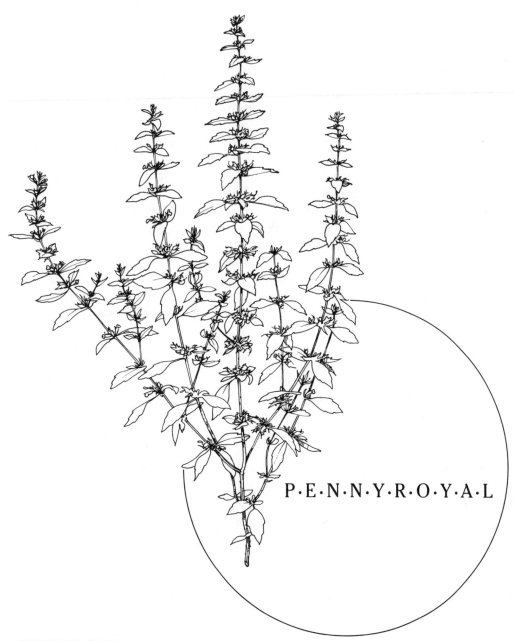

P·E·N·N·Y·R·O·Y·A·L

PENNYROYAL

Botanical: *Mentha pulegium, Hedeoma pulegioides*

There are two plants commonly called pennyroyal. They have similar healing properties, even though botanically they are distinct. The more famous one, *Mentha pulegium,* is a native of Europe and Asia, from where it spread to North America and other parts of the world. It is a ground-hugging mint; the only part of the plant that rises above ground level is its flower stalk. This plant loves rich, moist areas such as pond and stream edges, boggy grasslands, meadows, and irrigated fields. This species is often called English or European pennyroyal. It's a good herb to grow at the edge of a water garden.

The other plant (*Hedeoma pulegioides*) is a native of North America and grows in dry fields, hills, woods, and marginal areas. It grows about 1 foot tall, and its tiny lavender flowers bloom in the leaf axils. *H. pulegioides* is often called American pennyroyal or mock pennyroyal. It is stronger than English pennyroyal. This kind of pennyroyal grows well in the same sort of conditions as peppermint and spearmint.

Pennyroyal's fragrance is sharper and more acrid than that of spearmint or peppermint. However, it has many of the same uses in herbal medicine. It is stimulating, diaphoretic, cooling, carminative, and sedative. It can also cause abortions, so pregnant women should never use pennyroyal. (The oil is particularly to be avoided—several women have died as a result of taking too much pennyroyal oil for abortive purposes. Pennyroyal has been used, as have been peppermint and spearmint, for headaches, colic, intestinal pain from flatulence, chest congestion, and colds or flu. The fresh leaves of the plant can be rubbed on the temples or forehead to relieve headaches. An infusion of the leaves, made into a compress, is also used for this purpose. One old-fashioned remedy for treating cases of hysteria or nervous tension calls for the patient to soak in a relaxing bath to which an infusion of pennyroyal, lavender flowers, wood betony, and sage has been added.

Pennyroyal is a good insect repellent. Pennyroyal oil is a common component in many commercially available natural insect repellents. (Pregnant women should avoid these also, since strong oils can be absorbed through the skin.) The oil readily repels flies, gnats, mosquitoes, ticks, and chiggers. You can simply crush some fresh leaves and rub them on your body. If you plant pennyroyal near outdoor decks, patios or pathways, you can apply its insect-repellent properties quickly when needed.

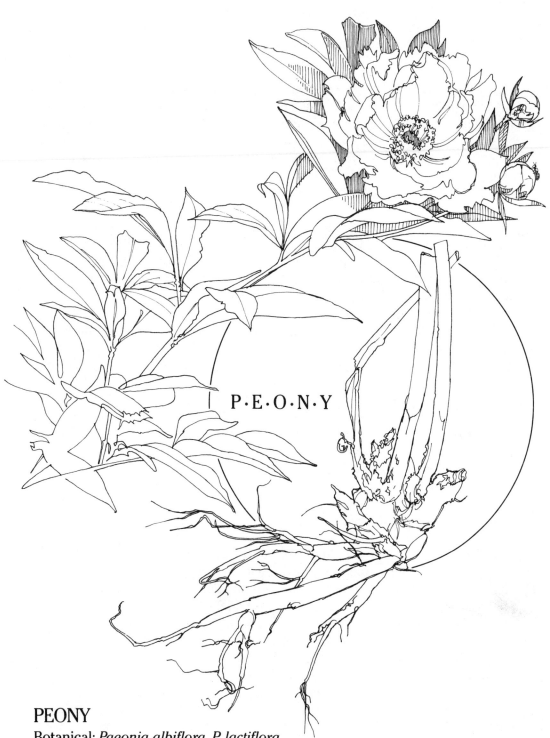

P·E·O·N·Y

PEONY

Botanical: *Paeonia albiflora, P. lactiflora*

The gorgeous peony has been immortalized in classical Chinese paintings, with its creamy pastel blossoms often accentuated by birds, butterflies, or clouds. In

China the peony is found wild and is also extensively cultivated. In the United States and Europe it is also highly valued as a garden ornamental. Peony flowers are large, delicate, and showy. Usually red, white, or pink, they bloom in May and June atop stalks rising from a lush, deep green clump of foliage. Although the flowers fade as summer begins, the foliage remains well into the first frosts of autumn, making an attractive low bush about 2 or 3 feet high.

Peonies are perennial and require little care once they are well established. They prefer a rich, loose soil and a location in full sun or partial shade. Prepare the planting bed a week or two ahead of time to allow the soil to settle, and enrich it with compost and bonemeal. Peonies are most often propagated by root cuttings, which can be planted from late August until the first hard frost. Select a piece of root that contains at least three "eyes" and set it with the eyes pointing up, 2 or 3 inches below the soil surface. Tamp down the earth and water thoroughly. Plants should be spaced 3 to 5 feet apart in order to provide ample growing room. Mulch the plants during their first winter. In the following spring they may need support for their branches, too.

Peony plants are usually left undisturbed, but after several years, or whenever the flowers begin to get smaller and the stems get too crowded, they should be divided. Division provides a good opportunity for harvesting some of the roots, which are the part of the plant used medicinally. Dig a circle 1½ to 2 feet around the base of each plant, and about 1 foot deep. Carefully lift out the whole clump of stems and let the plant sit undisturbed for several hours. Then cut off the foliage 2 or 3 inches above the crown and gently wash excess dirt from the roots. With a sharp knife, cut apart sections of the root. For replanting, leave at least three eyes on each section; for harvesting, select fresh, firm and unspoiled root material. Wash and slice the harvested roots into thin pieces, then dry them on screens in a warm, sunny place.

Peony roots are used in both Chinese and European herbology. Researchers in China found that they contain sedative and analgesic properties. Because of these analgesic properties, peony root has also been used by Chinese herbalists to relieve headaches, gastric pain, and bladder infections. In the Orient, peony root is especially valued for women. It is used to relieve menstrual pain and to support a healthy pregnancy and childbirth. European herbalists use peony's reputed sedative, antispasmodic property in treating convulsions and epilepsy, also. An infusion in the ratio of 1 ounce dried root to 1 pint of boiled water is made when using peony as a simple. In Oriental medicine, peony root is used in a great number of herb formulas.

While the lovely flowers are not usually used in a therapeutic way (except for their beauty), they can be used in making scented waters and lotions. Peony water is easy to make. Place ½ cup of fresh, macerated peony petals in 1 cup of cold water in a Pyrex pot. Let the mixture steep for 30 minutes, then heat it gently for 10 minutes.

Remove the pan from the heat and strain off the petals. Refrigerate the water and use it within one week as a face or body refresher. Peony water can be added to a soothing warm bath, too. The recipe in chapter 6 for Astringent Facial Wash also includes peony petals.

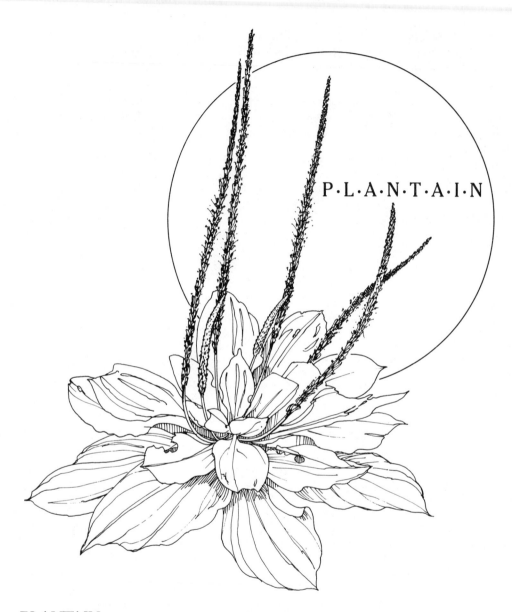

P·L·A·N·T·A·I·N

PLANTAIN (Broad-Leaved Plantain, Waybread, White Man's Foot, Snakeweed)

Botanical: *Plantago major*

Plantain is a humble perennial weed with an ancient reputation in both Oriental, European, and, within the last four centuries, in Native American medicine. The Indians called it white man's foot because the plant, with its rosette of ribbed leaves and its seed stalks somewhat resembling miniature cattails, seemed to follow the white settlers wherever they went. Today, plantain can be found growing wild throughout the United States along roadsides, in meadows, in the poor soil of marginal areas, and to the consternation of homeowners, in lawns. Plantain is a very prolific weed and seems to have always been gathered wild. In the regions where it grows, the problem has not been how to cultivate it, but how to keep it from spreading. Harvest the leaves just before the flower stalk matures and dry them in the shade on screens. For use in their fresh state, gather the leaves whenever they are needed and available.

The tiny mucilaginous seeds of the plant, often called psyllium seeds, were used as a bulk laxative in Appalachia. They resemble the seeds of another species, *Plantago psyllium,* found in Europe and Africa, which is used today in pharmaceutical laxative preparations. The tiny plantain seeds, combined in tea with flaxseed, are used in Chinese medicine for curing loss of sexual power in men, as well as for treating general debility.

Native American tribes gathered plantain seeds and mixed them with other grains for food. They also used the juice fo the plant for treating rattlesnake bites, hence the common name of snakeweed. European settlers used plantain for this purpose, too. Some Indian tribes used poultices of plantain leaves to ease the pain of wounds and to soothe rheumatic pain. In Europe, the plant has been used in poultice form also to soothe wounds, skin inflammations, burns, and insect stings. Internally, plantain leaves are famous among herbalists as an ingredient in blood purifying and diuretic formulas. In a simple infusion, the leaves have been used to treat diarrhea and as a local application for piles.

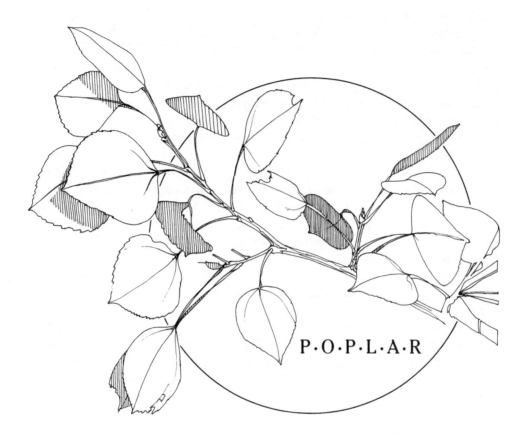

P·O·P·L·A·R

POPLAR (Aspen, Quaking Aspen)
Botanical: *Populus tremuloides,* and other species

Like most poplars and willows, the quaking aspen has been a highly revered medicinal plant. When the nineteenth century naturalist Henry David Thoreau was canoeing in the Maine wilderness, his Indian guide claimed to be a doctor of natural medicines and able to list a medicinal use for every plant Thoreau could point out. Thoreau wrote in *The Maine Woods:* "I immediately tried him. He said that the inner bark of the aspen was good for sore eyes ... "

This beautiful deciduous tree grows up to 40 or 50 feet tall, and its distinctive silhouette is narrow and symmetrical. It can be found in open woodlands and on hillsides throughout the cooler regions of North America. The trunk of the tree is a whitish gray or green color that turns darker as the tree grows older. Poplar's heart-shaped, dark green leaves turn bright yellow or golden in the autumn, contrasting exquisitely with stands of evergreen trees often found nearby. Poplar leaves are borne on very thin, flat petioles that twist and bend, making the leaves flutter in the slightest breeze and giving the tree one of its common names—quaking aspen.

Poplar trees will grow in many types of soil, but they do best in well-drained, loamy soil. They can be propagated by layering or cuttings (as described in chapter 5). Many species of poplar are available from nurseries, too.

The part most often used for healing purposes is the bark, which is gathered in the fall from large branches or the trunks of trees being pruned or removed from the landscape. You can also obtain poplar bark from small branches and twigs gathered in the spring.

Poplar has been used by herbalists to cure dysentery, fevers, diarrhea, loss of appetite, colds, and general weakness. Modern scientists have not substantiated poplar's effectiveness in relieving these conditions. The bark is made into a simple decoction of 1 ounce of the dried bark to 1 quart of just-boiled water. To make the decoction, follow the directions in chapter 6.

A decoction of poplar bark has also been used to treat urinary tract infections, irritations of the bladder and prostate gland, and weakness due to the stress of chronic illness. A tea has also been used both as a beverage and as an external compress to ease arthritic inflammations.

Poplar has traditionally been assigned astringent, diuretic, antiseptic, and slightly sedative qualities. It contains salicin, which breaks down in the body to salicylic acid, a substance related to the active ingredient in aspirin. Willow trees also contain this property, and the bark of white, black, or yellow willow is sometimes used in the same way that poplar bark is used.

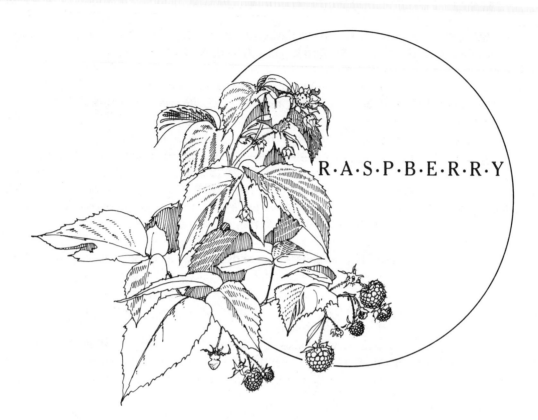

R·A·S·P·B·E·R·R·Y

RASPBERRY

Botanical: *Rubus idaeus,* and other species

    The raspberry, which is native to many parts of Europe, is a favorite in the garden because of its luscious red berries. The plant has a perennial root; it sends up erect, spiny stems (more correctly called canes) ornamented by slightly hairy, irregularly toothed leaves. The canes bear pretty white flowers followed by the deep red jewellike fruit.

    Raspberries are usually propagated from suckers taken from a mature plant. These are planted in the early spring in rich, loamy soil. The plants prefer a sunny location and slightly acid soil with plenty of potash. Adding wood ashes to the raspberry bed is a good idea. Raspberries are heavy feeders, and liberal additions of well-rotted compost should be dug into the soil to provide humus. Because their roots spread rather quickly, raspberry plants are usually spaced about 2 feet apart. If there are two or more rows, allow 4 to 6 feet between rows.

Plants are not allowed to bear fruit during their first year, because fruiting then weakens them. They will not flourish if grass is allowed to grow up around them, either. By the second year, the plants will produce delicious harvests of berries. Each year the plants should be pruned in the late winter. Old canes or stems are cut out, and when the new canes appear in the spring, they are thinned to six to eight per plant.

Raspberry is susceptible to several diseases. Fungus diseases discolor leaves and the affected part should be cut from the plant. Curling and red and yellow mottling of the leaves indicate mosaic disease. Diseased plants should be removed from the patch and destroyed. Iron deficiency from an overalkaline soil causes yellowing in the leaf veins and can be remedied by amendments that decrease soil pH, such as decomposing pine needles and acid peat moss.

Both raspberry leaves and fruits are credited with healing purposes. Leaves can be harvested after the plant's second year of growth. Pick them in the spring before the flowers have fully matured. No more than one-third of the leaves should be gathered from any plant—you don't want to decrease the plant's vigor.

Few people need instruction on harvesting raspberries, which are among the most delicious of all summer fruits. Containing modest amounts of vitamins A, B, C, and E, and calcium, phosphorus, and iron, raspberries are as healthful as they are delicious.

In both Chinese and in European herbal medicine raspberry leaf tea is a classic herbal preparation for pregnant women, which is administered to prepare them for childbirth. In the 1940s, British researchers isolated from the leaves a substance called fragerine, which was found to be a relaxant that reduces muscle spasms in the uterus. Today's researchers consider the clinical evidence inconclusive, but herbalists nonetheless find success with raspberry leaf tea in its traditional applications. In Chinese medicine, a cup of raspberry leaf tea is recommended to be taken one-half hour before meals to prepare for childbirth and to help prevent miscarriage.

Raspberry leaf tea is also believed to be excellent for relieving heavy cramping during menstruation, and it is sometimes mixed with other herbs in a douche for treating leukorrhea. The infusion has also been used for coughs, sores in the mouth, stomachache in children, and diarrhea. Raspberry leaves are considered to be astringent and to readily absorb moisture.

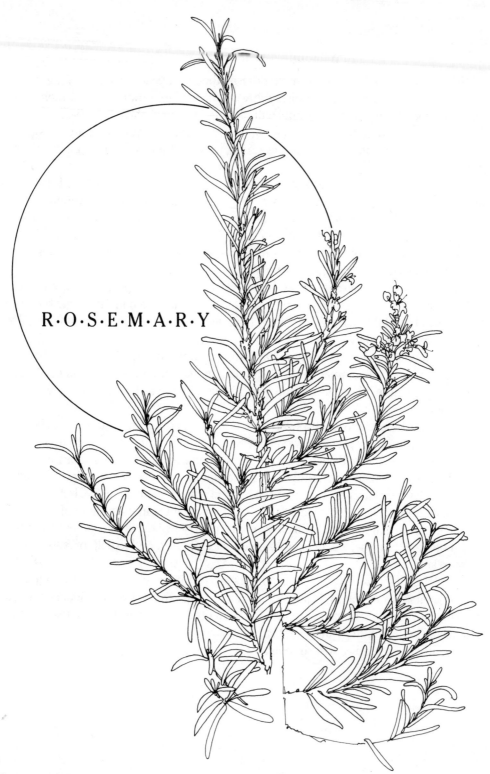

R·O·S·E·M·A·R·Y

ROSEMARY
Botanical: *Rosmarinus officinalis*

Rosemary, with its intense piny scent, was a token of loyalty and commemoration in olden days. For this reason it had a prominent role in several holy rituals, including Christian nuptials and burials. A bride's bouquet was likely to contain rosemary "for remembrance." Steeped in herbal lore, the fragrant herb was also a favorite of the gypsies who valued it for its beneficial effect on their skin and hair.

Rosemary is a woody evergreen shrub native to the chalky hills of southern France. It has small, narrow dark green leaves, which are almost needlelike and carried opposite one another on the stem. Tiny pale blue flowers grace the bush in summer. It can grow up to 5 feet high, if it is provided with a hospitable environment. For rosemary, this means a sheltered, southerly location with a light, well-drained, alkaline (chalky or sandy) soil. In this type of soil and situation, rosemary achieves the most aromatic and beautiful growth.

Rosemary can be grown from seed, but it's easier to start with cuttings. Seeds are sown 6 inches apart in shallow drills in the spring. When the plants are 2 to 3 inches high, transplant them to a holding bed with about 6 inches between plants. Then plant them out when they have grown to about 5 inches high. They should be set about 3 feet apart.

Most gardeners propagate rosemary from cuttings, considering them generally more dependable than the seeds, which do not germinate reliably. Six inch long cuttings can be made in either the spring or fall. Bury them in sandy soil, leaving one-third of the cutting above ground. Keep them in a shady location, water them carefully, and they will be ready for planting in about six months. During the bedded plants' first winter, cut back the stems by one-half their length. Then mulch the plants with leaf mold, making sure they are entirely buried, and cover them with burlap bags.

Rosemary's leaves and flowers are the parts used for healing purposes, and they are harvested from the second year of the plant onward. Cut back the stems just before the plant flowers, or during the flowering period if you intend to use the flowers, too. Harvest no more than one-third of the plant in a season.

In European herbal medicine, rosemary has been used for depression and other nervous diseases. Regarded as antiseptic and astringent, rosemary has also been used to release gas from the intestines, dispel mucus from the stomach, calm nervous stomach, and restore digestion. A simple infusion of the leaves alone or the leaves and flowers together is drunk several times daily.

In China rosemary became popular for treating headache, insomnia, and mental fatigue. A simple Chinese tea for headache includes rosemary, sage, and peppermint.

The Chinese recommend treating nervous stomach by adding a pinch of powdered ginger to a cup of rosemary tea and drinking it three or four times a day.

Like juniper and cedar, rosemary has cleansing and antiseptic properties when burned. In French hospitals during World War II, rosemary was combined with juniper and burned to help kill germs in the air. It has been used to purify sick chambers for centuries all over Europe. Its antibacterial properties are contained in the volatile oil it contains.

Rosemary can be used in a wash to alleviate dandruff, too. It is a traditional old-fashioned hair rinse for dark-haired people.

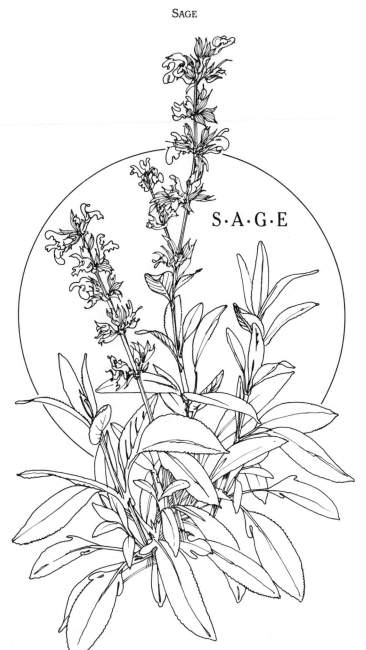

S·A·G·E

SAGE

Botanical: *Salvia officinalis*

"Why should a man die when sage grows in his garden?" So went an old saying during the Middle Ages. The ancient people who named this robust herb must have held it in the highest regard, for its name derives from the Latin verb *salvare,* to save.

Sage is an evergreen shrub native to the Mediterranean region. It grows about 18 inches tall and sends up numerous slightly woody stems on which its silver-green leaves are carried in pairs. The leaves are finely wrinkled and veined, and softly hairy. Sage's beautiful purplish flowers are displayed in whorls.

Sage can be propagated from seeds sown in late spring in sandy soil. When the seedlings reach about 3 inches in height, transplant them to stand 15 to 20 inches apart. Sage can also be propagated from cuttings. Cuttings should be about 4 inches long, taken in the fall and planted out the following spring.

The leaves are the part of the plant used for healing purposes. Harvest them just before the flowers begin to bloom, by cutting the plant back to about 4 inches above the ground. Dry the stems and leaves, then strip the leaves off the stems and store in airtight containers.

The leaves of plants in their second to fourth year of growth are considered the best for healing purposes, because of the strength and concentration of herbal properties. After the fourth year, the plant's potency markedly decreases, and for this reason, herb gardeners usually rotate older plants out of the garden at that time and introduce new plants.

The many species of sage all have virtually the same properties. Sage is one of those herbs that has been used to cure a multitude of ills. Its leaves contain a type of tannin, and its astringent properties have been demonstrated scientifically. Other properties are more controversial, but the list of use to which sage has been put by herbalists is long, indeed. It is regarded as a tonic that keeps the stomach, intestines, kidneys, liver, spleen, and sexual organs healthy. Sage is used as a stimulant to increase circulation and relieve headache, to break fevers, and to help reduce cold symptoms. The plant has a traditional reputation as an excellent nervine, strengthening the brain and nervous system, instead of sedating it as some nervine herbs do. The English herbalist Gerard wrote in his classic herbal:

Sage is singularly good for the head and brain, it quickeneth the senses and memory, strentheneth the sinews, restoreth health to those that have the palsy, and taketh away shakey trembling of the members.

Sage should never be boiled. When making an infusion of the leaves, put them in water that has just been boiled and removed from the heat. Hot sage tea has been used to bring on late or suppressed menses and to help lessen excessively heavy menstrual flow. Women who have been breast-feeding and want to dry up their milk supply sometimes drink cold sage tea. Sage also has a reputation for tempering sexual desire.

A strong infusion of the tea is considered useful in washing wounds, for sage does have antiseptic properties. Sometimes powdered sage is sprinkled on a cut or wound after it has been washed with the tea to stop bleeding and encourage healing. A gargle of sage tea is a well-known old-fashioned remedy for treating sore and bleeding gums, loose teeth, cold sores, excess saliva, sore throat, and colds. As an ingredient in herbal toothpaste, powdered sage acts as a disinfectant and strengthens the gums.

Sage tea or extract makes an excellent addition to the herbal bath. It also can be used in shampoos, soaps, and hair rinses, especially for dark-haired people. Sage is held to be generally stimulating and cleansing to the skin and scalp, soothing to sore muscles, and restorative to aging skin and hair, although again, these effects have yet to be proven scientifically. Sage does make a stimulating after-shave lotion, because it is styptic, astringent, and aromatic. (See page 312 for recipe for Sage and Lavender After-Shave Lotion.)

According to Chinese medicine, sage increases physical strength, mental equanimity and alertness, and body heat. It should not be used medicinally by those who are already robust, red-faced, always warm, happy and optimistic, which are all characteristics of a strongly sanguine constitution.

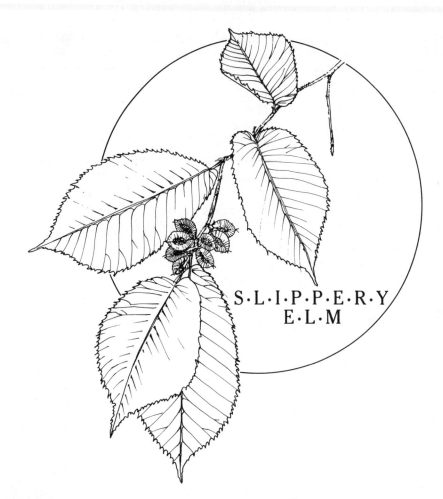

SLIPPERY ELM

Botanical: *Ulmus rubra*

The slippery elm tree can be found in the northern and central United States, growing in moist woods and bottomlands, and along the banks of streams, as well as on poor, dry soil. It grows to 60 feet in height and has deeply furrowed bark and dark green leaves 6 to 7 inches long and about 2 inches wide. The leaves are toothed, almost oval, rough on the topside, and fuzzy underneath. The buds at the ends of the branches often have orange tips.

Slippery elm trees can be propagated by cuttings, as described in chapter 5, or young trees can be purchased at nurseries. The tree is relatively adaptable and easy to grow, but it does best in moist locations, in soil that has been enriched with compost or leaf mold.

The pinkish white inner bark of the tree contains the tree's healing properties. You can collect it in the spring or fall, according to general harvesting guidelines in chapter 6.

Slippery elm bark provided one of the most versatile medicines for both Native Americans and the early settlers of this country. It is an extremely safe and gentle medicine for a wide variety of ailments, and it is still current in two of the major catalogs of drugs currently used and approved: The U.S. Dispensatory and the National Formulary.

Slippery elm's calcium content makes it a good calmative medicine for those with emotional or nervous problems. Herbalists have regarded it traditionally as an excellent food for convalescents: nutritious, easy to digest, and helpful to the stomach and intestines. Slippery elm "food," as herbalists sometimes call it, is made by mixing 1 teaspoon of powdered slippery elm bark with cold water to a paste consistency. The paste is gradually blended with 1 pint of boiling water until the mixture is smooth. (Slippery elm powder tends to form lumps, so you must add the liquid gradually.) Season the paste with cinnamon or nutmeg to give it a pleasant flavor.

Today, the most visible form of slippery elm is the old-fashioned lozenges sold in many health food and herb stores for alleviating sore throats and the coughs due to colds. Slippery elm lemonade is an old-fashioned remedy for treating colds and bronchitis. To make it, mix 1 tablespoon of slippery elm powder with enough cold water to make a paste. Gradually add 1 pint of boiling water, stirring constantly. Squeeze in the juice of half a lemon, add honey to taste, and drink.

People in Appalachia have used a tea made of slippery elm's inner bark as a laxative. Slippery elm's demulcent properties are thought to soothe sore intestines, allowing them to eliminate waste more readily. The powder is also used by herbalists in suppository form with a little powdered white oak bark, to treat mild cases of hemorrhoids (see the recipe on page 315).

Various Native American tribes gave pregnant women a tea containing slippery elm powder to assure an easy labor. Indian tribes have also used it in poultice form for burns, fevers, and respiratory infections. A poultice of slippery elm powder is also supposed to be good for treating wounds, boils, and other surface inflammation, such as mastitis.

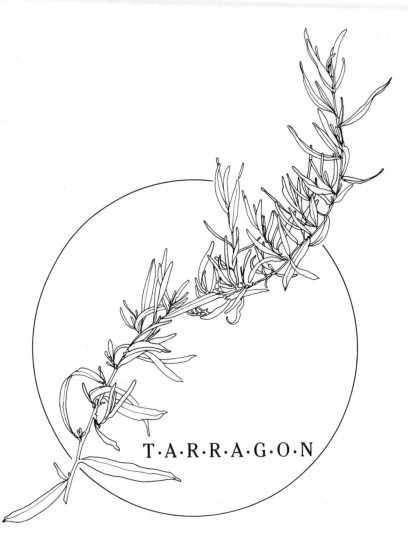

T·A·R·R·A·G·O·N

TARRAGON

Botanical: *Artemisia dracunculus*

In medieval times, pilgrims embarking on long journeys would stuff their shoes with sprigs of tarragon in the hope that the herb would impart stamina. Tarragon's common name seems to be a corruption of the French *esdragon,* which is in turn derived from the Latin *dracunculus,* meaning "little dragon."

Tarragon is a perennial member of the Composite family, the same family to which daisies belong. It has narrow, dark green leaves and small yellow flowers, and it grows about 2 feet tall. The herb likes a warm, dry environment with well-drained, fairly rich soil, although it will also grow in poor soil.

There are two major varieties of tarragon—French and Russian. French tarragon contains an aniselike aromatic oil that the Russian variety lacks, so it is the type preferred in both cooking and medicine. Unfortunately, French tarragon rarely produces seeds and it grows slowly from root divisions and cuttings. This is one reason why it is a bit expensive.

Tarragon is propagated from divisions or cuttings taken in the spring or autumn, according to directions given in chapter 5. Plant the rooted cuttings outside when they are established, in a warm, sunny environment. Side-dress your tarragon each year in the spring with well-composted manure. Tarragon has long fibrous roots and lateral runners, and it doesn't like to "get its feet wet." Some gardeners plant it on a slope so that it never is in danger of becoming waterlogged. But do not allow the roots to dry out completely, either. Mulching around the plant is a good way to help conserve soil moisture.

Mulch your tarragon plants heavily wherever there is a danger of heavy frosts. If you live where winters are severe, it is best to dig up the herb in autumn and pot it up to be kept indoors until the weather warms up again.

Tarragon is best if harvested just before it flowers. Cut it back to within 1 inch of the ground. Cooks use tarragon fresh or dried, preserved in vinegar, or frozen. Cut the plant into small twigs that you can handle, store, and use easily. For storage for medicinal purposes, tarragon can be either frozen or dried, although some of the aromatic properties dissipate when the herb is dried. To dry tarragon, hang the branches in bunches upside down in a warm, dark place as described under Drying Herbs, in chapter 6. Carefully strip the leaves from the stems when dry.

The "little dragon," as tarragon is still known in France, is famous in French cuisine, but not too many people known that tarragon has valuable healing properties in addition to its light licorice flavor. Tarragon does more than season rich French dishes like Lobster Thermidor or béarnaise sauce. Herbalists say that this herb contains digestive enzymes that help break down meat and proteins. It is also regarded as a mild, nonirritating diuretic that helps the system flush out toxins released from the digestion of meat and other proteins.

A simple infusion of tarragon leaves has been used to stimulate the appetite, relieve flatulence and colic, regulate menstruation, alleviate the pain of arthritis and rheumatism and gout, and expel worms from the body. The fresh leaf or root, applied to aching teeth, cuts, or sores, is said to act as a local anaesthetic.

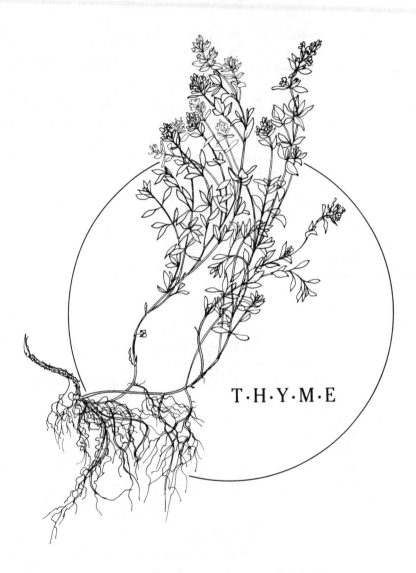

THYME

Botanical: *Thymus vulgaris*

In legend and history the thyme plant has been synonymous with courage and bravery. And the ancient Greeks associated thyme with elegance. The phrase "the smell of thyme" was an expression of praise for one's commendable style. The tiny elfin leaves and flowers of the plant appeal not only to people but to bees, too.

Thyme is cultivated extensively in Greece and other Mediterranean countries, where thyme honey is regarded as the very best.

Thyme is a hardy perennial herb with a woody, fibrous root, from which grow numerous hard-branched stems that reach from 4 to 10 inches high. Its tiny, elliptical, gray-tinted leaves are set in pairs along the stems. The little blossoms of the thyme are white or lilac colored. Thyme has a spreading habit, and the plant makes a delightfully fragrant ground cover or lawn.

Thyme is easily grown from cuttings or root divisions taken in the early summer. Cuttings should be 6 inches long. You can plant them outside in the spring in full sun, in a light, well-drained, lime soil. You can also propagate thyme from seed. Sow the fine seeds ¼ inch deep in light soil, about 2 inches apart. When you plant them out, space them about 9 inches apart. The plants will enjoy a side-dressing of well-rotted compost in the spring.

Thyme leaves are used for both cooking and healing purposes. Individual leaves can be picked as needed throughout the growing season. To harvest the whole plant, cut it back to about 2 inches above the ground just before it flowers in midsummer. Dry the herb according to the directions provided in chapter 6. The plant will bush out again after you harvest it, but don't cut back this second growth, or the plant will be less winter hardy. Thyme should be mulched well in climates with severe winters.

Like so many of the old-fashioned "simples" such as lavender and sage, thyme has long been acclaimed as a treatment for numerous ailments. Although the efficacy of thyme for these applications has not been documented in the laboratory, herbalists believe it works and still use it in traditional ways. For example, they consider thyme an excellent treatment for nervous problems such as neurasthenia, depression, or lack of energy. It is also used for disorders due to circulation, such as vertigo, migraine, and ringing in the ears. The ancient Greeks used thyme to calm convulsions and other spasms. For nervous conditions, a simple infusion of thyme is taken two or three times daily, and a hand or footbath using the thyme infusion can be enjoyed before bedtime, for about eight minutes. (See the directions on making footbaths and handbaths in chapter 6.)

From the fifteenth to the seventeenth centuries, when waves of plague ran across Europe, thyme was used as a germicide. In World War I, thymol, the oil extracted from thyme, was used extensively as an antiseptic to treat soldiers' wounds. Thymol was also used to purify the air of hospitals and sickrooms, especially in Europe several decades ago.

The antispasmodic qualities that are traditionally ascribed to thyme make it useful in alleviating asthma, stomach cramps, and whooping cough, according to the French herbalist Maurice Mésségué. Thyme tea has also been drunk by people at the onset of a cold, or to bring on and regulate menses. In a compress, thyme tea has been applied to soothe nursing mothers' sore breasts.

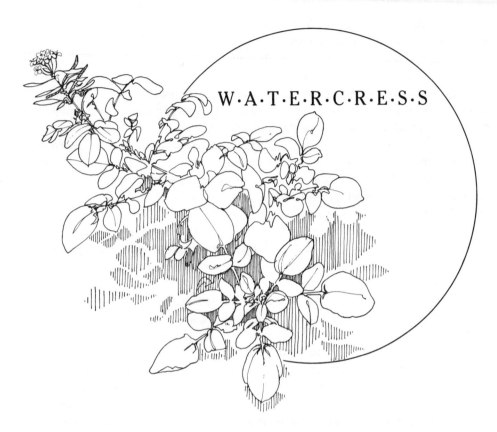

W·A·T·E·R·C·R·E·S·S

WATERCRESS

Botanical: *Nasturtium officinale*

It took the advent of America's new-style cuisine to elevate the likes of watercress (and other herbs, too) to new esteem. From the humble position of a seldom-eaten garnish to a starring role in much more elaborate culinary preparations, watercress has regained its well-deserved status through a type of cooking that considers your health as much as your palate.

American cooks now use watercress in many ways. It can be found in salads and dressings, herb butters and spreads, sandwiches, soups, and casseroles, where it adds a zippy, pungent flavor. While cooks value watercress for its taste, herbalists value the plant for its nutrients. Watercress contains a substantial supply of vitamins and minerals, including phosphorus, iron, calcium, sulfur, nitrogen, and vitamins A and C.

Watercress is a juicy, vivid green aquatic plant, introduced here from Europe. It grows in every state and throughout Canada in shallow creeks, ditches, along the edges of slow-moving rivers, in ponds, lakes, and brooks—wherever the water is clear, cool, and neither stagnant nor too fast-running. Watercress usually grows where the water is from 2 to 6 inches deep. You can often see large beds of watercress in country streams, its leafy stems protruding several inches above the water's surface.

You can easily bring watercress to your neck of the woods, if it doesn't grow there already. If you don't have a creek or pond, try making a small pool, or simply plant it in a tub filled with sand and water. You can even grow watercress in clay pots, placed in a tray of water. Just be sure to change the water every day to keep it fresh and clear. Easy to propagate, watercress likes a mixture of rich alluvial soil, ground rocks such as river sand or limestone, and peat or humus. Below the water's surface, watercress sends out many fine white roots. Any section of the plant stem with roots on it will take hold and begin a new patch when anchored in a suitable environment. This is how watercress survives in nature, as stream beds are constantly being altered by floods and droughts. It is also how watercress spreads so quickly once it is introduced, often traveling in advance of civilization on its way down an undeveloped river system.

The entire watercress plant is used by healers. Harvest it while the plant is flowering and dry it according to the directions given in chapter 6. This pungent, peppery plant can simply be included regularly in the diet. For more specific medical action, an infusion of the dried plant can be taken.

Because of its nutrients, herbalists have used watercress in a tea to tone the liver and cleanse the blood. Watercress is considered diuretic and is thought to aid in breaking up kidney or bladder stones as well. The juice of the fresh leaves has been used to treat acne, eczema, ringworm, rashes, and similar skin irritations and infections.

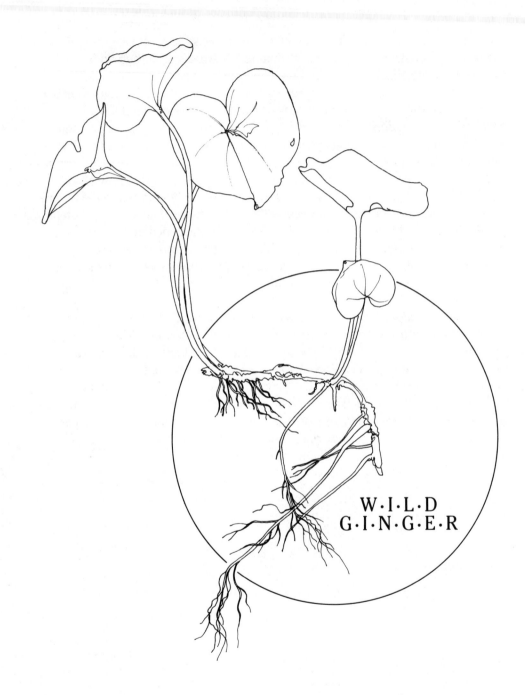

W·I·L·D
G·I·N·G·E·R

WILD GINGER (Canada Wild Ginger, Indian Ginger, Canada Snakeroot, False Coltsfoot, Black Snakeroot, Colic Root)

Botanical: *Asarum canadense*

This attractive little wildflower grows throughout northern United States and Canada, as far south as northern California and the Carolinas. It frequents shaded, damp woods in spots along creeks, bogs, and springs and in similarly wet, rich soils. Wild ginger is a creeping perennial that rises to modest heights of 6 to 12 inches and often spreads to form patches of dense ground cover. The plant usually bears two heart- or kidney-shaped, dark green leaves on each stem. A single, delicate bell-shaped flower, deep purple or reddish brown in hue, can often be seen hanging inconspicuously from between the two leaves. The leaf stems are a lighter shade of green, from ⅛ to ¼ inch thick, crisp in texture, hairy and round. They often originate from the underground rhizomes, giving the appearance of separate plants. A little deeper investigation, though, reveals a mass of tangled rhizomes and roots. These are ¼ to ⅜ inch thick, pale green to yellowish green, crisp, succulent, and slightly fibrous when broken.

Wild ginger plants for your garden will probably have to be obtained from wild specimens, since these lovely woodland plants are not, to our knowledge, available commercially. Before collecting specimens of wild ginger, though, it is important to know that in some areas it is considered a rare species. Formerly very common throughout its extensive North American range, wild ginger has dwindled due to a loss of habitat. Logging, housing developments, cattle grazing, and reservoir construction have all taken a toll on the fragile ecology of forest-shaded streams and marshes, where this plant finds a cool home.

Fortunately, the collection of wild ginger stock for your home garden doesn't need to pose a threat to wild populations of the plant. (But check local and state laws before gathering *any* wildflowers or rare plants.) The good news, according to herbalist and gardener Tom Ward, is that "just one section of wild gingerroot will grow and spread into a large patch, and the patch you take that cutting from will proliferate evern more abundantly."

Here's how to propagate wild ginger in your garden without disturbing a wild stand. First, gently brush away the soil around the base of an established plant. With a sharp knife, *very carefully* remove a 6- to 12-inch section of the underground rootstock with an attached new leaf bud or shoot. You may do this anytime during the growing season, but midspring is best if you want the plant to take hold and remain outdoors during winter. Take up a shovelful of the plant's native soil. At home, select a shaded site near a water garden or find another place in your yard where the ginger will be sure to get plenty of water or watering. Make sure the soil is rich by adding peat moss, leaf mold, and some finished compost. Plant the wild ginger stock about 2 inches deep in its native soil and cover it loosely with a mixture of soil and leaf mold. Then place a thin layer of sphagnum moss over the area and water well. Keep the ginger rhizome damp but not waterlogged. In several weeks the wild ginger should be at least partially tame and growing. This same procedure can be followed to grow the plant in a shallow rectangular or oval clay pot, such as those used for bonsai plantings. The pot must be wide so the rhizomes will have room to spread. The potted ginger can then be kept outdoors or brought into a greenhouse.

Harvest some roots from your wild ginger crop in the fall as the plant's leaves begin to die down. Wash the roots carefully and dry them whole in a shady, warm room. Store the dried roots in tightly covered glass jars, away from light. You can break the dried root into smaller pieces as needed or grind it to a powder.

Wild ginger tastes and smells much like its namesake, the tropical true ginger. Its traditional uses are very similar, too, but the two species are totally unrelated. Wild ginger's relatives are the Virginia snakeroot and numerous other *Asarum* species around the world. The indigenous peoples of America used virtually all these species for treating snakebite. The North American Indians also valued the wild ginger, or Canada snakeroot, for treating colds, chest congestion, intestinal cramping and flatulence, dyspepsia, colic, fever, nausea, and heart palpitations. A tea made of wild ginger was used to wash wounds.

Wild ginger has a spicy, pleasing fragrance that has found its way into some perfumes. The Native Americans and early European settlers savored its fragrant taste in meaty soups and stews, and in bean dishes. They believed the wild ginger's medicinal properties also imparted wholesomeness to these foods, aiding in the relief of flatulence and indigestion. Almost all native tribespeople believed that wild ginger, when used as a condiment, would prevent food poisoning and digestive problems.

A species of wild ginger native to Europe is assigned almost identical medicinal properties by herbalists there. In China, wild ginger is known as *Hsi-Hsin,* or "slender acrid." It is used in that herbal tradition as a diaphoretic, expectorant, diuretic, headache remedy, stomach tonic, and to treat coughs and chest distention.

Wild ginger can be nibbled in its fresh or dried state. You can make an infusion by steeping a small handful of the dried roots in 1 pint of boiled water for 20 minutes. The dried root can be powdered and added to hot water in the ratio of 1 teaspoon per cup. The fresh roots can also be made into a cough syrup. (Follow the directions for Herbal Syrups in chapter 6.)

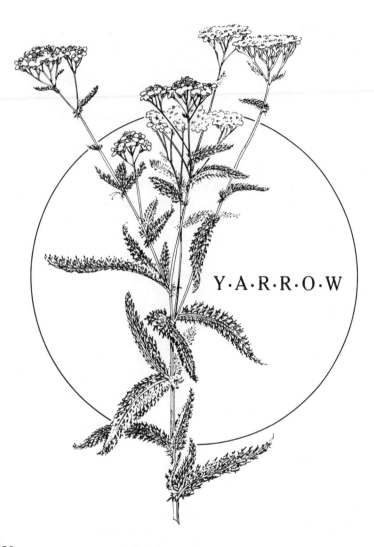

YARROW (Milfoil, Soldier's Woundwort)
Botanical: *Achillea millefolium*

   Mythology holds that yarrow was present on the battlefield with Achilles during the Trojan War, hence its Latin name *Achillea*. More readily verifiable is the plant's appearance–very feathery and fernlike–from which comes its nickname milfoil, a corruption of the French *milles feuilles,* or thousand leaves.

   Yarrow originated in Europe and Asia, but it is now fully naturalized throughout most parts of North America. It grows from 1 to 3 feet tall and is found in fields, meadows, and open woodlands, along roadsides, and in marginal areas. You can easily recognize it in bloom by the pretty, disk-shaped clusters of tiny white, daisylike florets atop its stalks, which look so refreshing in the midst of its green and brown-toned habitats.

There are also orange, yellow, and red-flowered varieties of yarrow, but the ones used most often for medicine are the wild white-flowered variety and sometimes the red-flowered type. Some gardeners say the wild white-flowered yarrow exudes a substance into the soil that is so strong that it prevents even yarrow from flourishing after a few years. They recommend moving the plant to a new location every year. Biodynamic gardeners, however, say that a few yarrow plants in the garden are beneficial to the soil and the garden's whole ecology. They recommend planting yarrow as a border to the vegetable or herb garden and believe it increases oil production in aromatic herbs. Yarrow helps to repel ants, flies, and Japanese beetles in the garden, and it attracts all sorts of beneficial predatory wasps and ladybugs. Planted near building foundations, it is supposed to keep termites away.

Yarrow is propagated from either divisions taken in the spring, or from seeds. Sow seeds on top of very fine soil and keep moist until germination occurs. When the seedlings are 3 inches tall, move them out to the garden bed. Yarrow plants are also available from many herb nurseries. Yarrow prefers a light, sandy soil, but it's a good idea to side-dress it with aged compost in the spring.

Harvest yarrow when the plant is in full bloom. The leaves, flowers, and stems are all used for healing purposes. Cut the leaves from the stems and dry them separately. Because they are so fine, you must dry the leaves quickly, or they will discolor. Be sure that your drying room is warm enough (90° to 100°F). You can leave the flowers on the stems and hang the stems upside down in bunches to dry. Store the flowers separately and cut up the stems into small pieces and store them. If you'd like to harvest the roots, dig them up when you harvest the rest of the plant. After scrubbing them well with water and a gentle brush, spread the roots on a screen to dry in the sun.

Yarrow is regarded as a very good vulnerary and styptic. In fact, its ability to stop bleeding earned it one of its old-time common names, soldier's woundwort. Fresh yarrow leaves have been mashed or macerated and applied directly to wounds. Sometimes the dried, powdered herb is sprinkled over cuts, gashes, punctures, or abrasions. A tea made from the plant's leaves, stem, or flowers is also believed to be beneficial to rashes, skin ulcers, and hemorrhoids.

Not too many people know it, but yarrow has also been used as an anesthetic. The root is the part of the plant that is usually used for this purpose. Backwoods doctors in the past sometimes performed surgery using only fresh yarrow roots, mashed in whiskey, as a local anesthetic. The fresh root or leaves of the plant is also sometimes applied to the gums or teeth to relieve toothache. Fresh yarrow seems to work better than dried yarrow for this purpose.

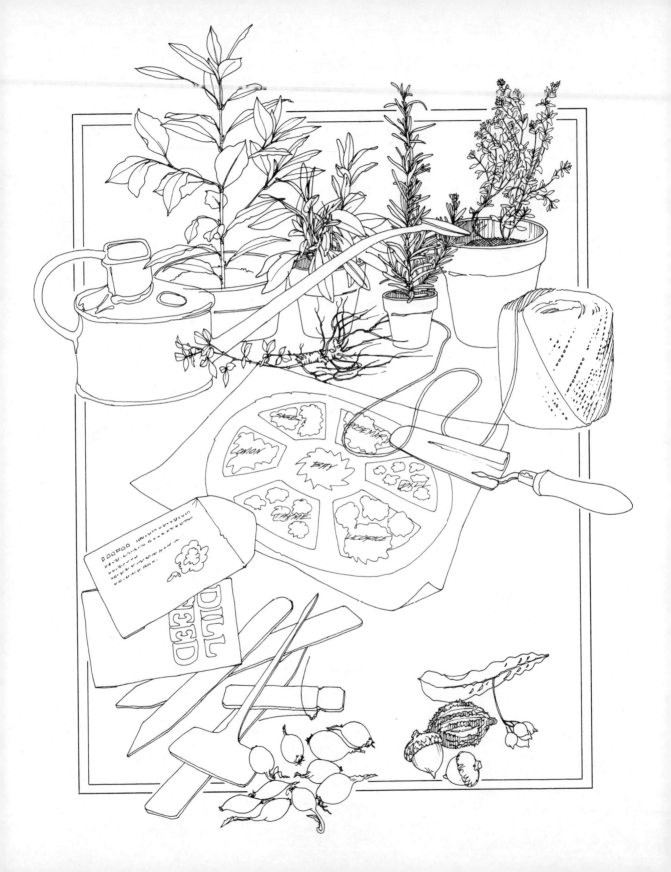

Creating a Garden of Healing Herbs

*M*ost gardens have definite boundaries that set them apart from other facets of the landscape. Within the garden areas grow neatly planted beds of flowers, vegetables, or herbs. From a holistic viewpoint, however, the entire landscape is a garden, a garden of healing. From this perspective, even the smallest garden is also a landscape, and the most expansive landscape is also a garden. Medicinal plants need not be limited by the fences, borders, edges, and rows that normally define garden space. They can spill over from these confines into the yard, the woods, and fields, and into the ponds, meadows, forests, and mountains that surround our homes.

Untaming the Herb Garden

Gardening is sometimes thought of as a way to improve upon nature's vast selection of wild fruits, flowers, vegetables, and grains. As they grow in the wild, or in the semiwild conditions created by natural farming (discussed later in this chapter), plants tend to be smaller, tougher, and more strongly flavored than cultivated varieties. Most of us prefer foods in their cultivated form. A salad made of wild lettuce is strong tasting and bitter, while one made with romaine, butterhead, or loose-leaf garden lettuce is light and tender and mild flavored. Cultivated carrots are large, sweet, and crunchy, but wild carrots are thin, strongly aromatic, and tough. Wild apples are almost always too sour; orchard apples are sweet. Wild roses are small and plain compared to ornamental hybrid roses, which are big and showy and of many different colors and forms. Perhaps bread can be made from the seeds of plantain, dock, and wild grasses, but it doesn't compare in taste or texture to a loaf of good homemade whole wheat bread. For most people, the sublime taste of wild strawberries is not enough to compensate for the tedious job of gathering them. We gardeners prefer the convenience of growing larger berries right at home. In fact, many of our most desirable foods are usually found growing in gardens.

Medicinal herbs are the exception to this rule, at least according to herbal healing tradition. In all parts of the world and throughout the centuries, wild herbs have been held in the highest esteem. Wild herbs have always been thought to possess stronger flavors and higher concentrations of minerals, vitamins, resins, oils, alkaloids, and other constituents than domesticated herbs. Cultivation is good for making vegetables more mild, but when it makes herbs more mild also, herbalists believe that it weakens their healing powers. This may be because herbs grown in the garden are raised as though they *are* vegetables. We pamper and coddle them, weeding, watering, and fertilizing all season long. But the horticulturist's goal of making sweeter, milder, more tender vegetables is the opposite of the herbalist's goal. The herbalist likes medicinal plants that are not necessarily fit to eat. A wild sage plant may be too strong flavored to use in cooking, but just right for an herbal formula. The qualities that make wild plants less desirable in the kitchen are the same qualities that make wild herbs *more* desirable in the medicine chest.

The Chinese say that wild ginseng—perhaps the world's most sought-after herb—is so valuable because of its unique natural habits. Traditionally, they say, the best ginseng plants grew in the Ever-White Mountains of northern China. Here, each ginseng plant developed slowly, often growing for decades or even centuries, reflecting the timelessness and endurance of the mountains themselves. The plants grew in virtual isolation, often only one to each mountain. This lone or "king" ginseng was believed to absorb the power or energy of the entire mountain it lived on. Thus, to the wild ginseng was attributed an

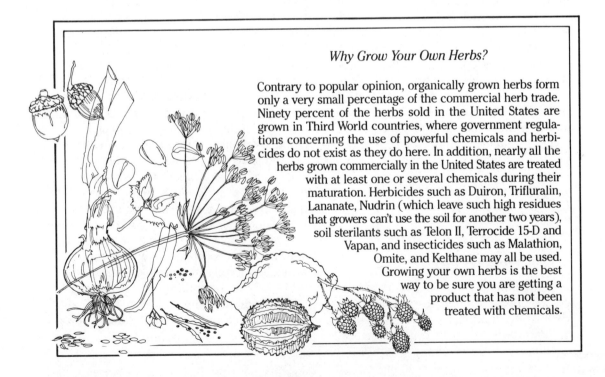

Why Grow Your Own Herbs?

Contrary to popular opinion, organically grown herbs form only a very small percentage of the commercial herb trade. Ninety percent of the herbs sold in the United States are grown in Third World countries, where government regulations concerning the use of powerful chemicals and herbicides do not exist as they do here. In addition, nearly all the herbs grown commercially in the United States are treated with at least one or several chemicals during their maturation. Herbicides such as Duiron, Trifluralin, Lananate, Nudrin (which leave such high residues that growers can't use the soil for another two years), soil sterilants such as Telon II, Terrocide 15-D and Vapan, and insecticides such as Malathion, Omite, and Kelthane may all be used. Growing your own herbs is the best way to be sure you are getting a product that has not been treated with chemicals.

efficacy far beyond that of its crowded cultivated relatives of the flatlands.

There are, of course, other reasons for the traditionally reputed superiority of wild herbs. The fundamental reason is that wild plants grow up naturally. They have to compete for nutrients, light, moisture, and space. Without the helping hand of a gardener only the strongest survive. Left to themselves, wild plants also tend to grow in places that are ideally suited for them, with just the right soil and growth conditions. In gardens, herbs will often grow under a variety of conditions, but in the wild, they are more temperamental about ecological factors. A particular species is found here but not there, or it migrates and changes location after a few years, depending on the successional patterns of the surrounding plant communities. In addition, herbs that grow naturally in the wild are considered more "pure" from the herbalist's point of view. For the same reasons that whole herbs are used instead of isolated purified constituents, herbs taken from natural environments are considered better than herbs grown in garden rows.

Having read this, you may wonder why you should bother to grow herbs at all. Well, for one thing, it is a whole lot more convenient. Sometimes it is difficult or impossible to find the herbs you need growing wild in your locale. And it is better to grow your own than to rely on buying commercial herbs from an unknown source. Also, herbs grown in a garden are still valuable as medicine. Although an herbalist might consider wild herbs ideal, cultivated herbs are still very good. It is a matter of degree and compromise.

Which brings us to the next question: Is it possible to have both the quality of wild

One way to plant an herb garden is in rows like the vegetable garden. This garden contains a row each of dill, borage, parsley, and cayenne.

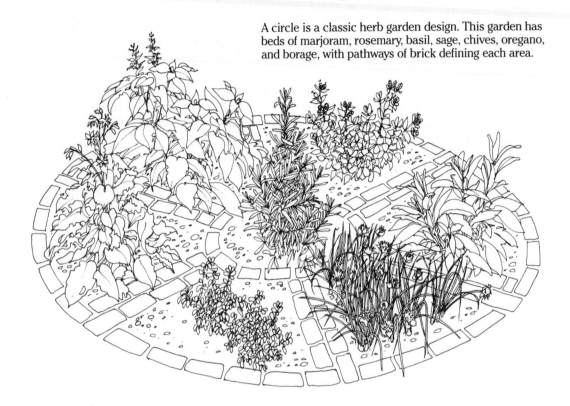

A circle is a classic herb garden design. This garden has beds of marjoram, rosemary, basil, sage, chives, oregano, and borage, with pathways of brick defining each area.

herbs and the convenience of cultivated herbs? We say it is, and what we are proposing is to tame the wild herbs and untame the domestic ones. What do we mean by untaming the herb garden? The process begins in the mind of the gardener with the view of creating a holistic design in cooperation with nature. It is a change in perspective, a reorientation toward gardening and growing plants. It is a process ideally suited to growing medicinal herbs.

There are four main stages of untaming the medicinal garden, and they can be practiced simultaneously, after being developed gradually over a period of years. The first stage is to grow herbs in beds of rows, circles, geometric or random patterns, in much the same way as vegetables are grown. The garden bed has a definite role in many landscapes. It is easy to plan and care for, easy to protect with fences, and easy to harvest from. These kinds of well-defined gardens are attractive and can be located close to the house for convenience and for the visual delight they offer. The particular design and layout of the herb bed can be as varied as the number of herbs being grown and the types of people growing them.

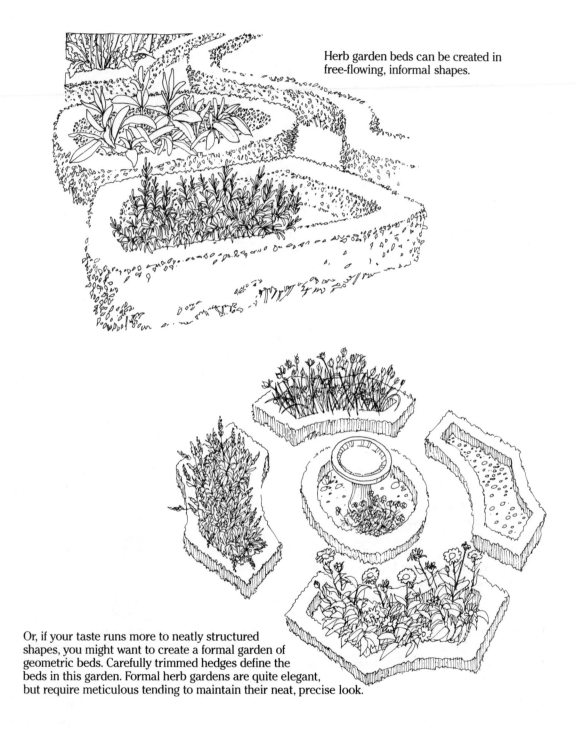

Herb garden beds can be created in free-flowing, informal shapes.

Or, if your taste runs more to neatly structured shapes, you might want to create a formal garden of geometric beds. Carefully trimmed hedges define the beds in this garden. Formal herb gardens are quite elegant, but require meticulous tending to maintain their neat, precise look.

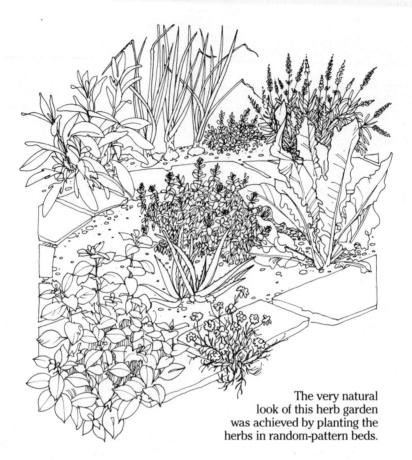

The very natural
look of this herb garden
was achieved by planting the
herbs in random-pattern beds.

The Backyard as a Landscape of Herbs

The next stage or element of the untamed herb garden is the integrated landscape. Here, design elements such as hedges, borders, ground covers and lawns, screens, pools, streams, walls, flower beds, orchards and trees are all seen as potential sites for growing herbs. The idea is to liberate your herbs from the conventional garden bed and spread them all around. Thus, a hedge becomes a bed of lavender or hyssop; borders are planted with mixed groups of herbs like borage, calendula, yarrow, and parsley, or singly with comfrey, mints, or aromatics. The lawn is replaced with plants like bearberry, thyme, pennyroyal, or German chamomile. For a screen, a grove of elderberry, poplar, slippery elm, and birch trees is planted along the edge of the property. A small pool of water is edged with wild ginger, chickweed, licorice, and horsetail, while a little stream draining the pool is planted with watercress. The front and top of a stone wall can be planted with Mediterranean herbs like sage, marjoram, rosemary, and thyme. In the

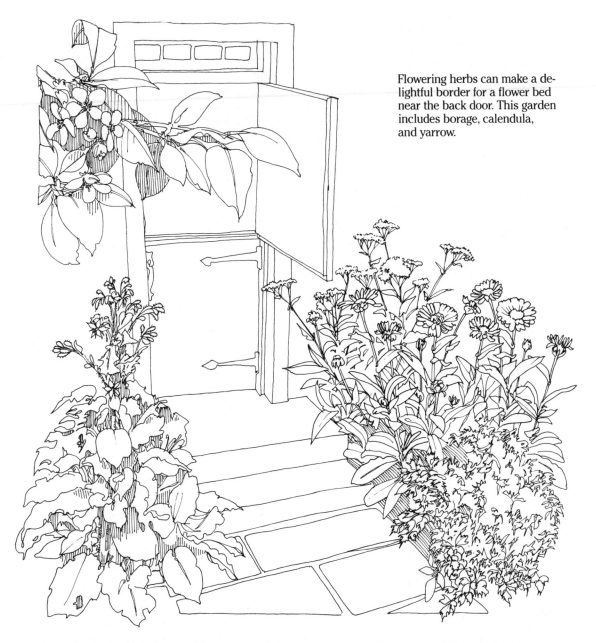

Flowering herbs can make a delightful border for a flower bed near the back door. This garden includes borage, calendula, and yarrow.

flower beds, healing flowers like peony, echinacea, yarrow, and elecampane are planted along with the more conventional ornamentals. A small orchard can include medicinal fruit or nut trees like apple and butternut and can also be home to herbs such as garlic, alfalfa, and clover. A stately basswood tree in the yard attracts bees to the landscape while

providing comfortable shade and a soothing floral tea. Other healing shade trees like
beech, bay, and oak can be planted, too, as
secret members of the medicinal herb garden.
Not generally recognized as "herbs," these
trees nevertheless are valuable as agents of
natural healing.

A landscape like this is naturally efficient because of its many "edges." In ecological terms, an edge is a place where one type
of plant community or geologic feature meets
another. Major edges commonly exist where
a forest meets a field or grassland, along the
banks of rivers and lakes, on the seashore, at
a mountain's timberline, or where a meadow
turns into a marsh. In smaller landscapes like

our backyards and lots, the design elements
described above—beds, borders, groves, walls,
lawns, and the others—create lots of little
edges. It is in these zones, small as they may
be, that life takes off and blossoms with diversity and richness.

The fully integrated medicinal landscape
makes use of vertical as well as horizontal
ecological edges. In fact, the distinguishing
feature of the integrated landscape is its use
of multiple vertical levels. This is in contrast
to most gardens, where just one "story" or
ecological level of growth is utilized: Whether
the crop is firewood, apples, corn, lettuce,
peas, or carrots, vertical space is taken up by
one and only one plant. In nature this is a rare

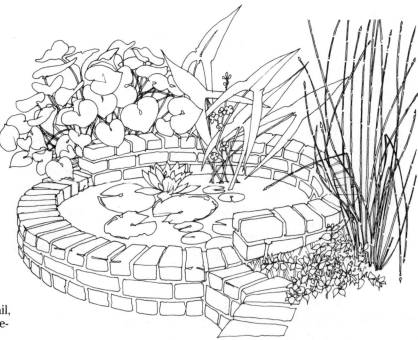

A small backyard
pool can be edged
with wild ginger,
chickweed, horsetail,
and other moisture-
loving herbs.

occurrence. Most natural systems have at least two, and usually three or more, vertical zones of growth. The first story is made up of grasses, ground covers, and low herbaceous plants and flowers. According to the botanical definition of the word, most "herbs" belong to this story. The next level, or botanical niche, is filled with taller herbaceous plants and low

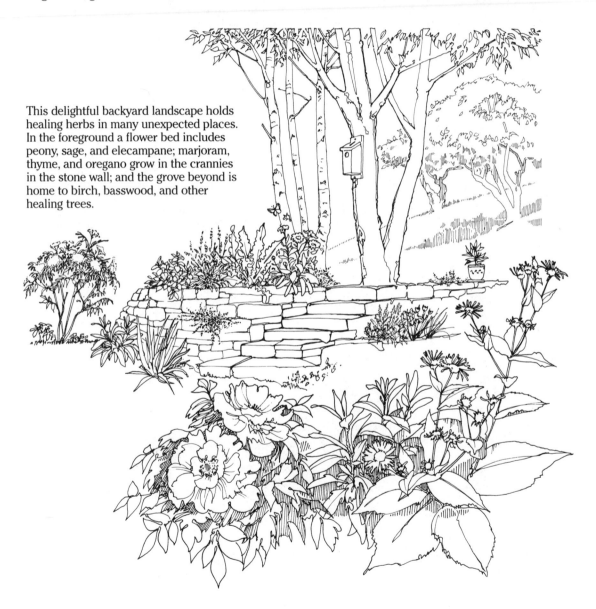

This delightful backyard landscape holds healing herbs in many unexpected places. In the foreground a flower bed includes peony, sage, and elecampane; marjoram, thyme, and oregano grow in the crannies in the stone wall; and the grove beyond is home to birch, basswood, and other healing trees.

shrubs and bushes. A third story is comprised of taller bushes, shrubs and vines and young trees. Mature trees form the upper story, providing shelter and support for the plants and animals below.

Most gardeners think of trees in terms of providing shade or blocking sunlight, depending on which of the two is desired. For the ecological landscape, though, trees are the primary benefactor. In vertical zones of growth, trees define the "contour" of the mature landscape. It is for this reason that trees are so important in planning an integrated landscape. In addition to being valuable healing plants in their own right, trees create the space for multiple levels of plant growth. They

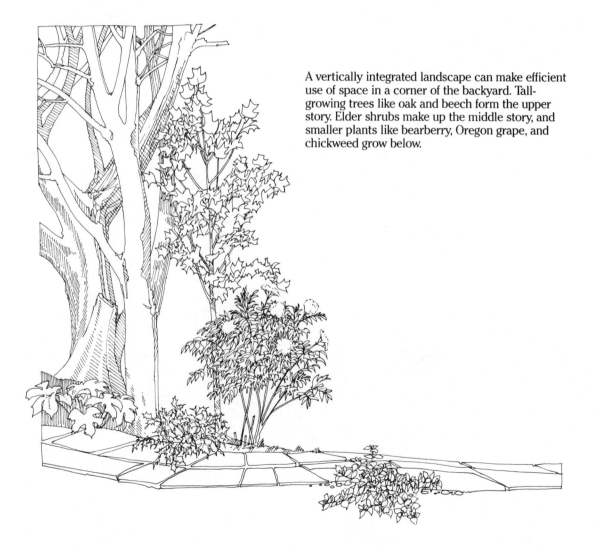

A vertically integrated landscape can make efficient use of space in a corner of the backyard. Tall-growing trees like oak and beech form the upper story. Elder shrubs make up the middle story, and smaller plants like bearberry, Oregon grape, and chickweed grow below.

also modify the environmental conditions—
the light, wind, precipitation, temperature,
and moisture in the soil and atmosphere. And
the presence of birds, animals, or insects in
the landscape is often due to trees, too.

To give you an example of an integrated
vertical landscape, let's say we have a small
stand of mixed medicinal hardwood trees in
the corner of a backyard. There are two oaks,
a beech, a birch, and a poplar. On the edge of
this little grove, and growing into it slightly,
are several elder shrubs. They make up another
story just below the other, taller hardwoods.
Underneath the trees, in the front of the grove,
there is one patch of Oregon grape and one of
bearberry. Growing under the Oregon grape
are little clumps of chickweed. In the back of
the grove, shaded by the taller trees above
and the shrubs in front, are several beautiful
clumps of goldenseal plants. And in between
the goldenseal a few ginseng plants are
flourishing.

The Semiwild Herb Garden

The integrated, planned landscape is only
the second stage of untaming the medicinal
garden. Next comes the semiwild area. This
could be a natural orchard with herbs growing randomly in the understory, as they do in
Masanobu Fukuoka's citrus grove in Japan
(see page 276 to learn more). Or it could be a
vacant field, an abandoned woodlot, a bog, or
swampy area, or any somewhat out-of-the-
way place. In the semiwild garden, size is not
as important as the ability to let nature take
its course. In the semiwild garden, domestic
herbs are allowed to revert back to their primitive habits, while native plants are allowed to
prosper and grow as well. If the semiwild
garden is a field, then an array of herbs like
catnip, mugwort, yarrow, burdock, dock,

chicory, anise, alfalfa, horseradish, mullein,
mustard, and nettles might be sown or planted
randomly, and then left to themselves. In woodland settings, ginseng and goldenseal are perfect semiwild crops. In a marshy area, plants
like licorice, horsetail, pennyroyal, wild ginger,
or spearmint can be set loose on their own.

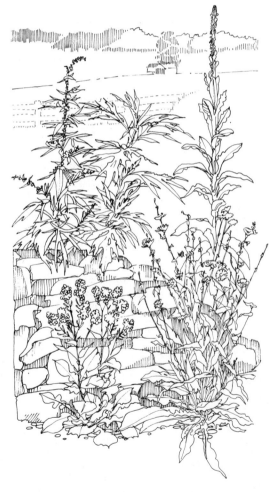

Naturalized clumps of herbs form a semiwild herb
garden in a sunny meadow. This garden includes
clumps of mustard, chicory, mugwort, and mullein.

In their natural state, most herbs follow definite patterns of succession. Some, like plantain, yarrow, chamomile, mullein, and dock, are important pioneers of new plant communities. They help to stabilize, enrich, and penetrate open areas that are too marginal for other plants. Herbs like catnip, gravelroot, blackberry, dandelion, wild sage, and mugwort will follow the early pioneers in colonizing new grounds. Alfalfa, clover, burdock, and the aromatic herbs come a little later, when the soil has been enriched further. And some herbs, like nettles, mustard, and holy thistle, are sure indicators of a relatively rich soil.

The semiwild garden often starts out with an array of herbs growing on their own. The types of native plants present can lend clues about the chances of success for other introduced species. For example, if a field contains only pioneer plants, the introduction of next-stage herbs may be moderately successful. But bringing in later-stage herbs and aban-

Ginseng plants
flourish in the shade of
a semiwild woodland garden.

Herbs from the Wild

The fourth stage of the untamed medicinal garden is made up of all the places where herbs grow by themselves. It is tempting to say this means the wilderness, but this is not quite true. The distinguishing characteristic is *wildness*, not wilderness. When Henry David Thoreau wrote that "in wildness is the preservation of the world," he was referring to the refreshing quality of freedom. Wild herbs are those which are fresh, which are free from the influence of cultivation. They can be found in many places—in fields and forests, in meadows and on mountains, along stream banks and ponds, in marshes, bogs or swamps, in isolated areas and on the edges of towns and cities.

Gathering herbs from the wild places is a transformation of the gardener's skill into the wildcrafter's art. It doesn't offer the rewards of patient nurturing and caring that come with garden growing. It is less controlled, less restrained, like the wild plants themselves. There is an element of the hunt, and the joy of discovery. Wildcrafting is a wonderful way to enjoy nature while reaping a harvest of healing herbs.

doning them to the untamed garden is probably a waste of time and plants. You need to get the soil in better condition before planting the later-stage herbs. On the other hand, a field filled with wild alfalfa, nettles, and thistles may be ripe for its next stage of succession: bushes and trees.

This third stage of the untamed medicinal garden doesn't have to start with an already wild area. It can easily be created from a very tame environment. In fact, many landscaped yards and gardens become semiwild with no difficulty at all, when left to themselves. But there is also a method to the madness. When a wild or abandoned area is "developed" as a semiwild garden, its rate of ecological succession can be increased. In one way, this is the goal of natural farming. Starting with a relatively simple and fragile ecology, the land is brought into maturity through the stages of succession. This kind of wild farming or primitive agriculture is also a very sophisticated way to grow natural medicinal herbs. The principles of natural farming as they apply to herb growing are discussed later in this chapter.

To gather wild herbs, you must know a few things that are not important to the stay-at-home gardener. First, you have to know where to find the plants. The easiest way to do this is to just begin to look. Although this technique sounds a bit simplistic, it forms the basis of wild herb collecting. There are many healing plants all around, but we don't know them because we never bother to look for them. So when you go on walks, rides, drives, or hikes, watch for herbs or herb habitats. Even if you don't see the herb itself, look for a likely place the herb might be growing. If you pass a cool, shaded brook in an open woods, and you have a hunch there may be some

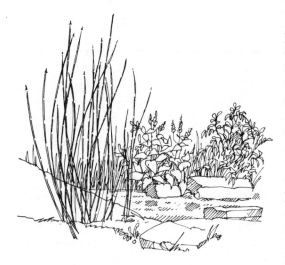

If you have a poorly draining spot on your property, you can plant a semiwild marshy garden with herbs like licorice, horsetail, pennyroyal, and spearmint.

wild ginger or horsetail growing there, stop and look to see if your guess is right. Take a little side excursion. Get into the habit of "hunting" for wild herbs where they grow.

Once you've perfected the art of looking around, *seeing* wild herbs is the next skill to develop. It is easy to be right in the midst of some herbs and not even notice them. If you've never experienced this it may sound a bit funny, but it's true. Herbs are often difficult to spot in their native habitats. There are two techniques that wildcrafters often use. One is to keep moving your eyes and head as you roam the herbal hunting grounds. The eye can focus better and see more clearly if its range and direction are changed frequently. Also, the moving fields of peripheral vision pick up more detail and allow the brain to put together a more intricate composite picture of the landscape.

Another gatherer's technique is to hold a picture of the plant in your mind. It will be easier to recognize that way. And when you find the first specimen in the field, concentrate on it for awhile. Look at it from several different angles. Notice how it blends in or stands out from the surrounding foliage. Then continue to contemplate the plant's appearance for awhile. If the herb is one that is hard to spot, this technique will pay off in making it easier for you to locate other plants. After you've trained your eyes to see, you'll be amazed at how many more plants of the same species are right around you. It's almost as though they just popped up from nowhere. Binoculars also help in spotting wild herb populations, especially in dimly lit woods, on open hillsides, and on distant riverbanks or the shores of ponds.

After you've found an herb, but before you collect any of it, proper identification is needed. This is absolutely critical when you are gathering plants for medicinal use, whether they will be taken internally or used externally. Of course, it helps to have a general sense of what the herb looks like before you set out the door. The easiest way to do this is to have it pointed out to you by someone else whose word is reliable. Books are also helpful. And unless you are totally familiar with the plant in question, by all means have it positively identified after you find it in the field. One way to do this if you have some knowledge of botany is to use the keys in a botanical text or field guide. *Don't underestimate the importance of proper identification.* Every year, well-intentioned people get sick or die by mistaking foxglove for comfrey, or by picking poison hemlock, thinking it is celery or water parsnips. *Never eat or drink a wild herb until you are sure of its identity.* Even then, if it is new to you, just take a little bit and watch your reactions. Allergies to herbs are not common, but they do exist.

The actual harvesting of wild herbs is done in the same way as domestic herbs, with one exception. It is more important to conserve and preserve a wild population of herbs than ones that grow in your garden. Carefully ascertain the relative vigor of the plant or plant community and gather only what you need. If an herb seems strong but is growing in an adverse environment—a windswept ridgetop, for example—then take no more than 10 percent of any one plant or stand. Another important note for wildcrafters: Check carefully to make sure that the land on which you're picking has not been chemically sprayed, as many areas are. Authorities who maintain the area can provide this information to you.

It helps to keep a journal of the wild herbs in your area. As you visit them through-out the year, make notes about their life cycle, appearance, surroundings, and locations. If you want to, you can plot your wild herb finds on a map. By keeping careful records, you can gradually develop an intimate knowledge of the healing plants that grow in your locale. This information will pay off when you make plans for harvesting the bounty of wild medicinal plants.

The only other cautionary note about wildcrafting is this: Make sure you are gathering the plants legally. Most local, state, and national parks have regulations prohibiting the picking of any foliage; wandering onto privately owned land to gather herbs is considered trespass. On private or corporate land, be sure to get permission from the owners before venturing forth into the field. On public state or federal lands, know what the laws are about picking or gathering plants. And never harvest plants that are designated as

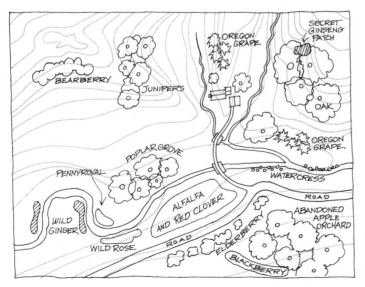

An example of a homemade foraging map showing the location of wild herbs that grow locally.

endangered species. Herbs like ginseng, wild ginger, and goldenseal are completely protected in some states.

The entire issue of gathering herbs on public land is one that is very vague and ambiguous. Technically, it is illegal to take anything out of the national forests without a permit. And yet, every year thousands of pounds of wild herbs are collected on public land and sold by professional wildcrafters. For example, every autumn tons of cascara sagrada bark are collected from public lands in the Pacific Northwest. The bark is sold to herb distributors and pharmaceutical companies for use in laxative preparations. It is an odd situation that falls into a legal and regulatory limbo: Federal agencies have no category for issuing permits to gather medicinal herbs, and they generally don't enforce regulations against it.

This poses two problems for those interested in gathering wild herbs from government land. Because of the lack of regulation, it is difficult to gather herbs legally. And because of the lack of enforcement of the regulations that do exist, the ecology of wild plant populations can be disrupted by overharvesting or improper harvesting. In order to remedy this situation, some herb growers, gatherers, sellers, and users in Oregon are organizing a wildcrafter's trade group. Herbalist Tom Ward says their purpose is to create professional standards of ecological wildcrafting. Through training and certification programs, Ward believes the group should be able to work with state and federal agencies in a management program for public lands. In cooperation with government specialists, the trade group would map wild populations of medicinal herbs and develop guidelines for harvest limits. In return, the government would issue collecting permits for certified wildcrafters. As with the administration of hunting and fishing permits,

fees for the harvesting permits would help pay for the expenses of running the program. As the prices of wildcrafted herbs rise along with consumer awareness of their quality, Ward believes the permit system would be economically viable. And for those not in it for the money, Ward envisions noncommercial permits. These would be for "head of household" type gatherers, who would have to pass a wildcrafting course before being issued a permit.

Ward believes that a similar approach would work well for herb harvesters seeking permission to gather herbs on private land. But whether you are certified as a wildcrafter or not, the important point is to establish a mutually beneficial relationship with the landowners around you. Because you are gathering only for your personal herb supply, perhaps offering the owner some of the finished herbal product will be sufficient return for the privilege of collecting on his or her land. Or you might offer an exchange of some other type, whether it be money, work, or a homemade loaf of bread. The important thing is to value the herbs themselves and the chance to collect the herbs from a wild place. Your respect and appreciation for the plants will be evident in the way you ask for permission to gather them. A little communication and a gesture of generosity go a long way in opening up new fields for gathering.

Planning the Herb Garden and Landscape

An herb garden can be located practically anywhere. If you are just starting out with herbs, you may want to make your first garden small and simple. In fact, you may decide not to have a separate herb garden at all for your first season. You could grow some

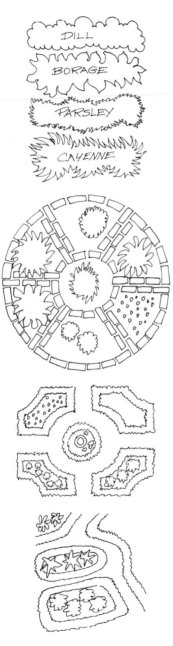

DILL

BORAGE

PARSLEY

CAYENNE

Drawing a plan on paper makes it easier to design garden beds. Shown here are plans for an herb garden planted in rows, a circular garden, a geometric garden and a garden of free-form beds.

herbs in a corner of the vegetable garden or in a section of a flower bed. You could tuck a few herbs into a window box or a container that sits on a patio. The thing to remember is that an herb garden can be as large or as small as your space, time, and level of interest dictate. Before you plow up the whole backyard to create an entirely integrated landscape of healing plants, perhaps you should try growing just a few and expand the garden gradually over a period of years.

If your intention is to create a separate garden for healing herbs, the choice of locations, shapes, and planting patterns is only limited by your imagination. Your herbs can grow in the front yard or back, or along the side of the house. You can plant them in straight rows, curves, blocks, or random patterns. The garden can be square or rectangular, round or oval. It can be triangular to fit in a corner, or gently curved to fill an irregular spot.

In the past, herb gardens were planted in intricate formal designs. If visions of an Elizabethan knot garden or a series of formal geometric beds patterned after an English estate dance in your head, you can work out that sort of elaborate scheme for your backyard garden, too. But consider that although formal herb gardens can be very beautiful, there is also an artificial quality about them. Somehow a garden of plants for healing seems more at home in a more relaxed setting.

If the untamed look of a natural landscape is not for you, you can still look for simple ways to provide shape and structure for your garden. For example, an old wooden wagon wheel laid on the ground could serve as a guide to designing a small round garden of wedge-shaped beds full of your favorite herbs.

After you've settled on a shape for the garden, the process of deciding which plants to put where is the same for herbs as for vegetables or flowers. In combining plants, you need to think about the growing environment and the characteristics of the plants themselves. Here are a few basic points to keep in mind:

The type of soil each plant needs. Does the herb grow best in a light, loose soil or a denser soil? An acid or alkaline soil? A sandy or humusy soil? Does it need soil that drains quickly or one that retains water and nutrients longer?

Light requirements. Does the plant need full sun? Partial shade? The deeper shade of a woodland environment?

Moisture. Will the plant need regular watering and lots of humidity? Or does it prefer a drier location? Would the plant do well in a damp or even marshy environment, like the edge of a pond?

Aesthetics. What is the basic size and shape of the plant? What is its height, growth pattern, texture, color? Will it visually complement the other plants you want to grow?

Uses. When is the plant harvested? (You don't want to complicate your life by putting a plant you'd harvest in fall in front of one that you'll want to pick in spring.) How is the plant used? It might be fun to plant a "headache" garden, or a garden of herbs for the bath, or a "stomach" garden.

The primary guide to keep in mind when planning any herb garden is that if you match the plant to the location, your job as a gardener will be much easier.

Planning a Backyard Landscape

When the garden is extended into the landscape, the planning process itself becomes more extensive. Landscape designers have always known that plants possess visual characteristics that make their selection and placement an art form. But modern landscape designers and environmental site planners also consider the way the landscape and the people or animals who use the landscape interact. These considerations of how plants in a landscape interact with one another, with the environment, and with the users of the landscape are becoming increasingly important today, as landscape planners place more emphasis on ecological factors in design.

In addition to their human uses as food, ornament, or medicine, growing plants provides tremendous benefits to the environment. Some of these benefits are oriented toward serving the needs of man in the landscape, and some serve the entire biosphere of life. They include:

Air purification and oxygenation
Erosion control and soil retention
Glare reduction
Wind deflection
Wildlife habitat
Climate modification
Fire protection
Soil enrichment
Articulation and definition of space
Privacy and pollution screening
Recreation and relaxation

As man is seen to be more and more *a part of*, and not *apart from*, nature, these potential benefits of landscape plants are considered together as part of a single overriding design goal: the direct and indirect enhancement of health values. If you view your landscaping as a process which considers all the benefits plants have to offer, you will be able to make the garden itself into a medium of wholeness and healing.

Assessing Your Backyard Site

The first step in designing an herbal landscape is assessing the site you have available. It's helpful to consider the history of the site—what it's used for now and what was there before you lived there, the type of soil and terrain, your regional and local climate, how much water is available, and what plants grow wild in the neighborhood. If your garden will be planted in a small suburban backyard, this analysis may be quite brief. The larger the landscape you're working with, the more complex are the natural factors affecting design decisions.

The key word in describing ecological conditions is change. Nature is always changing. In a geologic time frame, the earth's changes occur over gigantic time spans— thousands, millions, even billions of years. The creation of mountains and rivers, oceans, lakes, and plains are geologic events whose history awesomely dwarfs the lives of human beings. And yet it is this geology that determines or modifies the landscape's most basic features: geography, soil, water flow, climate, and plant communities. Although it may not be clear at first how geologic information can help in designing a backyard landscape, a little investigation will reveal its value. Geologic factors such as the type and depth of bedrock, whether or not a glacier has ever passed through the region, the presence or lack of lava or magma flows, natural biological barriers of water, mountains, distance or elevation, or corridors through them, and even the slow movement of continental plates all affect the ecology of a region.

The geologic features that most influence landscape planning are categorized under the term "physiography." This word refers to the appearance of the land, the physical form it takes. A physiographic study of a piece of land shows the presence of rivers and creeks, lakes and ponds, flood plains, marshes, swamps, springs, hills, slopes, ledges, and other natural land forms. With this kind of information, the landscape designer can begin to understand the basic constraints and resources of the land.

At this point in the design process, maps become an essential tool. For suburban sites, a simple sketch or plot outline will suffice as the base map. If you want to plant a large garden or landscape with healing herbs, an aerial photographic map or a United States Geological Survey (USGS) topographic map of the land is valuable. Aerial maps can usually be obtained from city or county departments of planning. Topographic maps are sold in some office or outdoor supply stores and in regional offices of the Bureau of Land Management or United States Forest Service.

Once you have a map or sketch of your parcel, make some copies of it. You will use separate maps to identify and plan different design elements, and you will inevitably use up some maps with mistakes and changes in plans. An alternative to the multiple map making process is to use pieces of thin tracing paper taped over the original map, or clear plastic sheets that can be written on. This provides a flexible system of overlays which places separate design elements in a composite picture. You might have one overlay for trees and shrubs, another for herbal lawns and ground covers, and another showing the location of a small pool or water garden. Or, if you plan to plant your herbal landscape over a period of years, you might have one overlay showing the areas you will plant this year, and separate overlays for years to come. The overlay method lets you look at one, several, or all of the design elements together. It also allows you to change single parts of the design more easily. Your local office, architectural, or surveying supply store can help you find the materials you need for making overlay maps.

With your basic map in hand, walk over your backyard, lot, or farm. For larger parcels of land, it is helpful to use a compass, stakes, and measuring tapes or cords to measure the dimensions of the features you will note on your site map. Draw in the natural features as you go. Some things to look for include:

Variations in soil types

Elevation contours

Degree of slopes and hills

Direction and amount of exposure to the
    sun in various spots

Flowing or standing water, including creeks
    and streams, ponds, marshes, bogs and
    springs, irrigation ditches and surface
    runoff channels, and signs of under-
    ground water

Wind direction and speed

Traffic corridors (the pathways traveled by
    deer, rabbits, farm animals, gardeners,
    children, bicycles, cars, trucks, etc.)

Plant communities (meadow, mixed hard-
    wood stand, successional field/forest
    border, orchard, flower beds)

Buildings and structural improvements

Many of these environmental factors will change throughout the year. Prevailing wind directions, for instance, often change from summer to winter, and even from morning to afternoon. A dry summer gulch may turn into a raging torrent in winter. What looks like a trickling spring in May could be a dry hole by August. It generally takes at least a full year of on-site observation to accurately map a location's physiography.

The gradual environmental changes that take place in a region are accomplished by a process called succession. If their natural progression is not interrupted, plant successions eventually lead to stable "climax" plant communities. If you can grasp the direction of ecological development, that is, if you can figure out at what stage of succession your backyard landscape is, you can enhance its natural tendency to achieve stability. You can plant early-stage herbs in the less developed spots or enrich the soil to accommodate the more demanding later-stage herbs. Or, if the natural stability of the ecosystem in your yard has been thrown off balance by human intervention, you can help to set it back on course. While you're walking about your property making notes on your map, think about the processes that created the landscape as it appears now. Whether or not your design fits in with nature's plan for the area will largely determine the success or failure of your gardening or landscaping project. And it will certainly determine how much work is required to maintain the plants.

To illustrate how principles of succession can be used in landscape design, let's take as an imaginary example a small backyard lot somewhere in New England. Research into the history of the site can take the form of either field or academic investigations, or both. A lot of ecological research is first done in libraries. Most cities, towns, and counties have historical societies that keep records of local events. You might be able to find out when the land in your neighborhood was first

KEY

This is a rough model of our yard in Portland, Oregon. Some of it came the way it appears, some we have already landscaped, and some is planned for the future. The front yard is very shallow and borders a moderately busy street. The herb design there is mainly for appearance, fragrance, and air, noise, and privacy screening. The backyard is larger and contains the herbs used for food and medicine. Notice it is an integrated, multipurpose plan that makes use of existing plants and features.

1. flowering plum
2. low variegated border or hedge of ornamental and fragrant plants, including rhododendron, azalea, rosemary, lavender, sage, barberry, hyssop, and peony. Along the sidewalk is a stone wall that holds the bank of the front yard. The herbs planted here are not used for tea or medicine, as they are too near the street. But they do mask the smell of traffic and add their own scents to the wind which comes predominantly from the east.
3a and 3b. instead of a grass lawn, patches of white and red clover and creeping thyme (4a) and chamomile (4b). The lawn is too small here to be used much, so these herbal lawns make it interesting and aromatic.
5. Japanese maple (large)
6. bed of mixed herbs and flowers, including echinacea, calendula, borage, yarrow, and roses
7. mixture of cedar and rhododendron bushes; a privacy and air and wind screen about 8 feet high around the three sides of the house
8. lilac bush
9a. 80-foot cedar tree
9b. 80-foot fir tree
10. low cedar hedge
11. flowering dogwoods
12. bed of goldenseal and ginseng, shaded by house and fence to the south, and fir tree (9b) and dogwood trees (11)
13. elder bushes
14. Oregon grape
15. apple tree
16. peach tree
17. cherry tree
18. blackberry patch
19. Oregon grape
20. lemon balm patch
21. mixed bed of medicinal herbs and ornamentals (like #6)
22. tall herbs and flowers—elecampane, sunflower, comfrey, echinacea
23. large flowering dogwood, dominates backyard (over 60 feet tall)
24. lawn of grass (and moss!)
25. sunken pool in a slight depression on top of a small knoll in backyard; fish and water lilies
26. horsetail
27. wild ginger
28. pennyroyal
29. large white or European birch trees

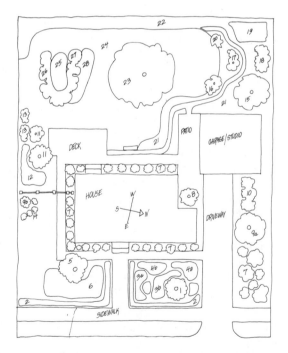

A homemade site map showing your house and property makes planning the herbal garden or landscape much easier.

cleared, whether the site was filled in or not, if there used to be an orchard that was taken out, and all sorts of other relevant information. Let's say you discover that your apparently solid backyard used to be a wet marsh. Checking a geologic map compiled by the local college, you learn there is an impermeable layer of bedrock covered with ten feet of clay. On top of that, your lot was made by adding several feet of landfill. A little further investigative digging reveals that the soil for the landfill came from a nearby open quarry. Looking at the geologic map again, you see that the landfill source is actually a glacial moraine. (That is, a deposit of rock, sand, and soil left by a retreating glacier.) The soil from a moraine is usually high in mineral nutrients but poor in organic matter.

This kind of historical information may seem abstract to the home gardener. After all, a simple soil test could determine what nutrients are present or lacking in your soil. But the ecological perspective adds another dimension to landscape planning. For example, let's say you want to make a pool of water in the backyard. By just looking at the surface soil's porosity, it would appear that a concrete basin is the only way to hold water there. But with the previously gained knowledge of your site, you realize that a little excavation will provide a naturally impermeable basin of clay on bedrock. What's more, by creating a shallow depression in the landfill around the pool, you will be able to easily simulate a bog or marsh for the planting of water-loving herbs like pennyroyal and licorice. Then the excavated dirt can be used to build drier hill contours, upon which herbs like sage, lavender, marjoram, and thyme can be planted.

Site-specific planning is, like nature itself, an organic process. Landscape planning starts with ecological factors, which are easily depicted on multiple or overlay maps. Then more human factors are applied over them, in a further refinement of the planning process. This method of environmental planning is championed by noted landscape architect Ian McHarg in his classic book, *Design with Nature*. Although McHarg's work focused on large areas like the New Jersey shore, Staten Island, and a Maryland valley/plateau region, his methods can also be used in smaller places like suburban yards, rural lots, and farms. Designing with nature is a process of merging the environment, the landscape design, and the people who will use the landscape, in order to maximize benefits and minimize disadvantages. (For further information on small-scale natural landscape design, see *Nature's Design,* listed in the Bibliography.)

Like the landscape itself, human values vary tremendously. It is this individual, subjective quality that makes landscape design a medium of artistic expression. But there are other qualities that make a good landscape besides what looks pleasing to the landscape designer's or gardener's eye. Landscape design utilizes both the forms and the functions of plants. One design system that allows personal preferences to harmonize with ecological priorities was developed by Bill Mollison, the founder of permaculture. His system is based on the use of "zones" and "sectors." In permaculture each lot, parcel, or farm is seen as a miniature ecosystem. Zones are used to map the flow of human energy within that system. Each zone refers to an area and also to the collection of functions that are most central to the life of that part of the landscape.

Zone 1 is the region where the most amount of activity occurs. It is the home, and the area immediately surrounding the home.

For someone who highly values the beauty of flowers, flowers are planted in zone 1. Another person who loves to pick fresh culinary herbs each day would place the herb bed in zone 1, just outside the kitchen door. Other possible uses of zone 1 include vegetable gardens, firewood storage, a driveway and garage, and family recreation areas like saunas or hot tubs, playgrounds, patios, decks, or pools.

Zone 2 is the region of activities that may require daily attention, but which do not need to be located right next to the house. Design elements in zone 2 might include chicken sheds, greenhouses, workshops, compost bins, windbreaks, orchards, and garden areas for crops that aren't harvested daily.

As one goes farther from the home, the permaculture zones change, according to the land and the land use of the area. Zone 3 is the border area, the back of the backyard, or the fields, ponds, or livestock grazing area of the small farm. It supports a mixture of human, plant, and animal activity, with an emphasis on the decreasing role of humans in the landscape. Zone 4 is the region of little intervention: it is the woodlot, the semiwild herb farm, the forest plantation. Zone 5 is the region of the least human intervention. It is the wilderness or wild areas that border some remote rural properties.

Theoretically, the zones should form concentric rings around the home. Actually, though, each site, each backyard, or parcel of land will have a unique zone pattern that may not resemble concentric rings at all. In fact, there is no standard permaculture design.

Sectors in permaculture are maps of interrelated design functions. Various factors such as sun exposure, wind direction, drainage, transportation needs, and wildlife corridors are incorporated into sectors. For example, the woodlot might be located in the wind direction sector of the landscape, so that it serves as a windbreak.

Permaculture is one approach to landscape planning that is in itself infinitely diverse. And there are also other systems of landscape design, each with a slightly different emphasis. But all forms of design with nature are based on respect for organic processes. In the following sections of this chapter we will look at some of the specific design elements that you can consider when you plan your herb garden and landscape.

Flowers in the Healing Garden

Flowers give beauty to the garden. Their striking colors and hues gladden the heart and uplift the spirit. Their lovely shapes and textures are a delight to behold, and their fragrant scents are delicious and wonderful. Flowers reach out to the core of our being with a touch of peace and purity, of beauty and joy, and of harmony. The impression of flowers in the garden landscape is in itself healing.

The healing influences of flowers affects more than the field of our senses, too. Many flowers are used directly in healing teas or syrups, baths or poultices, along with the other parts of plants. Several healing flowers are discussed in chapter 4. And flowers also have some special uses of their own.

Manufacturers of perfumes and colognes have known for centuries about the subtle effects of floral scents. That these fragrances have been used specifically for healing purposes has been less known. Called aromatherapy, the use of flowers and other scents in holistic healing is an ancient tradition in many cultures. It is based on the ability of delicate scents to sway the physiological, emotional, and mental moods of people. The use of perfumes to arouse sexual attraction is only one branch of aromatherapy. Flowers also embody many other influences, such as joy, peace, inspiration, clarity, strength, purity, and harmony. These sorts of meanings have been attributed to flowers by the people of many cultures. Shakespeare knew of them,

and his plays contain many references to the qualities attributed to various flowers.

One of the twentieth century's greatest experts on the subtle influences of flowers was known simply as "The Mother." Born and raised in France, she later emigrated to India and married the famous philosopher, poet, and teacher, Sri Aurobindo. Throughout her life, The Mother spent much of her time contemplating flowers. To her, flowers represented the simultaneous beauty of physical and spiritual existence: "Life must blossom like a flower, offering itself to the Divine," she wrote.[1]

The Mother assigned psychological and spiritual significances to hundreds of different flowers. She explained that a flower's significance is not something the flower itself creates. "There is a mental projection when you give a precise meaning to a flower," she wrote in *Flowers and Fragrances*. But each

A garden of healing flowers can be a beautiful addition to the backyard landscape. This garden mixes elecampane, lavender, chamomile, clover, and sage in a lively display.

SOME FLOWERS USED FOR HEALING

Flower	External Uses	Internal Uses
Apple blossoms	———	Infusion for sore throats and colds, as a diuretic.
Basswood flowers	Baths for insomnia, anxiety, nervousness, irritable children.	Tea as a nervine for insomnia, cramps, indigestion.
Calendula	Ointment for sores and wounds; lotion for bee and wasp stings. Powdered flowers used to soothe skin rashes.	Infusion to induce perspiration, treat toothaches.
Chamomile	Infusion/bath for irritable children.	Tea as a nervine and to relieve indigestion.
Red Clover	———	Infusion for colds, asthma, and bronchitis.
Elder flowers	Cosmetic water for skin; infusion for irritated skin; baths for anxious people.	Tea to induce perspiration, for influenza, sore throats, colds.
Lavender	Pillows for restful sleep; compresses to relieve headaches or cold symptoms; calming or antiseptic baths.	Tea as a nervine to soothe sore throats and colds, stimulate appetite, relieve flatulence.
Mullein	In oil, to treat earaches, bruises, piles.	Infusion for respiratory problems.
Peony	In skin wash.	
Yarrow	Tea for rashes, skin ulcers, piles, sores.	———

flower does have a "special vibration," an essence or quality that can "answer, vibrate to the contact of the projection . . . if you feel it, you get an impression which may be translated as a thought."[2]

Some of the plants discussed in chapter 4 were among those studied by The Mother. She attributed the following meanings to these flowers:

Aloe	Dreams
Basil	It fills the heart with joy
Calendula	Perseverance
Chicory	Idealism
Clover	Kindness of nature
Elder	Charm
Ginger	Strength and purity
Peony	Contemplative beauty
Sage	Aspiration for wisdom

The Mother often gave specific flowers to friends and students as personal aids to wholeness and healing. These flowers were meant to be gazed upon, their fragrances inhaled and their subtle impressions contemplated. It was, and still remains, a simple and direct way to appreciate flowers. But healers have also devised other mediums of flower therapy. Most notable among them is the use of flowers in homeopathic preparations. In the 1930s, an English physician named Dr. Edward Bach developed this healing use of flowers. A successful allopathic and homeopathic doctor, Bach came to view disease as a disharmony of the whole person, which simultaneously affects the body, mind, and spirit. Bach felt that physical health could be restored by creating inner harmony. For this, he turned to the harmonizing influence of nature's flowers.

Dr. Bach left his medical practice in 1930 and began experimenting with distillations of flower essences. He conducted experiments on himself to test the remedies. When he had finished, he had categorized 38 different flower essences. Today, the medicines created in Bach's forest and meadow laboratory are known as the Bach Flower Remedies. Taken in tiny doses over a period of months, the flower essences are designed to correct imbalances in the personality that lead to illness. The remedies, according to Bach, do not "cure" a disease directly. Rather, they work holistically. By increasing the person's inner strength and awareness, the flower remedies make it easier to focus on areas where change is needed. According to the system Dr. Bach developed, beech flowers cultivate tolerance, acceptance, and understanding of differences. Mustard flowers cultivate joy, serenity, and peace of mind. Willow flowers increase one's ability to accept responsibility and release

blame. Clematis increases the ability to be grounded and present, which leads to inspiration. As emotional patterns change in the ill person, new flower essences are given to continue the process of healing.

Today, the Bach Flower Remedies are very popular in Europe and have gained some popularity in the United States as well. New flower essence remedies are emerging, also. Richard Katz, founder of the Flower Essence Society, in Nevada City, California, is currently developing flower essences from a variety of plants. Some of these include:

Blackberry	Creative power of thought
Borage	Cheerful courage
Chamomile	Inner harmony and calm
Red clover	Decreases one's susceptibility to the emotionalism and hysteria of others
Sagebrush	Purification of what is inessential
Yarrow	Brings protection from harm by reliance on inner strength

Katz, who has worked extensively with the Bach Flower Remedies, calls the flower essences "health catalysts which can energize our own health process."

Herbs in the Perennial Garden

Perhaps the most dramatic of plantings is a border or bed of perennial flowers. Creating a perennial flower garden is a task that can take years to perfect. But when it is done, what a wonderful sight it is, as year after year flowers of varying heights, shapes, and hues bloom in succession from early spring to late autumn.

A border can be planted along a fence, wall, building, or property line. Borders can be planted on both sides of a path or can be curved around the edge of a lawn. In England, where the flower border originated, it was planted along the long side of the property to give a feeling of spacious depth. Sometimes, borders are designed with shrubs as a background. These not only provide a leafy backdrop for the colorful patterns of the flower border, but they also give support to tall flowers at the back of the border, which otherwise might lean or topple. Where the edge of a flower garden meets a lawn, it is a good idea to line the border with flat bricks set adequately below the surface level of the lawn. That way, when the grass is mowed, the flowers will be somewhat protected. Low-growing, flowering herbs like Roman chamomile or thyme can be planted at the front of the garden to ramble over the bricks.

Choosing flowers for the perennial border or bed is a very personal business, and the final arrangement certainly represents the preferences of the gardener. Flowers are chosen according to height, color, and time of blooming, so that the garden has a continuous display. Also, make sure that basic conditions of soil, light, water, and climate are met by the floral candidates of your choice. It is good to keep principles of companion planting in mind as well, especially if the flowers are to be used in health preparations. For such applications, you certainly do not want to spray the flowers with anything in order to keep back insects.

When arranging flowers in a border, most gardeners set the largest plants in back and graduate down to low-growing flowers in the front part of the border. For beds that can be seen from both sides, it makes sense to place the tallest flowers in the middle, with shorter ones on either side of them. Often, it takes several years of moving this and that flower clump into another location for the gardener to achieve the desired effect. Most plants make the best showing when planted in clumps of three or more. Flowers should not be planted in straight rows, but in groupings that create a rhythm and pattern when the final border is viewed.

Herbs are wonderful mixed into the flowering border. They add their own lovely flowers to the mix, and many of them also have insect repellent properties. Flowering herbs to try in your perennial garden include borage, echinacea, elecampane, hyssop, lavender, lemon balm, mints, peony, rosemary, and yarrow. If you live where the climate is warm, you can also grow aloe, ginger, and calendula (which will self-sow in mild regions) in your perennial beds and borders.

Trees in the Herbal Landscape

It is no accident that a great tree stood at the very center of the Garden of Eden. Trees are the oldest and largest living things on the planet and have held an important place in the mythologies of many countries. For people in the ancient world, trees embodied and symbolized what was substantial, enduring, majestic, useful, and even mysterious. Trees were revered and respected in ancient cultures. The Hebrews, for example, had injunctions against destroying the trees of those they conquered. And many old cultures held the tradition of the sacred grove, a healing place in which the natural qualities of various trees could be appreciated and used for rejuvenation.

SOME TREES USED FOR HEALING

Tree	External Uses	Internal Uses
Apple	———	Bark used to treat nausea and flu symptoms; fruit as a digestive aid.
Bay	———	Infusion as general tonic, to dispel gas.
Beech	Infusion to bathe skin irritations, burns, sores, swellings.	———
Birch	Oil as topical treatment for rheumatism; poultice for wounds and skin irritations; tea as antiseptic, scalp wash.	Tea as a diuretic.
Butternut	Bark to treat rheumatism, headache; leaves to treat sore muscles.	Bark as laxative; tea as a general tonic.
Oak	Decoction to treat bleeding gums, piles, as a footbath; poultice for wounds.	Decoction of bark to treat diarrhea.
Poplar	Compress for arthritic inflammations.	Decoction for general weakness, diarrhea, urinary tract infections.
Slippery Elm	Poultice to treat boils and wounds.	Eases intestinal irritations, sore throat, cold symptoms, nervousness.

In addition to the powerful psychological image they portray, trees play a vital role in our planet's ecology. They provide over half of the world's oxygen supply. They hold the earth in place with their roots. They are masters of transpiration, continually drawing water up from the ground through their roots, pulling it upward through trunks and branches, and sending it out into the air through their leaves. An acre of 40 apple trees can transport a remarkable 450 tons of water from the soil into the atmosphere in one month.

Trees can add a great deal more to the backyard landscape than just shade and fruit. A line of trees can define property boundaries or serve as a windbreak or privacy screen. Some trees offer fragrant blossoms in spring or brilliantly colored foliage in autumn. Trees can be appreciated for their forms and shapes, for the textures of their bark and leaves. Some trees bestow special favors, like the stately basswood with its masses of blossoms so beloved by bees. As the uppermost story in an integrated landscape, trees serve as visual anchors and support for the lower-growing plants. They provide a haven for birds, a place to climb or hang a swing. Trees are a wonderful addition to the healing garden.

Insects and Birds in the Garden

In the four directions were the four medicine mountains. Between the mountains were charming valleys with various beautiful flowers and lakes and pools with water. . . . The mountains were thickly covered with jungles of medicinal plants. To improve the medicines celestial birds and wild animals lived there joyfully without harming each other.[3]

The quote above describes the ideal medicinal garden, according to Tibetan medicine. Not to be found on this earth, it is like the Western version of the heavenly garden in which "the lion shall lie down with the lamb." In the gardens we humans plant, not all creatures are so beneficial for plants or for each other. We often find mixed blessings in the presence of insects and birds in the garden environment. But these creatures are not only unavoidable, they are also an indispensable part of our planet's ecology. Recognition of this truth has led many people to view farming and gardening as a process of nurturing the earth and its creatures, as well as growing food for people. As Henry David Thoreau said in his famous book, *Walden*, "These beans have results which are not harvested by me. Do they not grow for woodchucks partly? . . .

The true husbandman will cease from anxiety, . . . sacrificing in his mind not only his first but his last fruits also." This attitude yields fruits of its own, including patience, observation, and responsible stewardship of the earth.

A book about healing herbal gardens would be incomplete without mentioning bees. For gardeners who have the time and inclination, beekeeping provides a very rich *(continued on page 270)*

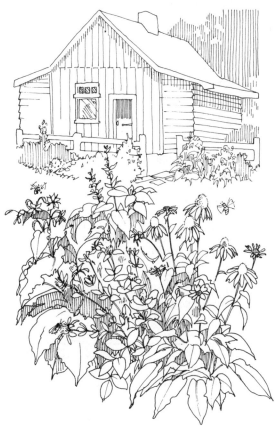

Flowering herbs will attract bees, which are beneficial in any garden or landscape.

Gardening Can Be Healing, Too

People who garden usually find it a richly rewarding experience. There are so many benefits that come from working with the earth and the plants. To many, it is a relaxing and calming pastime. It is a good form of exercise, and a creative act. It nurtures the sense of joy that comes from participating in the ever-changing miracle of life.

In a holistic sense, it is therapeutic to garden. But saying so is like saying that plants grow from seeds. Most gardeners intuitively understand the therapeutic value of their avocation. Recently, though, the idea that gardening is therapeutic has been attracting specialized attention. It has resulted in the emergence of a new field of holistic treatment called horticulture therapy. Horticulture therapy today is an exciting acknowledgment of the benefits that come from working with nature in the garden. It is an effective, simple way to bring joy and a sense of personal fulfillment to the emotionally ill and physically handicapped.

Horticulture therapy began as an independent discipline during the seventies, through programs developed at the Menninger Foundation in Topeka, Kansas. One of the movement's initiators, Andrew Barber, noted at a 1979 conference on horticulture therapy, that:

before psychiatry became a science, physicians prescribed gardening as therapy for emotional and nervous symptoms . . .

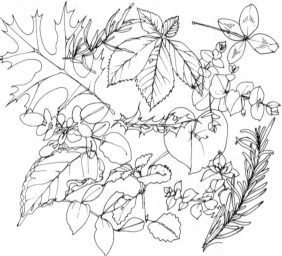

Horticulture provides a meaningful emotional experience because it deals with life and the life cycle . . . Another explanation of the powerfully therapeutic effects of horticulture may lay in the ease with which it lends itself to the projective tendencies in all of us. There is ready propensity for plants to become extensions of our human experience, almost as though they are extensions of our personality.

In his address to the conference, Barber also spoke of the primal nature of man's connection to the earth and the soil. "This intuitive understanding about the relationship between people and earth is perhaps why the most regressive patients often find their greenhouse or gardening activity the point at which their emotional renaissance begins," he said.

Many institutions and individuals are beginning to use horticultural therapy. It is popular in nursing homes, drug rehabilitation programs, halfway houses, nurseries, and school programs in many parts of the country. There are a number of pioneering programs in the Pacific Northwest. One, in the Snohomish Valley of Washington State, involves developmentally disabled adults. Becky Burns, the horticulture therapist associated with the program says:

> The average age of the gardening clients I work with is 40. Many of them have been institutionalized for many years. They have been dependent on the system and on others all their lives. Here in the garden the dependency roles are reversed, however. Many who cannot care for themselves take pride in the fact that a plant needs them. A lot of the clients wish they could have had children. Here they are finally able to care for and nurture a plant as if it were a child. They experience an emotionally meaningful relationship dealing with living plants and their life cycles.[13]

The people involved in this garden project not only grow, but also harvest and market their vegetables to local restaurants, receiving a salary for their work. For many, it is the first paying job they've ever had. This, combined with the healing power of working within the garden, has considerably raised many of the participants' self-esteem and spirits.

The healing power of the garden is not new, of course. About 2,500 years ago, Hippocrates discussed the relationship between cultivating the earth and cultivating inner wholeness. He wrote:

> Instruction in medicine is like the culture of the productions of the earth. . . . our natural disposition is . . . the soil; the tenets of our teacher are . . . the seed; the instruction in youth is like the planting of the seed in the ground . . . the place where the instruction is communicated is like the food imparted to the vegetables . . . diligent study is like the cultivation of the fields; and it is time which imparts strength to all things and brings them to maturity.[14]

But old truths put forth new appearances, according to the needs of the times. Now, horticulture therapy is emerging as an important new field for professional health care service. Colleges and universities across the United States offer degrees in horticulture therapy. Information on horticulture therapy as a career is available from Edmonds Community College, Department of Horticulture, 20,000 68th Avenue W., Lynnwood, WA 98036.

addition to the garden ecology. Bees provide the invaluable service of pollinating flowering plants. There are 5,000 species of bees in North America. Most of them pollinate only wild plants, but several hundred species pollinate cultivated plants. Over 100 different species of bees, for instance, pollinate alfalfa. Bees have a wonderfully beneficial influence on any garden.

Even if you don't want to keep bees, we still recommend encouraging their presence in the landscape. Basswood trees are especially good for attracting bees. Fortunately for the herb gardener, bees are very fond of the flowers of many herbs, including clover, borage, echinacea, thyme, comfrey, lemon balm, basil, catnip, chamomile, chicory, fennel, hyssop, lavender, marjoram, rosemary, anise, alfalfa, and mustard, to name only a few. Old hollow trees, abandoned sheds, and even commercial bee hives can attract and hold wild bee swarms, a bonus for the gardener who doesn't want to "keep" bees, but who appreciates their presence nearby.

Except for bees, beneficial insects are usually considered to be those that eat or destroy insects that are garden pests. The subject of insect pest control is vast and beyond the scope of this book. We will not go into the subject in depth, but suggest that you consult a good book, such as *The Encyclopedia of Natural Insect and Disease Control,* edited by Roger B. Yepsen, Jr., or *The Bug Book,* by John and Helen Philbrick. Both books are listed in the Bibliography.

The best approach to protection from insect damage is prevention. The value of prevention in the garden can be compared to the value of prevention in human health. Even though contagious diseases may exist in the environment, a healthy person is not as likely to catch them as someone who is run down and weak. While this approach to insect control is insufficient in the short run, especially for the gardener who is only beginning to work with poor soil or spare environmental conditions, it is something to look forward to and to work for.

Until the time when your garden obtains a full stage of health, you will probably want to use some specific organic or natural pest control methods. These should be used judiciously, and you may feel after a few years that it is actually more worthwhile to spend time building up the richness of the earth and diversity of plants and animals, than attempting to combat insects directly.

Birds in the Herbal Landscape

The old-time tradition of allowing free-roaming farm birds in the garden seems to be enjoying a revival in many areas. Many kinds of chickens will keep down garden insects without damaging crops. Small varieties, which don't compact the soil, and birds with small feet or a moderate scratching habit, are best for the herb garden planted in beds and rows. Larger birds are suitable for orchards and semiwild meadows or woodlots. Even geese and peacocks can be valuable in keeping down insects. In addition, geese are good "watch birds," and peacocks are beautiful. The decision to keep domestic birds, though, must take into account the gardener's ability to care for them properly. In even slightly rural areas, this includes protection from predators like skunks, raccoons, snakes, coyotes, bobcats, foxes, and predatory birds. As with protection of plants, the best method of protecting domestic fowl is prevention. For birds, this takes the form of well-built coops, perimeter and overhead fencing, and personal supervision of roaming and roosting cycles.

Probably the most efficient insect-controlling birds are wild birds. Recent agricultural research has shown conclusively that many songbirds significantly decrease insect populations in the small integrated garden. (They do not, however, have that effect on large monocropped areas, because of the absence of cover and the presence of chemicals.) Birds eat enormous amounts of insects and their eggs. In one feeding, a red-winged blackbird can eat 28 cutworms. A yellowthroat can eat 3,500 aphids an hour. A yellow-billed cuckoo can ingest over 2,000 webworms in one feeding. There is hardly a more effective form of natural insect control than birds.

Owls must certainly be mentioned at the top of the list of helpful birds. Not only do they eat insects, but they also control the local rodent population. Woodpeckers help control codling moth. Bluebirds will nest in holes in apple trees and have a voracious appetite for insects. So do wrens, and neither bluebirds nor wrens will eat fruit!

Try inviting wild birds into your garden by creating appropriate landscapes. Barn swallows, chickadees, tanagers, and many other birds will be attracted to your orchard and garden if there is enough plant variety, as well as sufficient cover in the form of trees and bushes. Smaller birds thrive in mixed edges and borders: hedges, small trees, berry bushes, shrubs, and meadows or pastures. Birds of prey like tall trees in undisturbed areas. A nearby woodlot or small grove of mixed evergreens and deciduous trees is ideal, especially if it is near a stream or pond. A natural corridor leading to more wild regions will help attract both large and small birds. Although wild birds will occasionally eat seeds and fruit, their net assets to a garden or farm far outweigh the potential crop losses from a varied bird population.

Building Nesting Boxes for Birds Why not set out some suitable birdhouses, to further attract birds to your orchard and garden? When building birdhouses, it is important to construct them so that the resident birds can get in, but their enemies cannot. This is not a problem with owls, but it is definitely crucial for the smaller birds, whose only slightly larger neighbors can sometimes be the death of them.

Screech owls' nests need a floor 8 inches square, with the entrance 9 to 12 inches above the floor. The entrance hole should be 3 inches in diameter. Place the nest in a tree 10 to 30 feet off the ground, or in the corner of a barn. Barn owls need nests with a floor about 10 by 18 inches, and the whole structure should be 28 inches tall. The entrance hole should be 6 inches in diameter, at least 4 inches above the nest floor. Hang the structure at least 12 feet off the ground.

Bluebird houses need a floor 6½ inches square. One important element: To protect the baby birds from predator birds, the distance between the entrance and floor should be 12 inches. Although most bluebird house designs call for a larger entrance hole, many bird fanciers say that an entry hole 1⅛ to 1¼ inches is big enough for the bluebirds and will keep out English sparrows. (The more aggressive sparrows will steal the nesting site from the bluebirds if given the chance.) Both bluebirds' and woodpeckers' nests can be cheaply made from hollow branches, with top and bottom sawed even and covered with a piece of wood. If you put a bluebird house on a post, sheathe the post with tin to keep away cats and raccoons, and make sure the house is at least 5 feet off the ground.

Farmer and writer Gene Logsdon suggests as a good resource on birds and their place in the garden and orchard, a book titled *The Bird Book* by Charles P. Shoffner, published in 1932 by Frederick A. Stokes Co. Logsdon was an editor of *Farm Journal* magazine at a time when that periodical championed the use of wild birds for protecting crops, and he has a lot to say about the beneficial role of birds in the garden in his own book, *Wildlife in Your Garden* (see the Bibliography). Although the Shoffner book he recommends is currently out of print, your local library may have a copy or can locate a copy for you. A retail or used book dealer can also search for an available copy.

Growing Methods

Three methods of organic gardening are especially well suited to herb gardens and landscapes into which herbs and healing plants are integrated. In this section, we will explore those three methods. Two of the methods are usually thought of as agricultural, but they are useful to herb gardeners who want to create an integrated and perhaps a naturalized or semiwild landscape on their property. Each of these systems requires careful observation as a prerequisite for success. From direct experience of natural cycles, the gardener is empowered with a deepening understanding of nature's play in the garden.

Biodynamic Gardening: Amplifying Nature's Abundance

Biodynamic gardening, developed in Europe in the 1920s and 1930s by Rudolph

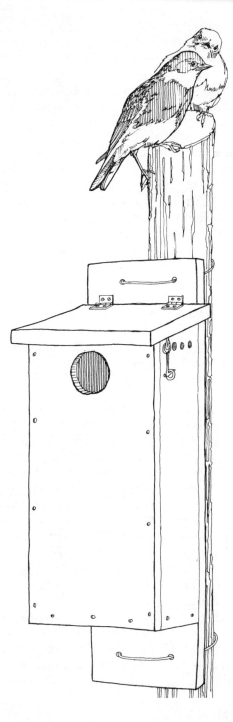

A bluebird house.

Steiner, is simultaneously a system of gardening, a philosophy, and a way of life. It was brought to this country by master horticulturist Alan Chadwick, who was tutored by Steiner himself. The philosophical basis of the method is the concept that "abundance is there naturally, we don't make it. It is simply there. We can destroy it, however. Giving as little as we can to get as much as possible results in a product devoid of totality and full of self."[4]

By aligning himself with the workings of nature, the gardener finds that "nature and creation flow through his work and bring about matters and cornucopias of produce about which he had no thought or vision when he began," according to Chadwick.

Those who have seen gardens created by these methods know the assertion is true. But how does it work? Biodynamic gardening is certainly an attitude toward nature and the garden, but it also employs a number of basic techniques. One of these is double-digging, which is done to create well-aerated, deeply cultivated soil.

Raised beds, from 3 to 5 feet wide and up to 20 feet long or longer, are another aspect of biodynamic method. On these raised beds, plants are spaced very close together. Because they grow in such proximity, the leaves of the plants mingle together to form a "living mulch," which helps slow the evaporation of moisture from the soil. While this system popularized the use of raised beds and intensive plantings, it did not invent them. Similar gardening techniques were practiced in Greek hillside agriculture 2,000 years ago, and in Chinese alpine agriculture as far back as 3,000 years ago.

As do gardeners in some traditional cultures, biodynamic gardeners plant by the moon. They also employ a sophisticated system of companion planting and use both weeds and herbs to strengthen and assist crops. Field sprays and compost preparations, developed according to indications in Steiner's foundational lectures, are an integral part of biodynamic gardening, too. Herbs are used in these preparations: yarrow, nettles, oak bark, chamomile, valerian, and dandelion. According to Steiner's guidelines, the preparations are supposed to correct imbalances in the soil, much as the tiny dosages of homeopathic medicine are believed to correct disease in the human body. Oak bark, for instance, provides "plenty of calcium," as Steiner tells us, "77 percent of the plant substance."[5] According to biodynamic techniques, chamomile is used to activate calcium and sulfur in the soil, while yarrow is employed to catalyze a combination of potassium and sulfur. Steiner characterizes the stinging nettle as a beneficial jack-of-all-trades, which brings the minerals potassium, calcium, and iron into the soil. Following Steiner's directions, the herb preparations are buried in the ground for specific periods of time and then applied to the compost heap.

Despite its apparent complexity, biodynamic gardening incorporates some features that make it particularly appealing to the grower of healing herbs. It uses a system of subtle elements and properties, just as do most natural healing systems. As Chadwick himself noted in one of his California lectures:

That life is partly governed by [subtle] forces . . . , and that the earth is a living thing, are both true statements, though many will vehemently deny them. Both are of supreme significance to our understanding of the garden. Without them, we reduce horticulture in general to mechanical tinkering, and cultivation in particular to the business of breaking clods of earth.[6]

(continued on page 276)

A Water Garden Surrounded by Herbs

Water gardens, whether formal or informal, are a wonderful addition to the overall garden design. They attract birds, frogs, and many other creatures that are beneficial to the whole environment. Small ponds and pools are a good way to catch and hold moisture where it is needed, in both the soil and air. Water in the garden helps to moderate temperature changes. Moving or standing bodies of water in the garden landscape also add a soothing, harmonizing influence that encourages a healthy state of mind.

Even the smallest garden can contain a body of water constructed in a large wooden tub or half-barrel, at least 15 inches wide and 15 inches deep. To make this type of miniature pool, bury the container in the ground and place a 6-inch layer of rich, well-rotted compost at its bottom. In this growing medium, you can plant either a water lily or water hyacinth. When you are finished planting, cover the compost with a layer of clean sand to keep the water clear. Then, add water to the tub gradually, running it down the side of the tub in a fine stream to assure that the bottom soil and sand is not stirred up. Total depth of the water should not be more than 2 feet for water lilies. When the little pool is surrounded with a ring of flat stones, it makes a pretty feature in the garden.

Water gardens are happy, relaxing places. They work best set into secluded areas of the garden. If there are no quiet, out-of-the-way places in your garden, try creating one with plantings of small trees and shrubs behind and around the water garden. When planning this type of plant screen, remember that trees and shrubs should be kept far enough away so that their leaves do not fall down into the water. The leaves of acacia, eucalyptus, and pepper tree are heavily acid and can injure pond fish, so they should be avoided entirely in the vicinity of the pool. Other trees' leaves may not be as harmful, but they can be unsightly as they fall into the water, obscuring its surface and making the pool difficult to clean. Don't avoid trees entirely, however. If there is a large oak, elm, chestnut, or

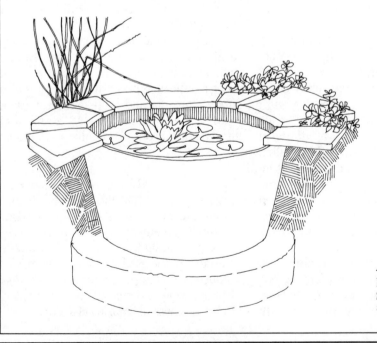

A simple water garden can be planted in a wooden tub or galvanized washtub that is sunk into the ground.

other shade tree on your property, consider designing the water garden in proximity to it. The relaxing shade of the tree nearby can add a lot to the water garden. A fence or hedgerow can help keep leaves that have dropped to the ground from blowing into the pond. Once you've selected a quiet, pleasant site, one which is exposed to the sun and has available water nearby, it's time to look at construction details.

The pool should have a rounded bottom. In sandy or gravelly soils, concrete is always used to create the pool's form. It can be wider at the surface than the bottom to prevent the concrete from cracking if the water freezes. Concrete is usually not needed with clay soils, though, because the impermeability of the clay acts as its own sealant. If cement is not used in clay soil, the bottom of the pool is compacted with a heavy tamper. Grazing animals like cows are sometimes used to trample and compact pond bottoms while the ground is wet.

When concrete is used in construction of a pool in clay soil, the pool is dug out 12 inches deeper than the desired finished depth. You should allow 6 inches for a layer of cinders for drainage, and 6 inches for the concrete. Flexible materials such as linoleum or benderboard can be bent several layers thick and then pegged or braced in place to create the irregular outline of the pool. The edges should be braced with reinforcing rods and wire mesh. If you plan a pool larger than 3 feet wide, use reinforced concrete throughout to prevent cracking. The walls should be about 4 inches thick. Tubs for planting water lilies are set into place and concete poured around them. Pockets or cups for shallow water plants can also be poured with concrete 3 to 4 inches below water level and filled in later with soil.

Pools, unless they are very small, should have an available supply of incoming water, from a spring, stream, well, or reservoir. (Regular tap water can be used, but it is best to avoid putting chlorinated water in the garden pond.) Plumbing can be kept simple. The piping for the incoming water and another pipe for overflow are all that is needed. In order to conserve water, some people design their pool so that they can simply recycle its water, using an electric pump and storage tank.

Ponds can be any length or width you choose, but they should be at least 18 inches deep, especially if fish are going to be stocked, or water lilies planted. If the water level is less than 18 inches, the water may overheat in summer, killing any fish in the pool. If it is more than 24 inches, it will be too deep for planting water lilies. Goldfish or mosquito fish, such as rice fish (*Dryzias latipes*) and gambusia (*Gambusia affinis*) add a good deal of beauty to the pond, the mosquito fish also act as natural controls for what might otherwise be a mosquito problem.

Marsh plants, bog plants, and aquatics all do well in the water garden. Marsh plants grow along the banks of streams or ponds, where they have plenty of moisture and a light soil. Purple loosetrife, purple cinquefoil, and chain fern are examples of marsh plants. Bog plants, including umbrella plant, bog bean, and skunk cabbage, grow in mucky soil with little drainage, where vegetation is decomposing. Some plants can be grown in either environment. They include sweet flag, narrow-leaved cattail, royal fern, great blue lobelia, crested fern, marsh fern, wild ginger, Egyptian papyrus, and marsh marigold. Many types of rushes are available for water garden plantings, too. Aquatic plants have roots which are submerged under the water. These include water lily, watercress, water horsetail, water poppy, and pickerel weed. Water-loving herbs like licorice, pennyroyal, angelica, and parsley can be used at the edges of the garden, too. A little farther away, plant ginseng or goldenseal. Some species of iris and bamboo also look very beautiful at the edges of ponds.

If you plan to keep fish in the pond, it will help to include some submerged plants that give off oxygen to the pool. Fanwort and loosestrife are two that are free-floating. They can be held in place by anchoring them to side pockets or water lily tubs.

At the water edge, set in marsh plants of varying heights, clustering them in several areas and leaving the rest of the border open, so that people can enjoy a good view of the water garden. The parts of the pond edge that are not planted with marsh plants can be edged with natural flat stones. In between the stones, plant aromatic herbal ground covers like creeping thyme or chamomile.

Biodynamic gardening is one of the only agricultural systems that recognizes the subtle element properties of nature and highlights them in the garden. Most other systems of agriculture completely ignore these special qualities. Or in cultures that do acknowledge the subtle element qualities, as do Native Americans, Chinese, and Tibetans, the people rely on nature itself to display them and value the wild places where pleasing displays of elements exist already. In many herbal traditions, such as in Tibetan medicine, herbs are almost always gathered in the wild rather than grown in the garden. But by using biodynamic gardening principles, the gardener can relate to the subtle factors of a plant's growth, as well as the plant's use in natural healing. For those who appreciate its philosophical view, and who enjoy the challenge of gardening in this way, the biodynamic approach can be very rewarding.

Permaculture

As we discussed earlier, the system of agriculture created by Tasmanian ecologist Bill Mollison is often referred to as a design process. Indeed, permaculture combines aspects of ecology, economic botany, horticulture, landscape architecture, forestry, animal husbandry, and hydrology, along with other less tangible factors. Permaculture is sensitive to the mutually enhancing relationship of the wild and the cultivated. It emphasizes perennial, native plants, intensive land use, diversity and richness in plantings, the integration of wild with cultivated species of both plants and animals, sensitivity to landforms and microclimates, and a long-range view of the garden and the entire place that is the garden.

The system is not relegated strictly to use on farmland, either. Bill Mollison, visiting and lecturing in New York City a few years ago, outlined ways to create roof gardens and vertical greenhouses up the south walls of high buildings. Permaculture is a design process which assesses each landscape and ecosystem in a systematic, individualized way. Taking into account the needs and wishes of the people in relation to the place, a map of resources and constraints emerges.

From the map of resources and constraints, using brainstorming, overlay drawings, or an experimental approach, a design begins to emerge. During its application, there is constant review of the design, based on how it's working in place. After some reassessment and renewed experimentation, a design usually stabilizes. Once the stabilized design is applied and enriched, the system begins to maintain itself to a higher degree. That's one of the goals in creating a sustainable landscape—to develop enough diversity and permanence that the system nearly maintains itself.

The other two systems we are discussing in this chapter, biodynamic gardening and natural gardening and farming, may never enjoy the broad-based popularity of a system such as permaculture. Both contain elements that are more philosophical in nature, and this tends to define their audience along those lines. But it is unwise to attempt to be prophetic concerning cultural trends. It seems more important to us to encourage all of these beneficial gardening systems. Each of these approaches, correctly applied, certainly creates wonderful natural herbal gardens and landscapes.

Natural Agriculture: "Do-Nothing Farming"

The third method that can readily be applied in creating backyard herbal landscapes is known as natural agriculture. Masanobu Fukuoka has been developing his system of "do-nothing farming" for the past 30 years, on family land on Japan's southernmost island. Since the publication in English of his book *The One-Straw Revolution*, Fukuoka's philosophical attitude and practical application have become one of the most discussed developments among organic gardeners interested in a holistic, regional approach to gardening.

Fukuoka gradually developed four principles in his natural farming system. They are: no cultivation, no chemical fertilizer or prepared compost, no weeding by tillage or herbicide, and no dependence on chemical pesticides. In the years he has been farming, the soil at the Fukuoka family farm has continuously improved in texture, fertility, and ability to hold water. Horticultural experts from all over Japan, and increasingly from other countries, come to see his work. "Technical experts have also come here, seen the weeds, seen the watercress and clover growing all around," Fukuoka writes, "and have gone away shaking their heads in amazement."[7]

Masanobu Fukuoka is perhaps the first applied agricultural ecologist. Believing (as do both biodynamic gardeners and permaculture designers) that the best control of plant disease and insects comes from a healthy environment, Fukuoka set out to create a garden setting as rich and varied as nature itself. In the process, he has invented a new way of relating to crops. It resembles the establishment of complete ecosystems, whose member species just happen to be food and medicine to man. His fields are miniature forests, with an actual organic soil that accumulates each year.

In orchards that have never been pruned, vegetables and herbs grow in the earth among the trees. In the orchard are not only fruit trees, but also acacia trees, which fix nitrogen in the soil, as well as pine and cedar trees. Fukuoka says:

> In growing vegetables in a 'semi-wild' way, making use of a vacant lot, riverbank, or open wasteland, my idea is to just toss out the seeds and let the vegetables grow up with the weeds. I grow my vegetables on the mountainside in the spaces between the citrus trees.[8]

Fukuoka's natural agriculture methods are ideally suited for growing the best cultivated or semicultivated herbs. But that is not his only goal. "Unless people become natural people," he writes, "there can be neither natural farming nor natural foods."[9]

And so Fukuoka continues to work the land, serving as an inspiration and teacher to young people who come from far and near to study and live with him.

Working with the Earth: Garden Soils

There is something deeply satisfying in improving the soil. There is certainly plenty of reason for this—the soil is one of our most precious resources. Because herbs are so varied in their soil preferences, it isn't possible to give guidelines on how to build a soil that's good for all herbs. We will discuss basic soil considerations here, but see chapter 4 for information on the soil and cultural needs of individual plants.

What are the characteristics of a good soil? It has excellent texture, structure, and porosity. A healthy soil smells wonderful, is spongy and crumbly, well textured and aerated. It is also full of beneficial soil life, and by its health it deters noxious soil organisms from inhabiting it, much as a healthy human body repels disease germs naturally. A healthy soil contains not only hearty populations of earthworms, but also such tiny creatures as bacteria, and such growths as actinomycetes, algae, fungi, and protozoa, whose complex interrelationships with each other and the soil itself make it clear that the living soil is a world in itself. All of these organisms have a part in decomposing organic material in the earth, and so enriching it.

Sandy soils and clay soils are less than good; they represent an imbalance of the ideal soil ecology. Few gardeners are presented with good soil when they first begin gardening on a piece of land. They have to work with the qualities of either sandy or clay soil and improve them. Clay soils contain a tremendous variety and amount of mineral nutrients, in most cases. But it is difficult for plants to utilize the nutrients in a clay soil, because the soil structure is so dense.

There are many techniques for lightening clay soil organically. One, recommended by gardening experts Bargyla and Glyver Rateaver, entails plowing rice hulls into the clay, working them down to a depth of 3 feet. The Rateavers recommend using enough rice hulls so that the soil resembles rice hulls with clay bits adhering to them. Then they suggest continued additions of organic amendments, until the soil is one-half organic material and one-half the original amended clay. Decomposition can be hastened, the Rateavers say, by spraying the amended soil with a tea made from manure and stinging nettles, soaked in pure water for a week or more, and diluted to a pale color. Commercially prepared bacterial cultures can also be used.[10] The following year, the land is tilled again, and a leguminous cover crop planted to enrich the soil by fixing nitrogen, and if it is a deep-rooted crop, by bringing nutrients up from the subsoil with its long roots.

Japanese farmer Masanobu Fukuoka regenerated a hillside of "bare red clay so hard you could not stick a shovel into it" by planting nitrogen-fixing trees, and by sowing a mixture of alfalfa and white clover. It took several years for the nitrogen-fixing plants to take hold; then he added deep-rooted daikon radish to the ground cover to help aerate the soil and make channels in it. Crop rotation and companion planting are also used to enrich and maintain the soil.

Sandy soil actually lacks nutrients, unlike clay soil, which has nutrients in a structure too compacted to allow absorption by plants. There is only one way to enrich sandy soil, and that is by continually adding organic materials such as kitchen wastes, manure, leaves, and green manure to it. These materials, and others listed in the composting section, will work wonders within two or three years' time. Although it is a lot of work, any committed gardener will agree that the result is well worth it when one day he gathers a handful of soil, which once was only sand, and finds it is now spongy, sweet-smelling, and alive with goodness.

Cultivation

There are as many notions of how to cultivate the soil as there are systems of gardening. Many gardeners use farm machinery to cultivate, but biodynamic gardeners think machinery is too heavy and compacting on the soil and prefer to till by hand to keep the soil well aerated.

Still other gardeners, who follow a no-tillage philosophy, think tillage itself is completely unnecessary and destructive. In *One-Straw Revolution,* Japanese master gardener Masanobu Fukuoka says:

When the soil is cultivated the natural environment is altered beyond recognition. The repercussions of such acts have caused the farmer nightmares for countless generations. For example, when a natural area is brought under the plow very strong weeds such as crabgrass and docks sometimes come to dominate the vegetation. When these weeds take hold, the farmer is faced with a nearly impossible task of weeding each year. Very often, the land is abandoned.[11]

But even such a staunch advocate of no-tillage agriculture as Masanobu Fukuoka agrees that unbalanced soils must be tilled once, at the beginning of their restoration. After this initial tillage, nitrogen-fixing legumes and trees, and deep-rooted plants are sown and planted to continue the job of regenerating the soil. Once humus is reestablished, the no-till gardener may choose to sow either in rows or in semiwild random-sown intercropping.

The biodynamic gardener will set to work "double-digging" the soil of his garden, carefully separating the topsoil from the subsoil while he does so. Double-digging is not really such a new idea. The ancient Greeks noted 2,000 years ago that plants flourished in the earth moved by landslides; the soil there was well aerated, loose, able to absorb warmth, moisture, and nutrients easily.

In the biodynamic approach to cultivation, breathability is important. As master gardener Alan Chadwick liked to say, when we cultivate the soil, what we are really cultivating is the air. Double-digging aims to cultivate deep (two spades deep, or about 24 inches is considered good), breaking hardpan layers and allowing the movement of subterranean moisture and gases upward, and the movement of moisture and gases from the air downward. For more information on double-digging, consult a reliable book, such as *How to Grow More Vegetables* by John Jeavons, or *Getting the Most from Your Garden,* by the editors of *Organic Gardening.*

Testing Your Soil for Nutrients and pH

Testing your soil for nitrogen, potash, and phosphorus, and to find out its pH level can save a lot of time and money. You can arrange for a soil test to be done through your local Cooperative Extension Service office. They can provide you with information on collecting the necessary soil samples from your garden and land.

If you learn that your soil's pH is too high, you can add a layer of decomposed pine needles, oakleaf mold, or acid peat moss. To raise the pH level, add dolomitic lime to the soil. Well-made compost is the most balanced substance you can add to the soil: a thoroughly aged compost helps to correct both acid and alkaline conditions naturally. When sufficient organic materials are added to the soil, plants tend to tolerate a wider range of acidic or alkaline conditions in the soil and still remain very healthy. The chart Organic Nutrient Sources lists other materials you can add to your soil to correct deficiencies of nitrogen, phosphorus, and potash.

ORGANIC NUTRIENT SOURCES

The materials listed here can be added to soil along with plenty of compost to boost the levels of the three major nutrients. Many of these organic materials also contain other minerals and trace elements in addition to the primary one they supply.

Nitrogen Sources

Animal manures
Blood meal or dried blood
Fish emulsion or fish meal (also contains phosphorus and potassium)
Cottonseed meal
Leaf mold

Phosphorus Sources

Bone meal (also contains nitrogen)
Rock phosphate

Potassium Sources

Granite dust
Greensand (also contains some phosphorus)
Seaweed (also contains some nitrogen and phosphorus)
Wood ashes (also contain phosphorus)

elements. The volcanic soils of the Cascade Range in Washington and Oregon, for example, are much lower in selenium than soils in other parts of the country. Medical research is discovering more essential health uses for trace minerals and elements all the time. So it is good "health insurance" to make sure your garden soil is rich in these vital substances.

Techniques used commonly by organic gardeners, such as composting, mulching, and applying soil amendments like seaweed and fish fertilizers, all help to maintain the presence of trace elements in the soil. There are also specific plants that act as accumulators of trace elements. When these "weeds" are intercropped, composted, or used as green manure, they are especially useful in regenerating the soil. Stinging nettle, for instance, accumulates sulfur, potassium, calcium, and iron. Chamomile concentrates calcium, sulfur, and potash in its tissues. Dandelion concentrates potash and zinc. Valerian increases phosphorus in its vicinity. In China, plants like these are placed directly on the soil for crop fertilization. Sir Albert Howard's famous Indore composting method, which is discussed on page 281, also uses green plants mixed with leaves, hay, and manure.

Trace Elements and Soil Deficiencies

Trace elements are naturally present in humus, and they are essential to a healthy soil. Many soils today are precariously out of balance due to overuse of chemical fertilizers and other improper farming procedures. And some soils are naturally low in certain trace

Composting

Any discussion of soil regeneration would be incomplete without a mention of compost. Compost is garbage heading toward a rebirth as humus. Grass cuttings, weeds, garden residues, such as vines and stalks, hay, leaves, sawdust, kitchen scraps (but not meat or bones), sewage sludge, manure, nutshells, and other organic wastes, such as leather dust, coffee wastes, vegetable pulp from a juice company, or brewery wastes, are all excellent candidates for the compost pile.

There are two basic types of composting: anaerobic (without air) and aerobic (with air). Aerobic composting is faster and is more commonly used. The three methods we will describe here are all aerobic methods.

The Indore Compost Method   Sir Albert Howard, whose agricultural research in Indore, India, served as a foundation for the organic gardening movement, developed a composting method that is regarded as the most classical aerobic technique. It is known as the Indore method. The compost can be made in either open piles or bins. Piles are usually made so that they measure 6 feet wide, 10 to 30 feet long, and 3 to 5 feet high. A 6-inch layer of plant wastes is set down as a foundation for the pile, covering the entire area over which the pile will be built. This layer can include leaves, sawdust, spoiled hay or straw, wood chips, or garden residue. After that, 2 inches of manure and animal bedding are added to the pile. A layer of topsoil about ⅛ inch thick follows next. Then lime, phosphate rock, granite dust, or wood ashes can be spread over the earth layer. The pile is watered, and layers are repeated in the order given until the pile is 3 to 5 feet high. It is important that the pile retain its aerating qualities. To provide ventilation, several pieces of wire netting formed into tubes are vertically in the center of the heap, about 3½ feet apart.

Within several days, the pile will heat up and begin to decay. It can be turned with a pitchfork in two or three weeks, and again about five weeks after being made. The compost will be ready to use in three months.

Compost in 14 Days   You can also make a compost that will be decayed enough to be applied to the garden about 12 to 14 days after the pile is begun. All the organic material must be well shredded in order for this method to work. The shredded materials are mixed together and stacked into a pile about 5 feet high, but no higher. The heap should be turned every two to three days, until the compost is finished.

Biodynamic Compost   The biodynamic compost preparations are made from six herbs: yarrow blossoms, chamomile blossoms, stinging nettle, oak bark, dandelion flowers, and valerian flowers. These preparations are inserted into the compost pile in order to help ripen the compost and increase its ability to hold nutrients. A teaspoonful of the appropriate preparation is inserted into a 20-inch-deep hole, slanting downward in the compost pile. The holes should be made halfway up the compost heap. The stinging nettle preparation requires 4 to 5 teaspoonsful, but each of the others requires a level teaspoon, not heaping. Then the holes are filled in and closed with organic matter.

Biodynamic gardeners like to locate their compost piles near an oak tree, because the oak provides a beneficial environment under its branches and allows the creation of good soil in its vicinity. Piles are located at least 6 feet from the tree trunk, to avoid creating the potential for disease in the tree.

Nitrogen Fixing

Of the three main elements needed for the soil's health, nitrogen has the most dramatic effect on plant growth. Plants cannot directly absorb the nitrogen mixed with oxygen in the air. Instead, they depend upon nitrogen-fixing bacteria in the soil to make it available to them.

The tremendous power of lightning flashes has the capacity to fix nitrogen in the soil, and some scientists theorize that it was this contact between lightning and soil that actually allowed the first life to develop on planet Earth. The reliable underground action of nitrogen-fixing bacteria is a much more common way to enrich a nitrogen-poor soil, however. Nitrogen-fixing bacteria flourish on the roots of over 1,350 species of leguminous plants, such as clover, alfalfa, vetch, peas, and beans. Some trees are also nitrogen fixing, such as acacia, red alder, and autumn olive. There are also nitrogen-fixing shrubs, which can be planted in hedges around gardens and orchards to increase soil fertility.

Cover crops such as clover and alfalfa are often cut and turned into the soil before they have flowered, releasing abundant nitrogen in a matter of weeks. This practice of green manuring is an ancient one and has been employed in many cultures. Sometimes, rather than turning the nitrogen-rich plants into the soil, gardeners make a mulch of them. Sometimes they add the cut legumes to the compost pile. Whichever way the plant is handled, the eventual result is the same: more nitrogen in the soil.

Some legumes can be sown in the late summer, and they will grow through winters where the temperature does not go below freezing. They include winter vetch, rough pea, fenugreek, sour clover, crimson clover, bur clover, and Austrian winter pea. There are many more legumes which flourish in the summer. Alfalfa is one of the most common. Some others are crotalaria, which can be used in poor sandy soils, in southern climates; red clover, good for cool temperate climates; lespedeza, used in southern climates a good deal; and cowpea and sweet clover, which grow almost anywhere.

Mulching

Spreading mulch over garden soil retains moisture, keeps down weeds, protects plants from too much heat in summer and too much cold in winter, and fertilizes the soil. Some gardeners have made mulching into a real art. Ruth Stout, a leading proponent of the no-digging method of gardening, used only mulch to fertilize and protect the soil in her garden, with great success. She used 6 to 8 inches of loose straw mulch year-round on her garden, pulling the mulch aside to plant, and then pulling it back around seedlings once they sprouted. The mulch layer, said Stout, is a "constantly rotting compost pile," which replenishes soil nutrients and keeps weeds down. If a soil has been depleted, most gardeners feel that it must be built up by digging in compost before beginning the no-digging mulch system.

Masanobu Fukuoka, who originated "do-nothing farming" in Japan, is also a proponent of mulch as a fertilizer and soil conditioner. He advocates a thick layer of mulch, as did Stout. What can be used for mulch? Practically any organic material – straw, shredded leaves mixed with straw, sawdust mixed with soybean meal, grass clippings, cornstalks, cocoa hulls, rice hulls, buckwheat hulls, cut up corncobs, alfalfa hay, and pine needles are some of the most used mulches. Mulch can be used to good advantage in the vegetable, herb, and flower garden, in fields, and in orchards. Many gardeners grow cover crops such as soybeans, millet, buckwheat, rye, vetch, clover, and alfalfa and cut them for use as mulch. Some gardeners also add a thin layer of seaweed or kelp to their mulch, as it is rich in minerals.

In fact, one thing to consider is the nutrient quality of the mulching material. Straw, corncobs, and sawdust are low in nitrogen and benefit from being mixed with leguminous mulch. Pine needles are acid, as are oak leaves, and do not make a good mulch for plants that need a neutral or alkaline soil. Strawberries like them, though, as do azaleas, rhododendrons, bearberry, and trailing arbutus.

Propagation Techniques for Herb Gardeners

There are four basic methods of propagating plants. They are growing them from seed, making root divisions, making cuttings, and layering. To be successful with any of these methods, it is wise to begin by observing the properties and the growth habit of the plant you want to propagate. The more you know about a plant's habits, the easier it will be to propagate it. Propagation methods for individual plants are recommended in chapter 4. In this section we will discuss the basics of how to do them.

Growing from Seed

Plant seeds are prodigious, long-lived, and very energetic. In nature, seeds are propelled out of plants by the force of seedpods bursting. They are carried on the hair of animals or in the bellies of birds or by the wind for long distances, seeking a new home. Some seeds can be planted almost as soon as they are harvested from their parent fruit. Other seeds go through a period of dormancy before they become viable and ready to germinate.

Some seeds need to be stratified in order to ripen and become viable. Stratification provides the cold temperatures that the seeds would ordinarily experience in nature over a winter dormant period. Seeds that require stratification must be cleaned, soaked for between 24 and 49 hours, packed in a moist medium such as sawdust or sphagnum, and refrigerated for from one to four months, depending on the species. Some seeds have even more elaborate dormancy requirements and need not just a period of cold temperature, but alternating periods of warm, cold, and warm temperatures. A third type of dormancy is provided by a very hard seed coat, which is impermeable to moisture until it is scarified, or nicked. Some horticulturists use a small file to scratch the seedcoat or drop this type of seed into simmering (not boiling) water to soften it. Even seeds that do not actually need soaking to germinate can benefit from a little soaking in lukewarm water. It livens them and prepares them for germination.

Most seeds germinate best in a neutral, porous soil medium. (A few plants, such as rhododendron, like acid soil for germination, but these are definitely the exception.) Materials such as sand, vermiculite (expanded mica), perlite (a volcanic product), peat moss (from swamps), sphagnum moss (from bogs), crushed granite, and sterilized soil are used in germination mediums. The medium should be light, but substantial enough to allow the seedlings to grow erect, with their roots held firmly. One good starting medium is mixed of equal parts of sphagnum moss and crushed granite. (Sphagnum moss is a favorite material for starting mixes, because it is very resistant to the fungus responsible for damping off in seeds and cuttings.) Seeds should be sown in rows at least 1 inch apart. Here is a general rule for determining how deep to plant: generally, the depth to which a seed is planted is equal to its vertical dimension.

Water the growing medium well before planting the seeds. Place the flat in a warm place, preferably around 70°F. Seeds need to be misted several times a day until they germinate. When they do, inspect the seedlings carefully for any signs of damping-off fungus. If plants appear damaged, separate them out carefully and destroy them. Biodynamic gardeners spray chamomile tea, which has been steeped a day or more, on germinating plants to prevent damping off. The spray should be applied in a mistlike manner to avoid damaging the tender growth.

The main perils in germinating seeds, aside from development of the damping-off fungus, are letting the medium dry out and not keeping the temperature warm enough. If you are careful to avoid these conditions, you should be able to help nature produce many healthy seedlings.

Biodynamic gardeners give their seeds baths in special herbally based preparations. According to proponents of the system, spraying seeds with weak solutions of the various biodynamic compost preparations speeds germination of healthy plants and inhibits development of fungal diseases. Biodynamic gardeners also advocate use of rainwater in watering seeds and seedlings. This is because rain, as it falls through the air, picks up trace amounts of nitrogen (remember, air is mostly made up of nitrogen gas). The biodynamic

experts say that seedlings can assimilate this nitrogen readily, and that it strengthens the newly sprouting plants. The use of rainwater, however, would not be a good idea where there is a lot of pollution nearby or in the direction of prevailing winds.

Biodynamic gardeners plant their seeds by the moon. They point out that subterranean moisture rises in the soil during the two weeks of the moon's waxing. At the full moon, the greatest amount of moisture is brought up in the soil by the gravitational pull of the moon. Seeds that take a long time to germinate are planted at the full moon, and for seven days after it. Seeds that germinate quickly, and also those that take a very long time to germinate, are planted two days before the new moon, and up to seven days after it. The goal is to time it so the seedlings are sprouting during the waxing moon. As John Jeavons writes in *How to Grow More Vegetables:*

> Both planting periods take advantage of the full sum of the forces of nature, including gravity, light and magnetism . . . The importance of the time of the month in planting seeds and transplanting is not so much in the exact day on which you perform the task, but rather in generally taking advantage of the impetus provided by nature.[12]

After plants germinate and have produced several leaves, the seedlings are ready for transplanting into small pots. If you decide to transplant into flats, be sure to space the seedlings at least 1¼ inches apart. Take care to handle these tiny plants carefully, without damaging the stem or new roots. A good potting soil can be made with equal parts of compost, sharp sand, and loamy topsoil. Let the seedlings grow in the pots for several more weeks to allow the new plants to extend their root system and produce new leaves. Then they are ready to enter their permanent bed.

Whether you purchase seeds or collect them from your own garden, they should be kept clean, dry, and cool, in a dark place. Stored this way, they should remain viable for years.

Division

Herbaceous (nonwoody) perennials are often propagated by crown division, in which a clump of plants is divided into smaller clumps and replanted. Crown division is often done in fall when the plants die back. But some plants are divided in early spring, before the season's new growth really gets underway. Dig up plants to be divided very carefully, and brush away the soil clinging to the roots so you can see what you're doing. Then pull the plants apart if they separate easily, or cut down through the topgrowth with a sharp spade or knife to divide the clump of plants into several smaller clumps. Hyssop, mugwort, oregano, and tarragon are all best divided by cutting the crowns apart with a knife. Onions, garlic, mints, and German chamomile can be separated with a spading fork after the plants are dug up.

When you are dividing plants, be careful to do as little damage to the roots as possible. Separate the divided roots carefully, and make sure each root has a shoot or stem attached. Replant the clumps and water them thoroughly. If you are dividing in fall, mulch the replanted clumps to protect the roots over the winter.

For plants that are more tender or that have long taproots, root division is the propagation method of choice. Root divisions are made by cutting the root into pieces, each of which has a bud from which new roots and shoots can grow. Root division can also involve separating offsets from an underground bulb, corm, or tuber.

Cuttings

There are a number of different types of cuttings: softwood cuttings, hardwood cuttings, stem, root, leaf, and leaf and bud cuttings. In order for cuttings to prosper, they must be taken from healthy plants at the correct time of year, set carefully into a good rooting medium, and kept moist and warm until they root.

Hardwood cuttings are the exception. They are usually made from the current year's growth of deciduous trees after the leaves have fallen. Making hardwood cuttings is a good way to create enough plants for hedges and windbreaks. The cuttings should be 6 to 8 inches long with three or four nodes, the topmost one about an inch from the top of the cutting. Bundle the cuttings together, bury them in slightly moist sand, and refrigerate them at about 50°F for a month. Then keep them at a colder temperature, just above freezing, until the spring thaw. After the last spring frost, the cuttings should be planted in a trench with only the top bud showing. Water them regularly and watch them carefully until they sprout. Don't leave your hardwood cuttings in the refrigerator too long or they might sprout before you get them planted.

Softwood cuttings, also known as greenwood cuttings, can be made from most plants, including those with hard wood. This type of cutting is made from the new growth of vigorous deciduous plants. The plant stem used as a cutting should break with a snap when

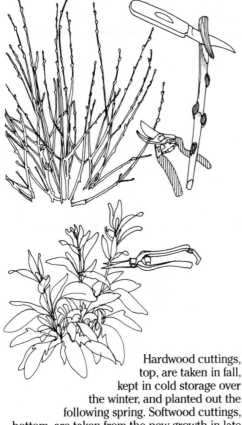

Generally, softwood cuttings are taken from ends of branches (they are then called terminal cuttings). As soon as the cutting is made, wrap the bottom of it in a moist paper towel or cloth and place the cutting in a plastic bag. Then, discard most of the leaves after carefully looking at the form of the cutting. Too many leaves will lessen the cutting's chances of rooting. When you are ready to plant, remove the cloth and set the cutting into a bed of sand or fine gravel that is moist. Be sure that it is able to stand erect, and that it is well supported by the rooting medium. Cuttings taken in the late spring or early summer should be well rooted by autumn. If the cuttings are from winter-hardy plants, they can be set out to harden and left to spend their first winter outside after having been transplanted into a medium made of equal amounts of sharp sand and topsoil, enriched with a small amount of compost. But if your rooted cuttings are in pots or containers, watch them carefully during cold spells—the soil in containers freezes sooner than your garden does.

Hardwood cuttings, top, are taken in fall, kept in cold storage over the winter, and planted out the following spring. Softwood cuttings, bottom, are taken from the new growth in late spring or early summer, depending on the plant.

Layering

Layering is a conservative way of making a new plant from an existing plant. It is most often used to propagate shrubs that are difficult to root. Unlike cuttings, in which the plant part is separated from its parent, in layering, a branch is encouraged to set roots by being bent down into the soil and held in place there, sometimes by means of a weight such as a rock. Layering has the advantage of being a very secure way of propagating a plant without injury to either parent or child. But layering also takes longer than rooting cuttings. Layering should be done in the spring before the buds open on your chosen plant.

bent. If it crushes between the fingers, it's too young. If it merely bends, it is too old. Softwood cuttings are made in late spring or early summer. The timing varies with the plant, and the best way to tell if the plant is old enough to withstand cutting, but still young enough to yield a goot cutting, is to test the stem this way.

Cuttings can vary between 2 and 6 inches in length. Make the cut at a 45-degree angle about ½ inch from a node to sever the cutting.

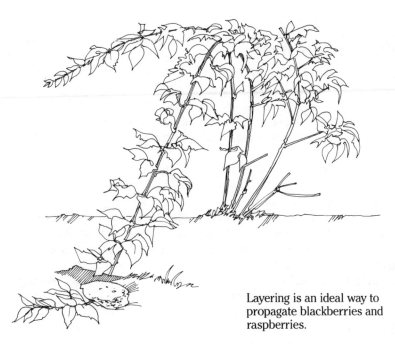

Layering is an ideal way to
propagate blackberries and
raspberries.

Choose a good strong branch that is long and
flexible enough to bend to the ground easily.
Actually bend it down to the ground and mark
the place where the new roots will set. Then,
carefully cut the bark from a small section of
the branch where it will be buried in the soil.
Be certain you do not injure the cambium
layer beneath the bark layer during this process. Add some peat moss, sphagnum, and
sand to the soil where you will set the branch
down to grow roots. Then hold the layered
branch in place in the soil, either with a small
rock or a forked stick. A thin branch can be
held down with hairpins. Some gardeners
prefer to effect their layering by building up a
small mound of dirt around the branch. Be
sure the tip of the branch you are layering
protrudes from the soil; it should not be
buried. Sometimes gardeners hold up the tip
of the branch by bracing it or tying it against
a stake.

The layered branch will be ready to dig
up the following spring. To take up the new
plant, carefully unearth it to preserve its new
root system and cut the branch just below the
new roots. Then plant it as you would any
new cutting. This is called simple layering.
There is also another type of layering, called
tip layering. It is a faster method of propagating
in which the tip of a branch is buried in the
spring. The new plant can be taken up and
separated in the fall.

A Few Words
about Planting Trees

Most trees are best planted in the fall, so that they have the advantage of the long, wet winter to grow into their new situation, rather than having to cope with midsummer heat and dryness soon after they are planted in spring. However, there are some trees that do better planted in spring, such as beech and birch, which have tender roots.

When digging a hole for your new tree, dig it deep enough to set the tree down a little farther than it rests in the container in which it is currently planted. Be careful not to plant the tree too deep, however. Make the hole big enough around to allow ample space for the tree's roots to take hold, before they encounter the more dense soil outside of the hole. A general guideline is to make the planting hole at least as wide in diameter as the crown of the young tree will be after a season's growth.

Set the tree into the hole on top of a mound of good rich topsoil. Do not leave the roots in a compact ball, but carefully straighten them out, while you arrange topsoil around them. To avoid air pockets, which are not healthy for the newly planted tree, soak the soil thoroughly with water when the hole is half-full. Gently rock the tree. Then add more soil and repeat the same process. Leave a depression, rather than making the soil level, to hold more moisture from rain or waterings in place for the roots. Gradually, the depression will fill in.

Make sure you water the tree very well after you plant it, and water it well each week, unless a heavy rainfall accomplishes the task for you. It helps a good deal to provide a nutritious mulch of well-decayed compost, straw and leguminous plants around the base of the new tree. Mulch is especially important when trees are planted in clay-bearing soils and exposed to hot, dry weather. The care and attention which you shower on your trees will bear fruit in the future.

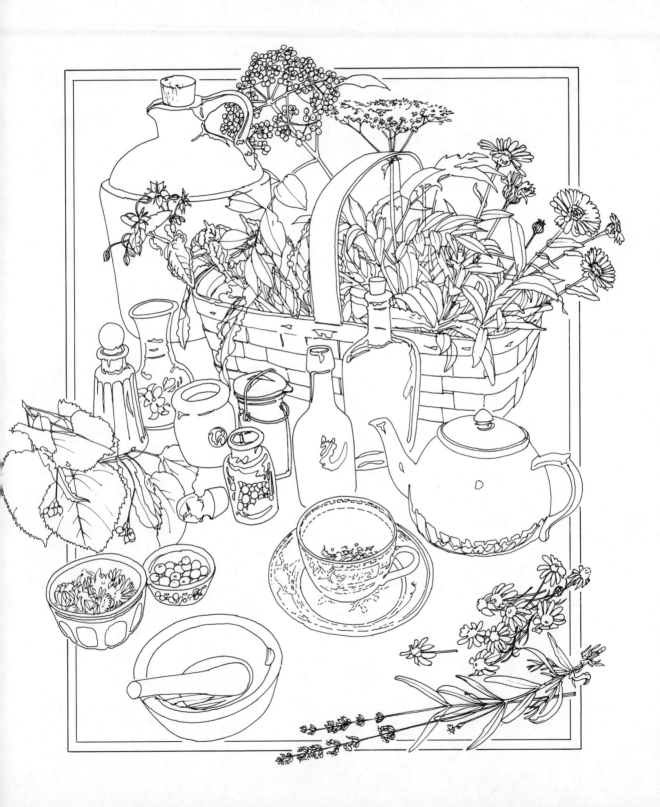

Good Things from the Garden: Gathering and Using the Herbal Harvest

athering the harvest is one of life's greatest joys, rich in meaning and satisfaction. It is the culmination of a nurturing relationship between the plant and the gardener, and the wind, rain, sun, birds, insects, soil, and everything alive within the soil itself.

When the harvest happens to be herbs, it is especially wonderful. The pleasures to the senses while gathering herbs is in itself a rich harvest. What a delight to gather basketsful of deliciously scented lavender spikes, in the wonderful light of a summer morning as their aroma fills the air. How refreshing it is to harvest mint growing at the edge of a cool stream, as you wade under a canopy of trees. The crisp leaves and aroma of the plants are a prelude to the herbal preparations that will preserve each herb's qualities. Dappled patterns of light on the water, the lush green leaves, and perhaps a blue sky—nature is generous in her backdrop for your rewarding toil.

When the fresh spring wind encourages the sleepy world of nature to awaken, and

cottony clouds scud across a deep blue sky, the harvest consists of twigs and small branches such as those of the birch trees. In summer, brilliant orange calendula blossoms overflow your basket, while you cautiously compete with the persistence of bees for the blue starlike flowers of borage plants nearby. In autumn, with winter's chill already in the air, it's time to dig up the roots of the bitter echinacea, the pungent horseradish, and the fleshy elecampane. Throughout the year you can relive the pleasant memories of sights, scents, and sounds evoked by your harvest as you make and use your herbal preparations from the garden.

Of course, the first step in making herbal home products is proper harvesting. In addition to harvesting at the right time and using the right technique or method, proper harvesting means maintaining a positive mental attitude. For many years, only the Native American herbalists spoke about the importance of one's attitude in gathering healing plants. But with the publication of books such as *The Secret*

Life of Plants and *The Findhorn Garden Book* in recent years, many people are coming to place more value on their relationship with plants. This is because plants seem to be sensitive to the thoughts and emotions of those around them. Science may never know for sure whether plants are creatures of feeling, or whether they are even able to respond as conductors tuned to the minds of humans. Although it is a controversial subject, some researchers claim to have shown that plants respond positively to positive thoughts, and negatively to negative thoughts. Marcel Vogel, for example, a senior research scientist with IBM, has conducted many experiments which seem to show the relationship between human thought and plant growth. His work is described in *The Secret Life of Plants.*

Whether or not you believe your plants will benefit from a positive mental attitude on your part, there are some other qualities that will help you in more tangible ways. Patience, sensitivity, and observation are among the harvester's most valuable tools. With these qualities the gardener comes to recognize the best times and methods for gathering each herb. This is important if you wish to maximize the healing qualities of plants you harvest. Each part of a plant is more energetic at different times during the year, and even at different times during the month and day. Spring is the best time for harvesting leaves and buds. That is when they just begin to form, so they have the most vigor. Barks and twigs, such as those of the apple, beech, birch, oak, and slippery elm, are also collected in the spring, when the rising sap enriches those parts with nutrients and minerals. In the summer, flowers, fruits, and berries appear, and are then the plant's most vigorous part. Harvest roots in the autumn, when the plant's sap goes back down to them. Some barks may also be harvested in the autumn.

A plant's energy circulates and has highs and lows, just like the energy of any other living organism. In the early hours of the day, the sap ascends to the plant's upper parts, and in the evening it descends again to the roots. So daytime is generally the best time to harvest the upper parts of plants, and evening is the best time to harvest roots.

The special characteristics of each plant are something you can learn best by observing nature carefully. When exactly in the spring should you gather the herb leaf? A very general answer is that gathering should be done before the plant begins to form flowers. Some generalizations such as this are possible, but harvesttime also depends on your region, the microclimate in your garden, and the weather conditions in any given year. There are so many variables, the best you can do is become sensitive to growing conditions and watch your plants. When you spend time in the garden, pay attention to the clues the plants themselves give, day by day.

In addition to developing an awareness of the general seasonal disposition of plants, and their daily changes, many herbalists today still consider the old lore concerning cycles of the moon and planets, and their effects on herbs' healing properties as they decide when to harvest. According to this traditional gardening wisdom, herbs should be gathered when the moon is in its crescent stage. French herbalist Maurice Mességué reminisced about his father's advice to him on gathering plants:

On the evenings when he said, "There's only a sliver of a moon tonight," this told me that the next day we'd be out gathering plants. "My boy, remember, never when there's a full moon; moonlight saps their strength. For plants to be at their best they need plenty of sunshine and very little moonlight."[1]

This preference for gathering herbs in the last seven days of the lunar cycle has a logical explanation. As John Jeavons explains in his book on biodynamic agriculture, *How to Grow More Vegetables*, plants exhibit the strongest growth of both leaf and root during the first seven days of the moon cycle, when decreasing lunar gravity increases root growth, and increasing moonlight produces leaf growth. In the second seven days, as the moon goes toward fullness, leaf growth is especially fostered and root growths slows down. Finally, during the last seven days of the lunar cycle, or the waning crescent moon, root and leaf growth both decrease, and plants enjoy a period of rest before the next cycle of growth. It is during this resting period that herbs should be gathered. They will have reached their monthly cycle of maturation, and they will last longer in a preserved state.

General Guidelines for Harvesting

No matter whether you are harvesting leaves, stems, or flowers, always gather them on a sunny day after the dew has evaporated off the plants, but before the full heat of the day has filled the garden. For plants with volatile oil, such as mints and lemon balm, just before noon is a good time to harvest. By then the oils have had a chance to reach the leaves, but have not yet been drawn off by the day's heat. Rain washes away some of the aromatic oils from many herbs, so after a rainstorm wait a day, preferably two or three, before harvesting in order to let the plants' oils collect again.

Unless it is time to harvest the entire plant, think of your harvesting as a pruning of the plant or the herb patch. To allow most plants to survive after selective harvesting,

never pick more than one-third of their available harvest, or better yet only one-fourth to be safe. And if you are at all uncertain about how much selective harvesting the plants can tolerate, start out by taking only one-tenth. Be sure to observe the herbs during that season and the next, noting well the effects of the harvest.

The plants you gather should be healthy and should not be picked from any place where they have been exposed to noxious fumes from cars or chemicals used in agriculture. You have more control over this aspect of harvesting if you have grown your plants at home than if you are collecting from the wild. Foragers must not only be careful of trespassing on private property and disturbing the habitat when collecting wild plants, they must also be very skilled at avoiding wild places that have been sprayed with herbicides or pesticides. Avoid picking herbs from

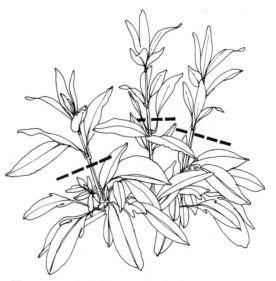

Harvest one-fourth to one-third of a plant by pruning the tips or culling whole stalks.

alongside highways, next to farm fields (unless you know the farm is organic), marshes that may have been sprayed for mosquitoes, forests that may have been sprayed for gypsy moths in summer, and even close to your neighbor's fence if he used herbicides on his lawn.

With tender, nonwoody stemmed herbs, gathering of leaves, stems, or flowers can be accomplished easily with scissors or a sharp knife. Plants with tough or woody stems will require small pruning shears at gathering time. Generally speaking, it is better for the plant you are harvesting, as well as for the final dried herb, if you harvest whole branches or stems, rather than stripping off leaves and leaving the stripped stems and branches on the plant. Herbs with flexible stems such as mint, oregano, pennyroyal, and lavender are easy to pick whole and strip later when they are dry. When you strip the dried herb from its stem or branch, try to keep the leaves as whole as possible. This helps preserve their healing properties longer. When you are harvesting hairy or prickly plants like comfrey, borage, nettles or mullein, wearing heavy gloves will make the experience much more pleasant.

You can also harvest material from plants with more woody stems, and parts of trees, as long as you are careful to harvest the parts as if you were pruning the plant. Some plant parts, such as oak leaves or elderberry leaves, may be easier to harvest by picking each leaf separately, but as a general rule, the harvesting-by-branch method works best. If you intend to use only the herb's leaves, hang the harvested stems or branches upside down in bunches for a few days. This will bring the sap present in the stems or branches into the leaves. Then, you can spread the leaves on screens in thin layers until dry, as described on page 298. If you will use the whole branch no hanging is necessary.

Harvesting Roots and Bark

You will find the task of digging up the roots of herbaceous plants, such as dock, dandelion, or comfrey, a simple one if you have properly prepared their growing bed. In cultivating long-rooted plants, you should create a deep bed that is porous and well aerated, so that you can easily harvest roots by hand. For uncultivated plants growing in soil that is compacted, digging up roots is more of a challenge. A shovel with a long, thin blade is helpful. Dig a hole straight down and to one side of the root. Gradually remove soil on the side of the hole toward the root. Then simply pull the root sideways into the hole. This method will damage the root less than the common practice of digging down all around the root and then pulling it up. This is especially true when the root is deeper than one shovel-length.

Gatherers who appreciate ease more than hard labor like to find their dock or dandelion roots on the edges of fields that have just been turned over, or in fields planted with other crops, where these herbs have invaded as weeds. Then, pulling the loose plants from the soil makes harvesting a simpler job. It is also easier to dig roots out of the side of a hill or bank than from level ground.

Often, the healing parts of trees come from the inner bark of their roots, trunks, or branches. This presents more of a problem to the conscientious harvester, because removing the bark from standing timber disfigures and injures the trees, and digging up roots can be equally traumatic. Although some people may take sections of trunk bark from living trees we do not recommend it. An obvious solution is to use the bark of branches that may need pruning anyway, rather than ruining a strong living tree.

Unfortunately, the bark from the trunk is more efficacious than the bark from branches, and the bark from roots is more potent than trunk bark. So another way to avoid cutting down healthy trees is to find trees that are being cut down anyway, or if you are harvesting from your own orchard or woodlot, select trees that need thinning or removing. Likely

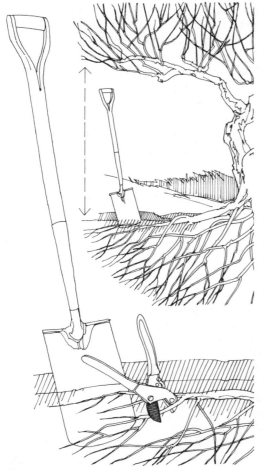

When you harvest root bark, be careful not to cut the tree's main roots. Instead, choose a moderate-size root and cut it out cleanly with pruning shears or a saw.

candidates for root or trunk bark include orchard trees that are too old and are being removed; young trees that need thinning; trees that must be removed because they are in the way of a road, house, power line, or scenic view; and trees that have been injured by lightning, cars, animals, or weather. (Notice we didn't recommend using bark from trees injured by insects. If a tree is ruined by insects it probably is not very healthy to begin with and would not make the best source for medicinal bark.)

You can gather the root bark safely from healthy trees if you do it as though you were giving the tree a mild root pruning. To collect roots from a living tree, dig down at the outermost edge of the tree's root range. The roots' circumference will fall roughly parallel with the circumference of the tree's branches. Root bark, like trunk bark, gets thicker as trees get older, so very young trees will not provide much. When harvesting for root bark, be very careful to avoid cutting main roots. Find a moderate-size root (the smaller the root, the less potent it is) and cut it out cleanly with pruning clippers, an ax, or a saw.

The twigs and small branches of any tree whose bark is used for healing purposes can be used instead of the trunk bark. These are cut in the spring when the sap rises. Treat it as a pruning. Strip off the small branch's inner bark and cut it into small pieces before drying. Simply chop and dry the tiny twigs as described later in this chapter.

Usually it is the living cambium layer of roots, trunks, and branches that is used in herbal healing. The methods used to expose this soft inner bark may vary with each tree. But to begin with you can scrape, chop, cut, or pry off the coarse outer bark. Several implements come in handy for this task. A knife with a strong, sharp blade and point is

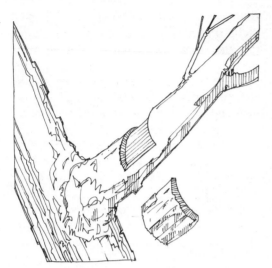

When harvesting bark, remove the coarse outer bark to expose the inner layer. It's best to collect bark from healthy branches that need to be pruned anyway.

good for scraping bark off roots that are not very thick and hard. A small, sharp hatchet can separate chips of inner bark from the heartwood of the branch you have harvested. A broad chisel and a hammer can also be used to chip off inner bark. A machete, if you know how to handle one, can be used to remove outer or inner bark. A crowbar or small spade is useful for prying off outer bark or strips of inner bark. A drawing knife is good for scraping strips of inner bark.

Whatever implement you use, be sure it is not only sharp, but easy to handle, and comfortable to hold. After removing sections of the outer bark, cut down through the cambium layer with a knife or chisel, depending how hard and thick the wood is. Then remove this inner bark in strips, squares, or chips, whichever is easier. Cut the bark into small

Some tools used to collect bark from branches and roots include a drawing knife, small hatchet, broad chisel, pruning shears, pocketknife, spade, and machete.

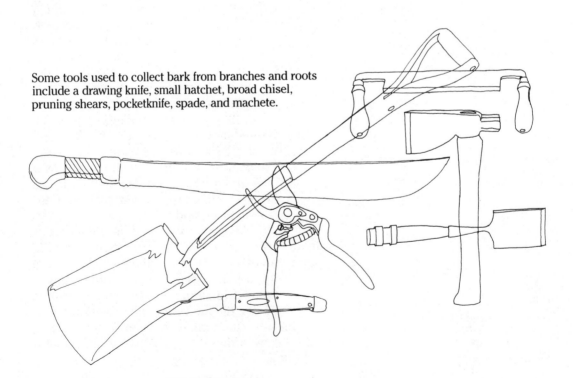

pieces before drying it (as described later) in the shade or in a warm place for several weeks.

Whether you are gathering plants in your herb garden or backyard, in the woods, or on a neighbor's land, consider the carrying containers for your harvest. The containers should be clean and lightweight, and they should allow plenty of airflow through them. Flexible baskets with handles or shoulder straps, double canvas bags that hang over the shoulder, and clean drawstring bags made of burlap or other cloth are all good choices.

After harvesting plant parts, try to limit their exposure to sunlight and prepare them for drying as soon as possible. If you are using a vehicle to transport the harvest, protect the herbs from wind, dust, or heat. For example, if you transport your herbs in a pickup truck, cover the bed with a tarp. If you pile them in a car, keep the windows open to keep the temperature down and prevent premature drying, but cover the herbs with a light cloth to shade them from the sun.

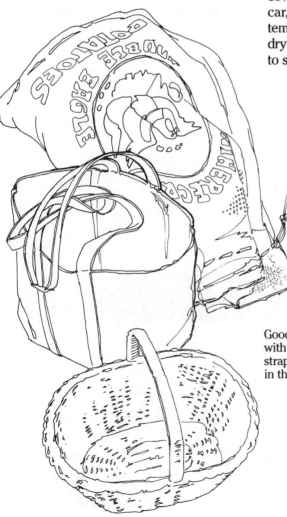

Good herb-gathering containers include a basket with a handle, a sturdy canvas bag with shoulder straps, and a clean burlap bag with a drawstring in the top.

Drying Herbs

Properly dried herbs retain a noteworthy amount of their original color, aroma, and healing qualities. Drying herbs correctly is not really that difficult, but it does demand some careful attention to each plant's attributes. The first step, as we've already pointed out, is to take the plants out of the direct sunlight as soon as you've finished gathering them. A general rule of thumb that many herbalists, including those working with both European and Oriental traditions of herbal medicine follow, is to dry warming herbs in the sun and cooling herbs in the shade.

Make sure that leafy herbs you've cultivated are kept clean of soil when you harvest them. A layer of mulch in the garden helps keep plants clean and free of mud from splashing rain. Wash herbs only if they really need it, because prolonged washing will affect their quality. If you do need to wash your herbs, wash them quickly and efficiently under cold running water. Allow washed herbs to dry well before placing them on a drying rack (see page 300) or hanging them. Gently pat them dry and place them in a cool, airy place to rid them of all moisture before beginning the drying process. If it is not possible to let your herbs air-dry naturally outdoors or in a warm attic, a heater can be used to maintain a steady, even temperature between 95° and 100°F.

The leafy parts of most herbs with volatile oils, such as mint, lemon balm, anise, dill, fennel, and lavender, dry best at temperatures between 95° and 100°F. Commercial herb processors often use much higher temperatures, but the patient home gardener can afford to dry herbs the way they should be dried: slowly and steadily. When herbs are drying, the flow of air over and around them is as important, or more important, than the

heat. Greater air circulation makes a lower drying temperature possible. Herbs containing volatile oils should be dried in the shade, *not* in the sun, where their oil would decompose or vaporize.

Flowers are much more fragile than other plant parts and are especially vulnerable to damage from water. Protect them from water after gathering and dry them in drying room or dryer with a temperature around 90° F. If it is too hot or too cool or not airy enough in the drying room, flowers will discolor and lose their subtle qualities completely.

Roots and barks should be carefully washed and brushed of dirt. Chop them before you dry them, into pieces 1 inch thick or less with a small hatchet, cleaver, or knife,

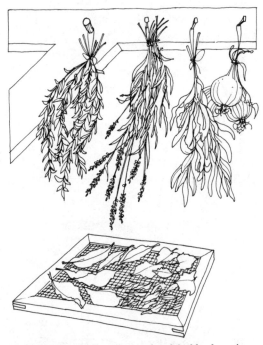

Herbs with volatile oils can be dried by hanging them upside down in bunches or by spreading the leaves in a single layer on a screen.

depending on how tough the root is. You can cut up large amounts of bark *after* drying if you have a compost shredder or a chipper. Generally, for the small-scale gardener, though, it is easier to chop bark before drying. Most roots can be dried in the sun, but sometimes, depending on the herb's properties, this is not desirable or possible. For example, if a root is gathered in October, there may not be enough sunlight to dry it properly. In this case, dry the roots indoors in a drying room or dryer. Roots can also be dried in a food dehydrator, which will speed up the drying process by at least three to four times.

Herbalist Maurice Mességué describes the importance of the drying process to the healing power of herbs:

Many plants are best gathered in the summer solstice, around midsummer day, as our forefathers knew. The weather should be neither too damp nor too dry . . . The actual drying of plants is of prime importance, for on this depends the extent to which plants retain their effectiveness. It is all a question of touch. Plants should be neither too dry nor too fresh and never completely dehydrated.[2]

Mességué suggests an initial drying in a shady, well-ventilated place, and hanging the herbs upside down in bundles from the rafters, as we have also suggested. This old-fashioned method is certainly the most picturesque way to dry herbs, and it is also very effective in bringing essential oils into the leaves.

If you are drying herb seeds such as anise, caraway, or fennel, place the whole herb branches or stems in large paper bags. Hung upside down with their umbels toward the bottom of the bag, the herbs will drop their seeds neatly into the bag's bottom. Another way to dry herbs in paper bags is to cut a hole in the bag's bottom and stick the herbs' stems through. Cut a few ventilation

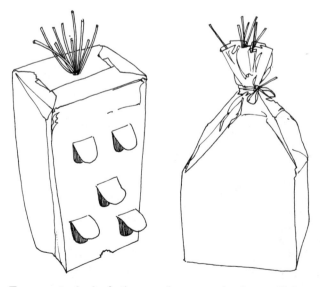

Two ways to dry herbs in paper bags: one that keeps off dust and one that saves seeds.

holes in the sides of the bag before placing the bunch of herbs in it. Then, hang the bag of herbs from a rafter and you've got a well-aerated arrangement that will keep the herbs clean as they dry.

Drying Racks

A good drying rack is very useful for the gardener who plans to dry quantities of herbs for medicinal use. You can construct a simple herb-drying rack with several levels, such as the one illustrated here. Window screening can be used both to maximize airflow and to support the herbs drying on racks. Fiberglass screens are suitable but avoid metal ones. You can also make screens from broad meshed cloth, such as muslin or burlap. Benches similar to those used in saunas, but made from thin strips of hardwood from ½ to 1 inch wide, are also good drying platforms if whole branches or large herbs are being dried. Leave ½ to 1 inch of space between each slat. Do not finish the wood with any stains, varnishes, or oils. Whether you use racks, screens, or benches, be sure to lay out the herbs in thin layers so they dry evenly.

Drying Rooms

It is prudent to determine beforehand how much drying space you will need, based on quantities of herbs and the cycle of harvest times for each herb. To dry about one-quarter acre's worth of fresh herb materials, you will need a drying room with about 200 square feet of flat drying space. An attic, if it is clean, is a good place to put the drying rack of herbs. You can also place the rack in a sauna (as long as no one uses it as a sauna). The entire wall of a shed can be converted to an herb-drying area by building drying racks onto its walls. Barns or sheds can be good herb-drying places, but they have a few potential drawbacks. The usually loose construction intended to allow plenty of air circulation may also allow dirt and insects to enter. And if the weather turns wet there is no way to keep out moisture. A more sophisticated drying setup involves construction of, or conversion into, a forced-air drying room or shed. You can use rafters, screens, or racks (as described above) in the drying shed or spread the herbs on a raised "floor," a framework of beams covered with permeable sisal cloth. Air is forced into the shed with a centrifugal fan mounted on an outside wall of the building, near floor level. Place a screen and filter over the fan intake to prevent insects and dust from entering. The room also needs an open-and-close exhaust vent near the ceiling. For

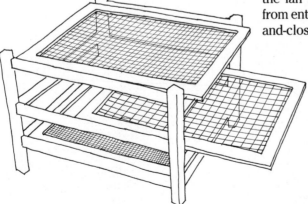

Here is a simple three-level rack for drying herbs.

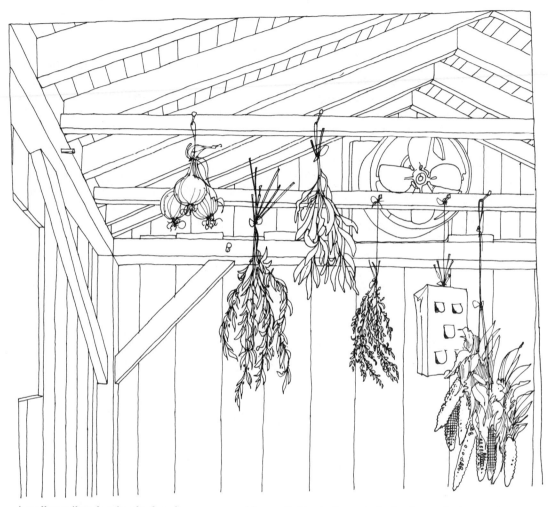

A well-ventilated attic, shed, or barn can provide a suitable drying area for herbs, and a fan can be installed to increase air circulation.

this you can use a window screen, a hatch, or a circulating vent.

The fan that blows air into the heating room can also contain heating elements to provide warm air. Although this may not be necessary in the middle of summer, it will help when nights are cool and in the spring or autumn. For large rooms, a propane or natural gas forced-air heater is more efficient than an electric fan-heater. You can use wood heat if you regulate it carefully. You can also build a solar hot air collector on the south side of the drying shed. There are many ways to do this, ranging from an actual greenhouse-type construction to simply supporting some black plastic over the ground and ducting the airflow into the fan. Do not use a greenhouse for supplying drying air, though, if it is full of plants, as the air will be too moist. But if your greenhouse plants spend the summer outdoors, you can use the greenhouse to dry herbs in summer.

If you don't have a greenhouse you can construct a simpler solar hot-air device with a length of the plastic hosing used in clothes dryer exhausts. Mount the tubing on a 4 by 8-foot sheet of plywood. Loop it back and forth in horizontal rows with the intake end on the bottom. Spray-paint the exposed surfaces flat black. Screen the intake end and attach the top end directly to the round opening in a "squirrel cage," or small blade fan, using duct

tape. Lean the plywood up against the south side of the drying shed, positioned so the fan exhaust can be ducted into the shed. On a low fan speed, during a warm, sunny day, this type of dryer will raise ambient air temperatures about 10°F. This is just right during the summer if outside temperatures are in the 80s. On hotter days, simply turn up the speed on the fan so the air passes through the tubing more quickly.

You can make a cool-air vent in your heater by cutting out a portion of the tube near the fan, replacing it with duct tape around the edges. (Be sure to cover this opening with

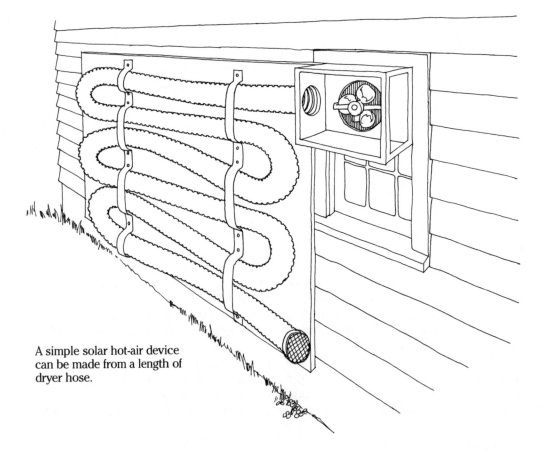

A simple solar hot-air device can be made from a length of dryer hose.

screening, also.) To open the vent, simply peel off the tape on three sides. A thermometer inserted into the shaded side of the tube just before the fan and sealed with tape or caulk, will allow accurate temperature readings.

Whatever type of heat you use with a fan in a drying shed, it is imperative that you regulate it carefully. If there is no heat source with the fan, then turn off the fan in the late afternoon to avoid any chance of blowing the cooler, moister air of evening into the shed. If there is a heat source with your fan, you really should have a thermostat to help you regulate the amount of heat the fan generates. If there is no thermostat, you will have to inspect the fan frequently and judge the heater for effectiveness.

How Long to Dry

Drying time for herbs varies with the particular plant and the part of the plant being dried. Flowers should be light and well dried, but not so dry that they crumble into powder with any handling. In general, leaves should be brittle enough to break between the fingers, but not so dry that they crumble. Stems and stalks should be breakable between the fingers, also, and not bendable. Bark and roots should be dry enough to snap if they are thin, or chip easily with the blow of a hammer if they are thick. With a little experience, it is easy to know when herbs are dried properly. The product should smell, taste, and look much like the original fresh plant, except that it is dehydrated. An herb that is green and fragrant when fresh should also be green and fragrant when dried. Be careful not to judge your dried herbs by the appearance of store-bought herbs. The latter are usually several shades lighter, browner or yellower than properly dried herbs should be.

Storing Home-Dried Herbs

Heat, light, air, and bacterial action can all dissipate the healing properties of herbs. So can plastics and metal. So you must protect your dried herbs from these factors with proper storage. For short periods of several weeks or so, you can store herbs in a wax paper bag that is in turn placed inside a brown paper bag. For longer storage, a tightly capped glass jar, preferably made of dark glass to protect herbs from deterioration caused by light, is superior. The type of canning jars that have glass lids that close with metal clamps to form an airtight seal are best. If metal lids are used, place a piece of wax paper over the jar before screwing down the lid. Do not use soft plastic jars or bags to store medicinal herbs because not all plastic is approved for food use, and the container you chose may have a residue that will taint the herbs. Even if it is approved for food, plastic may encourage condensation inside the container that will hasten decomposition. Plexiglas containers are acceptable for herb storage. You can also store herbs in fiber drum barrels (such as the kind that hold bulk dried goods in natural foods stores), air-tight wooden boxes or bins, and wooden barrels.

It's a good idea to figure out the approximate amount of herbs you will dry before you make the first harvest, so you know how much storage space you will need to accommodate them. Otherwise if you dry a lot of herbs, you will notice that they soon take over your cabinet space. Plan to keep small jars of dried herbs in the kitchen or medicine chest for regular use, but find a convenient larger space for the bulk storage jars or containers that hold the entire harvest. This not only saves cabinet space in the kitchen, but it also ensures the freshness of the stored herbs. Opening and closing a big container of herbs all the time only hastens spoilage.

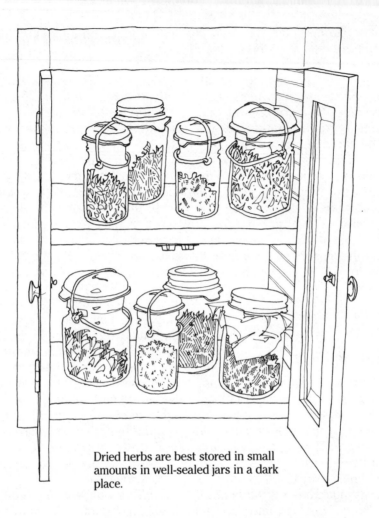

Dried herbs are best stored in small amounts in well-sealed jars in a dark place.

The best places for long-term storage of herbs are dry, dark, and cool. Household pantries and cupboards may be dry and dark, but they are not always cool. Garages and cabinets in the house near the ground floor often stay cool, but be sure they are moisture-free if you store herbs there. Also make sure that there are doors in front of shelves to keep out light.

It is very helpful to label your herbs carefully with the name of the plant and the date of harvesting. You may wish to include other details of cultivation or harvest, such as phases of the moon and weather conditions at the time of harvesting, seed or stock source, type of fertilizer or growing methods used, location of the growing plant, and methods and duration of drying.

How long can dried herbs be kept and still retain their healing properties? We follow the advice of a Native American herbal healer, Oh Shinnah Fastwolf, who uses this rule of thumb:

All medicinal plants are kept only as long as their corresponding growing cycle. For example, if an herb seed takes two years to mature, the seeds are kept no more than two years. If a flower blooms every year, it is kept for one year, only. For the actual details, that's all there is to it. It's that simple.[3]

The Chinese tell an imaginative story of how the ginseng hunters kept their roots fresh. The "man root," as ginseng was called, had arms and legs. These were bound with cord to immobilize the herb. Then little slivers of bamboo were placed in appropriate "acupuncture" points. The idea behind this treatment was to sedate the root, thereby preserving its life-force while it was transported to market.

To prepare herb leaves for teas, the traditional mortar and pestle works well. Grind or break the leaves into small pieces first. You can rub soft, leafy herbs such as mint or sage between your palms, or through a ¼-inch mesh screen. To powder leaves and small pieces of roots, use a mortar and pestle, *suribachi* (a Japanese-type mortar and pestle, which has fine ridges inside the bowl that aid the grinding process), or an electric blender or coffee grinder. Put large pieces of roots through a flour mill first before powdering them. Some people use only the flour mill to break or powder roots and find that they can get a fine enough product this way. If you do large-scale herbal gardening, you can use a *clean* compost shredder to break up large amounts of herbs, but we recommend this method only if an electric machine is used. The fumes from a gasoline engine will contaminate the herbs. There are also some ingenious devices powered by hand, foot, wind, and water that are sometimes used for shredding organic materials.

How to Cut, Rub, and Powder Herbs

There are a number of ways to process herbs further once they are dried, either before you store them or just before you use them. We recommend storing herbs in their whole state as much as possible and cutting or powdering them in small batches as needed. The more surface area an herb has exposed, the sooner it will be affected by decomposing factors like air and light. On the other hand, further processing at the time of use is done to expose the greater surface area, making the herb's medicinal constituents more readily available.

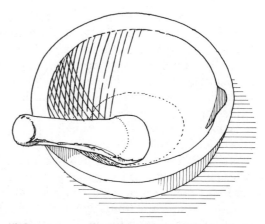

A Japanese *suribachi* has ridges on the inside to facilitate the grinding of herbs.

You can sift herbs with large mesh screens (such as a ½-inch mesh) that separate small herb pieces from stems and unbroken leaves or pieces of root. Simply change the size of the mesh to determine the size of the finished product. Pour or place the herbs on top of the screen and put a basin or clean cloth under the screen. Shake until most of the herbs have sifted through, then pick out the debris left on the screen. Repeat this process in small batches until most of the stems or unbroken pieces have been removed.

Commercial herb dealers may use agricultural machinery for cutting, sifting, chopping, or powdering leaves, bark and roots, but for home use these are usually not necessary. However, if you wish to process large amounts of herbs, some herb companies (such as Green Mountain Herb Co. in Colorado) will cut and sift or powder quantities of herbs that you send them, for a slight charge.

Making Healing Infusions and Decoctions

There are many different ways that you can use herbs to enhance your health. Probably the most common way to take herbal medicine is in a tisane, or herb tea infusion. Drinking a medicinal tea is different from simply drinking herb tea as a beverage, however. Medicinal teas are usually stronger. They often require 1 ounce of the dried herb per pint (2 cups) of water. Commercially prepared herb tea bags contain only about one-seventh that amount of tea per pint of water. Drinking commercial herb teas may be enjoyable and relatively healthy, but they will probably not have the same healing effect as specially prepared medicinal herb teas. Drinking small amounts

of potent medicinal herbal beverages will have much more noticeable effects than that of commercial herb teas. As Michael Tierra, N.D., says in his book *The Way of Herbs:*

There is an important difference between beverage teas, which use only a small amount of the [mild] herb, and medicinal teas, which use much larger amounts. Too many people are drinking herb teas to cure their ailments thinking that a sprinkle of herbs in a cup of boiling water will do the trick. In general this is not the case.[4]

The container in which you prepare medicinal herbal beverages is important. Pyrex glass, Corning Ware or similar heatproof glass are the best materials because they do not impart any of their own qualities to the herbal preparation. Earthenware is also good—its use is very traditional among many Chinese herbalists. Safe alternatives to these include containers made of *unchipped* enameled steel, or stainless steel. Avoid vessels made of aluminum and cast iron as these materials can taint herbal preparations. There are some unusual vessels that have traditionally been used to prepare some herbs, too. For example, in China, ginseng was traditionally boiled in a silver kettle. French herbalist Maurice Mességué's father used a copper tub for giving chamomile baths:

"Look, my boy," he would say, "that's copper, it's finer than gold. It's red like that because it has been a mirror to the sun and the fire, and you are going to have a bath in it."[5]

Be especially careful not to use heavily chlorinated tap water or water that is very high in mineral content for making medicinal preparations. Pure springwater, good well water, or distilled water are the best to use. They are free of chemical additives, and springwater and well water themselves contain very healing qualities. In the Native American tradition, pure springwater is a highly esteemed medicine. Since it is so healing, it is naturally a fine foundation for any herbal preparation used in healing. For cosmetic preparations, soft water is very good.

As a general practice, when you wish to substitute dried herbs for fresh herbs in a recipe, you should decrease the quantity of each herb by half. Similarly, if you want to substitute fresh herbs for dried herbs, double the quantities called for unless the recipe directs otherwise. Fresh herbs contain much more water than dried herbs, and so they are proportionately less potent.

Infusions

Infusions and tisanes are medicinal beverages made by steeping herbs in hot water until their useful qualities are extracted. Made from the delicate parts of herbs, such as leaves and flowers, infusions or tisanes are rather simple preparations. First, bring a pint of water to a full rolling boil in a medium-size pot then remove it from the burner. Immerse 1 ounce (about 2 cups) of the dried herb in the boiled water and cover the pot tightly. Let the infusion steep for 10 to 15 minutes, depending on the herb's potency and how strong a tisane you want to make. The herb will soak up about ½ cup of the water, leaving you with roughly 1½ cups of beverage. One pint of tisane—if you drink ½ cup three times daily—should be more than enough for one day.

"Sun tea" infusions made in the summer sunlight are often as strong as those made with boiling water, and they are fun to make. Sun teas made with very aromatic herbs that contain lots of volatile oil, such as pennyroyal or birch, can yield tisanes even stronger than infusions made with boiled water. To make sun tea, use the same amount of dried herb and water as for a regular infusion, but place the dried herb in cool water in a covered glass jar. Place the jar outdoors in the sun and let the mixture infuse there for three to four hours.

There are many types of herbal tisanes, yet exploration in herbal healing may reveal still more. Some of the most time-honored and popular tisanes still in use today are those made with chamomile, peppermint, linden flowers, and sage. Both chamomile and linden flower infusions are used for their soothing, sedative qualities. Peppermint tisane is well known as an aid for upset stomachs, as a soother for headaches, and as a fever-breaker. Sage is regarded as both tonic and stimulating in tisane form. For centuries, people have taken it to strengthen the brain and nervous system.

While these four herbs are among the best-known simples for tea, many other common herbs have been used to relieve complaints arising from minor coughs and colds, fever, sore throat, headache, tension and nervousness. All the teas we are talking about here can be made in either infusion or decoction form, according to directions given for making infusions or decoctions in this chapter.

Teas for Colds Whenever we feel a cold coming on, we head for the kitchen, cut some thin slices of gingerroot, and make a pot of ginger tea. With the addition of lemon and honey to taste, ginger tea is a tasty and effective beverage, either for warding off a cold, or treating one that has already set in. Other people swear by teas made from slippery elm, horehound, garlic, or thyme. The European herbal tradition has many well-known, old-fashioned herb teas for treating colds. One

Making an Herbal "Coffee"

Most people don't think of coffee as an herb, but it is, and a very strong one at that. In terms of its pharmacological properties, coffee is considered stimulant, diaphoretic, laxative, and diuretic. You can make substitute coffee beverages with herbs to avoid coffee's harmful effects. Roasted and ground dandelion and/or chicory root is often used for this purpose. In fact, the French often add chicory root to their coffee, and recently a major producer in the United States has been marketing freeze-dried coffee with chicory root added. Many commercial coffee substitutes also use dandelion or chicory root as a base, adding other ingredients such as roasted and ground sprouted barley, carob powder, roasted ground beets, malt powder, and flavorings such as cinnamon, nutmeg, vanilla, or orange peel.

    You can make your own beverage at home to suit your taste with any of these or other ingredients. To make a coffee substitute based on dandelion or chicory root, gather young, tender roots in the spring. Wash and dry them carefully, spread them in a Pyrex or earthenware pan, and then roast them whole in a slow oven, about 180° to 200°F, for one to four hours or more, until the roots are thoroughly dry. Turn them occasionally so they dry evenly. Allow the roots to cool at room temperature. You can grind the roots and store them in jars, or store them whole and grind them as you use them. Use the ground roasted dandelion or chicory as you would real coffee, brewing it according to your favorite method. If you grind the roots to a very fine powder, you can dissolve them directly in hot water and drink without filtering.

    The following recipe is a tasty coffee-substitute beverage that you can make at home. You will need 5 parts roasted chicory and/or dandelion root; 2 parts holy thistle; 1 part sarsaparilla root; 1 part Irish moss; 1 part ho shou wu (also called fo-ti, and available in natural foods stores) or ginseng root; ½ part licorice root; ½ part dried orange peel.

    Grind all ingredients to the same coarseness as coffee for the brewing method you prefer. The holy thistle may tend to remain in larger fibers. If you don't like the hint of licorice in this brew, you can use powdered malt instead.

    You can drink this beverage black or with milk. It looks like coffee and tastes close to coffee, and it has similar effects without being addicting.

calls for equal amounts of hyssop and hore-hound, in a simple infusion. Another calls for an infusion of equal amounts of elder flowers, basswood flowers, sage leaves, and yarrow flowers. An herb tea made of equal amounts of peppermint leaves and elder flowers is another traditional cold remedy. Both peppermint and elder encourage perspiration, a common way to break fevers. The soothing qualities of licorice make it a good tea ingredient for sore throat, cough, or chest congestion. Slippery elm's demulcent qualities soothe sore throats, too.

To treat excessive mucus due to colds and flu, herb teas with expectorant qualities such as ginger, thyme, cayenne, and garlic are all helpful. In addition to teas, many people also use herbs in vaporizers or take them in capsules, to decrease mucus. Both marjoram and eucalyptus tea infusions can be put in a vaporizer to help eliminate mucus. (Make sure the infusions are strained well.) Capsules made of equal amounts of cayenne and slippery elm powders, taken along with herb teas such as ginger, peppermint, or thyme, have been taken to decrease mucus during bouts of cold and flu. Garlic tea, and capsules of garlic powder are also sometimes used, as is ginger tea.

Lavender, marjoram, and sage teas make effective gargles for use during colds and sore throats. Teas made of herbs that contain salicylic acid, such as birch or poplar, may help to alleviate fatigue and aching muscles that accompany flu. A strong infusion of peppermint is probably the best-known herbal remedy for breaking fevers. But infusions of gravelroot, holy thistle, yarrow, and poplar bark have also been used for this purpose.

Teas for Headaches and Tension Herbs can sometimes remedy common headaches, depending on their cause. Herbs that increase circulation, such as bay leaves, cayenne pepper, holy thistle, and peppermint, can help alleviate headaches due to poor circulation. Herbalists say that toxins in the blood can contribute to the cause of headaches, too, by interfering with proper assimilation of oxygen and nutrients in the brain. To relieve this problem, echinacea, Oregon grape, plantain, or burdock can be added to an herbal infusion. Eucalyptus, goldenseal, and ginger are considered to be good remedies for headaches due to blocked sinus passageways.

Poor posture, misaligned vertebrae, improper reading glasses or the need for them, and a host of other factors can also cause headaches. But probably the single greatest cause of headaches is nervous tension. For these kinds of headaches we recommend only mild herbs, such as the old-time simples discussed in chapter 2, whose healthful and calming properties have been recognized and used for centuries. Chamomile flowers and linden (or basswood) flowers are two of the herbs best known for promoting a relaxed feeling. Borage, catnip, marjoram, cabbage, or lavender teas all are used to help lessen anxiety and encourage relaxation. Lavender tea, especially, is a well-known European remedy for nervous headaches and is one of our favorite nervines. Sage is also regarded as a useful nervine, because it is thought to strengthen the nervous system while it calms and soothes. Ginseng, to which is assigned some circulatory and stimulating properties, may be of help to people who get headaches when they try to break the coffee-drinking habit. (Note: People with high blood pressure should not take ginseng, and it shouldn't be used with caffeine.)

Nervines can also be administered in the form of a footbath or a relaxing full body bath. See the information on herbal baths, later in this chapter.

As with other types of medicine, the use of herbs for healing must be tailored to each individual. There will probably never be an herbal cure-all headache remedy. Even aspirin and caffeine, both of which originally were derived from naturally occurring plants, do not work for everyone.

Decoctions

Decoction, simmering herbs in water, is the most effective method for drawing the healing elements from coarse plant parts such as bark, roots, stems, and heavy leaves. To make a decoction use the same proportion of herb and water as you would to make an infusion—1 ounce of dried herb to 1 pint of water. The heavier herb parts require a higher heat than that used for infusions. Add the dried herbs to water that has been brought to a boil in a medium-size pot. Keep the water just below boiling for about 30 minutes and let the herbs simmer gently. Some treatments may require heating for up to one hour, but 30 minutes is the general rule. Chinese herbalists use a slightly different method to make decoctions of roots such as ginseng and other strong herbs. They cook the herbs at a slightly higher heat until half the liquid volume has evaporated.

Some herbal formulas combine roots, bark, and the more delicate leaves, buds, or flowers in one remedy. In this case, the strained decoction made from coarser parts is poured over the leaves or flowers, covered, and left to steep for 10 to 20 minutes.

Herbal Baths for Gentle Healing

The herbal bath, a very old form of medical treatment, is a safe and effective way to use herbs for healing. Besides being healing, herbal baths are enjoyable. Baths can relax the ill person, as the healing qualities of the herbs permeate the body through the skin. If you doubt the efficacy of herbal baths, try pressing a slice of garlic against the sole of someone's foot. After a short while, smell his breath—you should smell the garlic. Conversely, if you have eaten a lot of garlic, you can remove that odor by taking a long, hot bath. The bathwater will then smell like garlic instead of you.

Today, many herbalists throughout the world use herbal body, hand, and footbaths for various purposes. To make an herbal bath, make an infusion with 1½ to 1¾ cups dried herbs and 1 quart water, following the directions given previously for infusions. Add the infusion to your bathwater.

Soaking in an herbal bath can help you relieve tension and stress, invigorate a fatigued body, rejuvenate the fluid content of the skin, and help relieve skin irritations. In addition, there are many specific applications for herbal baths. For example, in her book *Jeanne Rose's Herbal Body Beauty Book*, this well-known herbalist recommends herbal baths to help remove cellulite deposits. The baths are taken in conjunction with diet and massage of the affected areas with herb oils. The use of the herbal bath is not limited to minor ailments. The well-known Japanese herbalist and traditional physician Naboru Muramoto, in his book *Healing Ourselves*, describes the use of the ginger bath for treating arthritis and other problems of the joints. Maurice Mességué emphasizes the healing quality of both hand and footbaths in his book *Of Men and Plants.* He includes treatments for heart disease, asthma, emphysema, impotence, jaundice, rheumatism, ulcers, and many other conditions. Although the treatment of such serious ailments is beyond our scope in

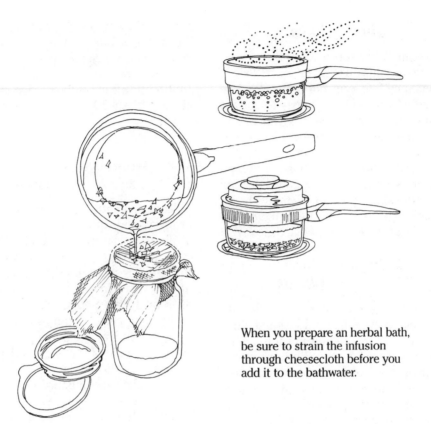

When you prepare an herbal bath, be sure to strain the infusion through cheesecloth before you add it to the bathwater.

this book, certainly herbal bathing can play a very broad supportive and therapeutic role in holistic health care.

Magic Waters Beauty Bath

Famous French beauty Ninon de L'Enclos remained lovely into her seventies and attributed her good fortune to the use of "magic waters," which were composed of a handful (about ½ cup) each of dried lavender flowers, dried rosemary flowers, chopped comfrey roots, and thyme. This actually equals 2 cups of herbs in the original recipe, but you can reduce the mixture to 1¾ or 1½ cups, and make an infusion in 1 quart of water.

The lavender in the bath is to help reduce puffiness in the skin, the rosemary flowers are energizing and astringent (if you cannot find them, use rosemary leaves—the effect will be more stimulating than that of the flowers), the comfrey root is emollient and rejuvenating, especially to aging skin, and the thyme is antiseptic and mildly deodorant. You can also add some rose petals to this bath, both for their fragrance and their hydrating powers.

Calming Baths

You can make a very relaxing herbal bath by pouring an infusion of either linden flowers or chamomile into your hot bathwater. Use the general formula for infusions–1 ounce of dried herb to 1 pint of water–given earlier. Both of these baths are considered excellent for calming restless or nervous children and have been used for that purpose in Europe and America for centuries. Of course, adults can benefit similarly. Other calmative herbs such as catnip, lemon balm, mullein, and slippery elm can also be used in this way.

Baths for Aching Muscles and Joints

Sage and mugwort baths are classic remedies to help relieve aching muscles and joints. A very good bath preparation for aching muscles consists of 1 ounce burdock root, 1 ounce mugwort, 1 ounce comfrey leaf, and 1 ounce sage. Infuse these in 1 quart of just-boiled water and steep for ten minutes, then pour into the bathwater. Poplar bark is also a good herb to use in baths for stiff joints.

Ginger Bath

A ginger bath is used to help promote circulation. In Oriental medicine, ginger baths have been used traditionally to treat arthritis and bursitis, as well as gout. Two pounds of grated ginger are placed in 1 gallon of water and heated but not boiled. Keep the water very hot for ten minutes, then strain off the ginger and add the liquid to a hot bath.

Lotions and Washes

Some of the most sensual and delightful ways to use herbs are in refreshing lotions to use after shaving, with a massage, and for cleansing. Lavender is one of the most preferred scents in such preparations. Herbs that are demulcent, astringent, aromatic, styptic, or antiseptic are good choices for after-shave lotions or washes. Here are some recipes for you to try.

Wonderful Wake-Up After-Shave Lotion

This aromatic after-shave is styptic, astringent, and stimulating. To make it, halfway fill a large jar that has a lid with 3 parts fresh sage leaves, 1 part fresh yarrow flowers, and 1 part fresh or dried lavender flowers. You can also add either 1 part eucalyptus leaves or 1 part peppermint leaves for a mentholated scent. Fill the jar to the top with rubbing alcohol or grain alcohol. Shake the mixture a couple of times every day for two weeks, then strain and discard the herbs. Add water to dilute the mixture to the desired strength, and enjoy as a refreshing, healthy after-shave lotion. For dry skin, add 1 to 2 tablespoons of glycerine or almond oil to the mixture. This herbal essence also makes a fragrant alcohol rub that is relaxing and refreshing.

Sage and Lavender After-Shave Lotion

This freshly scented after-shave lotion is delightfully invigorating. To make it, combine 2 cups witch hazel extract (which is available in most drugstores), 2 tablespoons apple cider vinegar, 1 ounce dried lavender flowers and 1 ounce dried sage in a large jar with a lid. Close the jar and let the mixture steep for one week, shaking it daily. Then strain off and discard herbs and bottle the lotion.

Medicated Skin Wash

Here's a medicinal skin lotion that can be used for anything from taking off makeup and cleansing oily skin to alleviating discomfort from skin rashes and irritations. In a large bowl, combine 2 pints of witch hazel extract and 1 pint of rubbing alcohol. Add 1 ounce each of chopped dried burdock root and calendula flowers, and ½ ounce each of dried beech bark, sage leaves, yarrow leaves, and chopped echinacea root. Let the mixture steep, covered, in the bowl or a jar, for one week. Stir it daily. Strain off and discard the herbs, add 1 cup of rosewater to the liquid and store the wash in bottles in a cool, dark place. This lotion is also good for washing cuts and scrapes.

Chamomile-Fennel Wash

This wash is gentle enough for even an infant's delicate skin. It is especially soothing for dry or puffy skin. To make this wash, combine ½ ounce each of dried chamomile and fennel with 1 cup cold water in a medium-size pot. Macerate the herbs with a wooden spoon to release their properties. Let the mixture steep for 30 minutes. Then cook the herbal water gently over low heat for 10 minutes. Strain off and discard herbs. Apply this wash warm to your skin.

Kathi Keville's Flowers in Your Hair Rinse

Herbs can enhance hair until it is truly worthy of being called our crowning glory. The properties of herbs that make them so useful in the form of teas, baths, and other preparations are the same properties that can be used to improve the health and beauty of the hair. Herbs with astringent qualities help to reduce excessive oils in the scalp and hair. Demulcent herbs soften the hair and nutritious herbs feed it, while aromatic herbs bring their wonderful fragrances. The simplest hair rinses are those made with herb teas. Chamomile and rosemary rinses are the best known of these. Chamomile is used by blondes to enhance their hair's lightness, and rosemary is favored by brunettes for its darkening properties. Hair rinses can also be made by combining a number of herbs. This hair rinse, created by California herbalist Kathi Keville, contains a skillfully blended selection of herbs and herbal properties and is enriched with agar-agar.

To make Flowers in Your Hair Rinse, measure 4 quarts of mountain springwater or filtered rainwater into a large heatproof glass or enameled container. If you cannot obtain either of these kinds of water, bottled springwater or distilled water will do. Add ½ ounce each of dried burdock root, wild cherry bark, comfrey root, and myrrh gum powder to the water. Cover the pot and simmer gently over low heat for 45 minutes.

Then, add 1 ounce each of dried chamomile flowers, lavender flowers, rosemary, calendula flowers, lemon grass, and nettles. Turn the heat as low as it will go and cook the herbs for 15 minutes more. Remove mixture from heat and allow to steep for at least 20 minutes.

Sterilize and have ready enough bottles with tight-fitting corks to hold the hair rinse (the recipe yields about 4 quarts). Strain the tea into another pot, large bowl, or clean container to remove the herbs. Add 1 teaspoon of agar-agar powder or 1 tablespoon agar-agar flakes (agar-agar is a transparent, nutritious, seaweed gelatin available in many natural food stores or in Japanese or Chinese grocery stores), along with ½ cup of apple cider vinegar, for every quart of "tea." Bring to a boil and cook for three minutes.

Using a funnel, pour the finished hair rinse into the prepared bottles and cork the bottle tops. Let the hair rinse cool. It will gel as it cools. Melt some paraffin and dip the well-corked bottles upside down in the paraffin to cover and seal the cork of bottles you plan to store or give away as gifts. A fancy label is all you need to finish a very special herbal present for family and friends.

Use the rinse in small amounts. It is concentrated, and you don't need very much to replenish your hair. On shoulder-length hair or shorter hair, one palmful of rinse is sufficient. On longer hair, two palmfuls should be enough. There is no need to rinse the Flowers in Your Hair Rinse out of your hair after applying. The herbs will keep on working as long as you leave them on your hair. Store the rinse in the refrigerator and use within one month, once the paraffin seal is broken.

Insect Repellent

A number of herbs, such as pennyroyal, eucalyptus, calendula, and lavender, are natural insect repellents. Steeped in alcohol, they make pleasant, nonchemical repellents. They do not work for long periods of time on all people's skins so reapply them regularly, but discontinue use if irritation occurs. The coolness of the alcohol makes their application in summer heat a pleasant task. To make a repellent, combine ¼ ounce each of pennyroyal, eucalyptus, calendula, and lavender with 2 cups of rubbing alcohol in a closed glass container. Let the herbs infuse for seven days, shaking the mixture daily. Then, strain and discard the herbs and bottle the repellent with a label listing its ingredients and the date made.

Bee Sting and Insect Bite Lotion

For those times that the bugs get to you, here is a lotion to apply: In a large bowl, combine 2 pints of rubbing alcohol with 1 ounce dried echinacea root, 1 ounce dried plantain leaves, ½ ounce yellow dock root, and 1 *bulb* of chopped or pressed, peeled garlic. Cover the bowl with a plate or plastic wrap and let the mixture stand in a dark place for one week, shaking it daily. Strain and pour the mixture into a dark or opaque bottle. Apply it as a wash and/or a small poultice, using a piece of cotton gauze.

Sunburn Lotion

In a large mixing bowl, combine 1 pint of witch hazel extract and 1 pint of rubbing alcohol with ½ ounce each of dry beech leaves, borage, comfrey, and birch twigs or leaves. As the herbs become hydrated again, macerate them gently in the bowl. Let the mixture stand for one week, covered, in a bowl or a jar, and mix daily. Then strain and discard the herbs. Place the liquid in an electric blender with 1 cup of aloe gel and 1 tablespoon of almond oil. Blend well, then bottle and store in the refrigerator. The lotion should keep well for one summer, but use or discard it before the next year's season. Shake well before using.

Suppositories

Herb-based suppositories can relieve pain in mild cases of hemorrhoids or vaginal infection. Astringent herbs such as oak bark, yarrow, or raspberry leaf, demulcent herbs such as slippery elm, and antiseptic/antibiotic herbs such as garlic, echinacea, or goldenseal are used by herbalists in making suppositories. One simple suppository recipe calls for equal amounts of powdered slippery elm bark, goldenseal root, and white oak bark.

Making suppositories is not difficult. Mix the powdered herb with vegetable oil or water to form a dough. Shape the dough into cylindrical strips, about ½ inch thick and 1 to 1½ inches long. Coat one end with cocoa butter to aid insertion. Or you can make the entire suppository with a base of cocoa butter instead of using oil or water. If you do use cocoa butter, refrigerate the suppositories until firm, then allow them to warm to room temperature before using.

Use suppositories at night before going to bed. Protect bedding and clothing from discharge with a towel, especially if the suppository is mixed with oil or cocoa butter.

Slippery Elm Suppository for Hemorrhoids

This is an effective and quick-acting treatment for mild hemorrhoids. For serious cases you should of course see a doctor. Combine 5 parts slippery elm powder with 1 part white oak powder. Moisten the mixture with enough water to make a dry, doughlike paste. Form the paste into 1-inch oblong spheres. Allow the suppositories to dry until firm. To apply one, moisten its entire surface, coat it with vegetable oil, and insert.

Tinctures

Until about 50 years ago, there were hundreds of tinctures listed in the United States Pharmacopoeia (the official listing of pharmaceutical raw materials and recipes in regular use, which is issued annually by the United States government). Although tinctures are no longer readily available to the general public, they remain very useful to the herbalist. Tinctures are an excellent medium for preserving and concentrating the healing qualities of herbs.

Tinctures are effective in very small amounts, because they are so concentrated. Several drops to 1 tablespoon is the general dosage, depending on the tincture and the ailment. We recommend caution in the use of tinctures, because they are so potent. They can be very effective, if not overused.

Do not confuse the concentrates called "fluid extracts" of herbs, available commercially today, with tinctures. These fluid extracts are even more potent than tinctures—often ten times as strong. Despite the potency of herb tinctures, pioneer homeopaths experimented freely with them, noting and recording the physiological reactions in themselves to each one. Much of our current knowledge of herb tinctures stems from their courageous research. These early herbalists theorized that if a tincture caused a certain condition in themselves, the homeopathic remedy made from the tincture would also "cure" that condition in a sick person.

To make a tincture, combine 4 ounces of the powdered or finely cut herb with 1 pint of spirits such as brandy, vodka, or gin in a large jar or jug with a secure-fitting lid. (Never use rubbing or isopropyl alcohol, or methyl or wood alcohol, both of which are poisonous!) Shake the mixture several times daily, over a two-week period. By the end of this time, the herb will have released its properties to the alcohol. Let the herb settle, then strain off the liquid into another clean bottle for storage. Many herbalists put up tinctures at the time of the new moon and finish them on the full moon to take advantage of the natural drawing power attributed to the waxing moon.

The classic book *American Medicinal Plants*, written in the 1800s by botanist and homeopathic doctor Charles Millspaugh, gives directions for making tinctures of many common American herbs. It makes interesting reading.

Making Herbal Syrups

Honey-based herbal syrups are a simple and effective way to preserve the healing qualities of some herbs. Syrups can soothe sore throats and provide some relief from coughs and colds. Some serve as laxatives or general tonics.

To make an herbal syrup, combine 2 ounces of dried herb with 1 quart of water in a large pot. Boil that down until it is reduced to 1 pint, then add 1 to 2 ounces of honey. If you use fresh fruit, leaves, or roots in making syrups, you should double the amount of herbs. Using these general guidelines, you can make herbal syrups with just about any herb. See the specific recipes, also. Store all herbal syrups in the refrigerator for up to one month.

Dried licorice, fresh gingerroot, and elderberries are all well-known ingredients for cough syrups. Another old-fashioned cough syrup recipe calls for horehound.

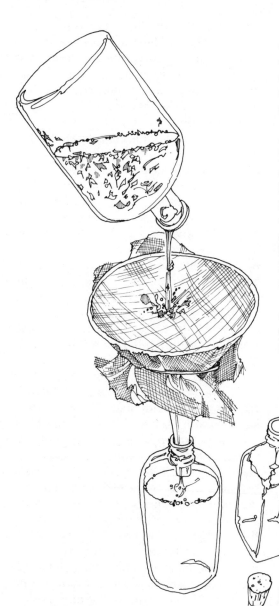

After two weeks, a finished tincture is strained into clean bottles and capped or corked.

Horehound Cough Syrup

Make an infusion of fresh or dried horehound leaves according to the directions under Infusions, earlier in this chapter. Allow it to steep for only ten minutes, though. Then strain off the leaves and measure the remaining liquid. Add twice as much honey as liquid, mix well, and bottle. To soothe a cough, take about 1 teaspoon at a time, about four times a day.

Borage Syrup

Borage has soothing, demulcent qualities. You can make borage syrup by juicing the borage leaves and stems in a vegetable juicer. Mix 1 cup of this mucilaginous juice with 1 cup of honey and bring to a boil. Remove from heat and bottle. Take about 1 teaspoon at a time four times a day.

Elderberry Syrup

European herbalists recommend this syrup for colds and constipation. To prepare it, simmer 1 gallon of fully ripened elderberries with ½ cup water in a large soup pot until soft. Strain the berries, saving the liquid. (You can puree the berries in a strainer and add the pureed pulp, if you like.) Add ½ ounce grated fresh ginger and 18 whole cloves to the liquid. Boil for one hour uncovered. Strain and discard the spices and bottle the syrup when cooled. The syrup is taken in 3- or 4-ounce doses. Pour enough syrup to fill a wine glass halfway. Then add very hot water to fill the glass entirely. Add honey to taste and enjoy!

Garlic Syrup

Herbalists use this syrup as an expectorant. Bring 1 pint of water to a boil in a medium-size pot with a cover. Remove the water from the heat and add 2 ounces finely chopped garlic. Cover the pot and allow the mixture to stand ten hours at room temperature. Strain and discard the garlic. Add 4 tablespoons honey and 1 tablespoon vinegar. Then bottle and store the syrup in the refrigerator. The syrup is taken by the teaspoonful about four times a day.

Licorice Syrup

You can make a simple licorice syrup by filling a Pyrex or enamel container with pieces of the fresh or dried root. Cover the roots with water and simmer for three to four hours. Strain and discard the roots and bottle the syrup in a sterilized bottle with a tight lid. You can add 2 tablespoons of honey for each cup of the syrup before bottling it. The honey adds to the existing demulcent and emollient qualities of the herb, and also acts as a preservative for the syrup. A teaspoon or two of this syrup can be used every few hours for alleviating sore throats, coughs, and lung congestion.

Compresses, Poultices, and Plasters

Compresses, poultices, and plasters are methods of applying herbs to the surface of the body to ease various imbalances. Herbalists around the world have for many centuries applied herbs in this way to stimulate, soothe, relax, and nourish the bodies of those they treated.

Compresses consist of towels soaked in herbal infusions or teas and applied to an area of the body in order to soothe, stimulate, or otherwise energize. The herbs used for compresses can be those with stimulating and warming properties, or those with soothing and cooling qualities. A stimulating herb such as cayenne or ginger is used in a compress to increase circulation and energize areas of the body that are congested or debilitated. A soothing compress can help dissipate excess heat or nervous energy, or calm swelling from sprains or bruises. Compresses, as well as poultices and plasters, should be applied in a warm room, in order to keep the recipient of such treatments comfortable.

To prepare a compress, immerse a clean washcloth or hand towel in the herbal infusion. Keep the tea steaming hot, between 150° and 180°F. Hold the cloth with the thumb and index finger of both hands, taking hold of its opposite corner. When the cloth is hot, wring it out by twisting it from the corners (see illustration) and apply it as hot as possible to the affected part of the person. If the washcloth or towel is too wet, it may burn the skin, so wring it out well and quickly, wearing rubber gloves if necessary.

Once applied, cover the hot compress with a dry towel and prepare another compress. The first compress will cool in two to

To apply an herbal compress, dip the towel in the herbal infusion and wring it out thoroughly. Then place the warm compress on the part of the body being treated and cover it with a clean, dry towel.

three minutes and will need changing. Replace it with the second compress and keep alternating the cloths this way.

Compresses are usually applied for 10 to 30 minutes, and the hot cloths are changed every few minutes throughout the treatment. But the duration of the treatment will vary, of course, with the herbs used and the condition of the person. Generally, you can stop the compress application when the treated skin becomes uniformly flushed, or if a tingling sensation or feelings of relief develop. This general procedure can be followed when making and applying most compresses.

A poultice consists of dried, powdered, or macerated herbs that are moistened with hot water or herb tea and applied directly to the skin area to be treated. A clean towel, cloth, or bandage placed over the poultice will hold it in place. Poultices are effective for drawing out infection and foreign bodies and relieving muscle spasms and pain. Whenever using poultices and plasters, make sure that the cloth covering the poultice is warm, and that the person is comfortably warm.

A sprain, bruise, or broken bone may require a cool cloth to ease the pain and swelling before the doctor arrives. Cool compresses made with cooling herbs such as aloe, borage, or comfrey leaf will help keep down swelling on such occasions. (Do not use comfrey *root* in this instance, because it is warming, not cooling.)

A plaster consists of herbs set within the folds of a cloth, usually cheesecloth or muslin. You can make an herbal bandage or mini-plaster to use for small injuries when an antiseptic and healing effect is desired. Sprinkle a little goldenseal root powder and comfrey root powder on a piece of gauze, and apply it with surgical tape over the injured area. Be sure that the cut is very clean before you apply the herbal bandage.

Ginger Compress

Chinese and Japanese healers use the ginger compress extensively. In his book, *Healing Ourselves,* Naboru Muramoto describes the benefits of a ginger compress:

The ginger compress is the typical symbol of "clean" medicine. It makes few demands of its user and takes only a few minutes to prepare. It is painless and even rather pleasant, costs little . . . and accomplishes a lot. In fact, one could write a book simply recording case histories of its successes.[6]

According to Muramoto, the herbalist can use the ginger compress effectively to relieve pain, improve circulation, and combat inflammation. Use 2 quarts of water and 5 ounces of grated fresh gingerroot. Remember, do not boil the water when making the tea, but keep it very hot, about 158°F. Strain the ginger tea through a cheesecloth strainer. Squeeze any remaining juice from the cheesecloth by twisting the cloth carefully. Apply the compress according to the general instructions given above.

Slippery Elm Compress

Naturopathic doctor Michael Tierra cites the effectiveness of the herbal compress in his book *The Way of Herbs.* Tierra relates a tale of a time when he applied a compress of slippery elm to a member of his family who was ill in the hospital. The patient was suffering from postoperative shock and displaying extreme weakness and severe diarrhea. The next morning, the diarrhea and dehydration had improved and the patient was able to eat again. Slippery elm has been described as encouraging muscle relaxation, and the herb, a mild calmative, has also been used as a specific for the intestines. These herbal qualities combine with the relaxing properties of the heated compress to help the ailing person. To make a Slippery Elm Compress follow the general directions above for compresses.

Slippery Elm Poultice

Slippery elm is used in poultice form, too, to soothe inflamed skin surfaces, burns, bruises, and wounds. Just work the herb powder into a paste with some warm water and apply it to a cloth, then to the affected area. It is considered an effective remedy for treating mastitis, too.

Burn Poultices

The best poultice for minor burns is made simply with the liquid, gellike contents of the aloe vera leaf. (For instructions on harvesting the gel for this use see the entry on Aloe in chapter 4.) You can also make effective burn poultices with the fresh, macerated leaves of beech trees, blackberry, borage, plantain, or comfrey.

Poison Ivy Poultice

The Native Americans used the fresh bark of beech trees as a poultice for skin irritations, especially poison ivy. To make this poultice, fill a jar with pieces of the bark, pour in boiling water to cover, and let the infusion steep for 20 minutes. Strain and discard the bark and allow the infusion to cool. Then apply the tea to the skin and cover it with cheesecloth.

Comfrey Poultice

A comfrey poultice is a traditional treatment for cuts, burns, skin ulcers, boils, hemor-

rhoids, sprains, and fractures. You can make this poultice in two ways.

One method is to place the chopped leaves in a pot with enough water to cover them. Boil the mixture briefly, allow it to cool, and then place the strained leaves in between two layers of clean gauze. Apply this poultice to the affected area. A similar poultice may be made by using fresh roots, which are pounded or ground. Fresh or dried leaves or roots can also be used in a hot compress.

Mustard Plaster

The mustard plaster was a popular home remedy until recent times. It was used to treat fatigue, tiredness, and overall weakness. In making this classic treatment, enough powdered yellow or black mustard seed is mixed with water to make a paste. The paste is painted onto a cloth with a small brush. The plaster cloth is placed over another cloth, which is laid on the affected part of the body. A third cloth should cover the plaster. Check the treated area every five minutes for skin irritation and remove the plaster immediately if any develops. You can dilute the plaster with some rye flour if the ill person has sensitive skin.

Burdock Plaster

Oriental medicine treats gout with a poultice of fresh burdock leaves. The leaves are bruised with a mortar and pestle, or other pounding implement, and applied to the affected area, then covered with a warm cloth.

Cayenne Plaster

A plaster of cayenne and bran is a good treatment for colds and chest congestion, or simply to invigorate a tired and fatigued person. To make the plaster, combine 4 tablespoons of cayenne powder with 2 cups of bran and mix in enough hot water to make a spreadable paste. Spread this paste between two layers of cheesecloth. For chest congestion, apply the plaster to either the chest or back and cover with a warm towel. For treating fatigue, put the poultice over the kidney area in the lower back and cover it.

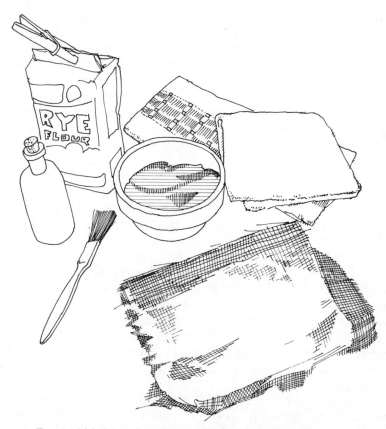

For an old-fashioned mustard plaster, a paste made of ground mustard seed and water is painted onto a piece of cheesecloth, which is then placed on top of a clean cloth.

Liniments

A liniment is a medicated herb liquid, perfect for soothing strained and aching muscles, as well as sprained and inflamed areas. Cayenne, myrrh, and goldenseal are herbs commonly used in making liniments.

All-Good Liniment

You can apply this liniment to soothe bruises, sprains, minor scalds, burns, and sunburn. In a large jar or jug with a tight-fitting lid, combine 2 ounces myrrh gum powder, 1 ounce goldenseal powder, and ½ ounce cayenne powder with 1 quart rubbing alcohol or 1 quart apple cider vinegar. Let the mixture stand for seven days in the closed jar or jug, shaking daily. Then strain and discard the herbs and bottle the liniment. To treat aching muscles or sprains, rub the liniment on the affected areas with your hands. For minor burns, scalds, or sunburn, simply pat the liniment onto the affected area with a clean, soft cloth.

Herbal Oils

The aromatic and healing qualities of herb oils make them very versatile. The essential oil can be extracted from any herb, using one of the three following methods.

Macerate 2 ounces of dried herb, or double that amount of fresh herb with a mortar and pestle. Combine with 1 pint of olive oil, or other pure vegetable oil, such as almond, sunflower seed, or sesame. Then, let the mixture stand in a warm place, covered for three days. Strain and discard the herb and bottle the oil.

Another method involves gently heating the herbs. Combine the herbs and oil in a pot large enough to hold them. Heat the mixture gently, uncovered, for 1 hour, allowing the oil to get no hotter than 200°F. Strain and bottle when cooled.

You can also extract herbal properties with alcohol (use the method described in tinctures, page 315). Combine approximately ½ cup of the herbal tincture with 1 pint of oil in a medium-size pot and gently heat. The amount of tincture used varies with the strength of the tincture and the desired strength of the oil. The alcohol will evaporate gradually, leaving just the herbal oil.

Commercial herb oils are usually prepared by direct steam distillation in large batches. Steam distillation can be done at home, but the equipment and techniques are somewhat specialized. For those who want to experiment in home distillation, we recommend personal guidance from a trained expert as the best method of learning. Local high school or college chemistry classes may be well equipped to teach safe and effective methods of distillation.

You can use any of these methods to extract the oils of a wide variety of herbs. Rose petals, lavender flowers, mint leaves, rosemary, jasmine, calendula, and sage leaves and flowers are just a few of the herbs that yield delightful oils. Actually, almost any medicinal property of an herb can be made use of in an oil preparation.

Massage Oils

An invigorating massage oil can be made by macerating equal parts of bay and eucalyptus leaves and grated fresh gingerroot. Prepare the oil as described above and use it for massaging sore muscles, bruises, strains, and older sprains.

To make a cooling oil to apply immediately to swollen joints, bruises or burns,

To make lavender oil, pure olive oil is poured into a pint bottle which contains 2 ounces of macerated lavender.

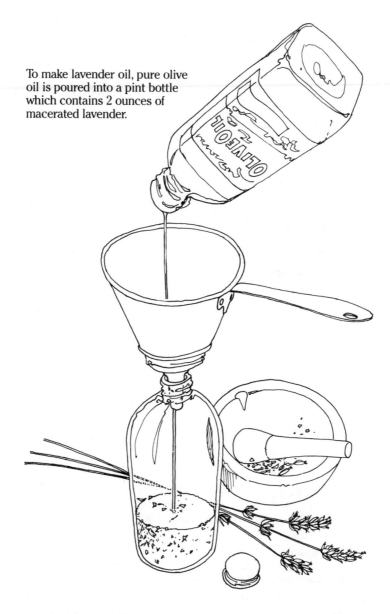

macerate equal parts of fresh borage, comfrey leaves, aloe vera, and peppermint and prepare as described above. You can also make a calming, analgesic, and slightly sedative massage oil with equal parts of lavender flowers, peony root, poplar bark, and slippery elm bark. If you wish, substitute birch twigs and leaves for poplar bark, and raspberry leaves for peony root. Or, use all of these herbs together. This recipe is very useful for relieving the type of subtle, almost imperceptible spasms that follow muscle injuries or strains. It is also considered good for chronic tension, menstrual cramps, and joint pains.

Bath Oils

There are many herbs that make wonderful bath oils. One that we particularly like, an all-flower bath oil, is made by the tincture method (described on page 315). To make it, fill a wide-mouth jar with equal parts of lavender, peony, sage, yarrow, calendula, and basswood flowers. Since this tincture is not for internal use, you can then pour in rubbing alcohol to fill the jar. Let the mixture stand for one week in a cool, dark place. Then for each pint of alcohol used, combine 1 pint of oil with the mixture in a large open bowl. Place the bowl in a warm place, for one day, allowing most of the alcohol to evaporate. Then strain out the liquid, squeezing the flowers as dry as possible. Store the oil in a cool spot. In general, add about ½ cup of this oil to a standard-size tub of bath water. Add more if you like, but you will deplete your store of bath oil quite fast.

Moisturizing Oil

One of the very best moisturizing oils comes from the yellow flowers of mullein. Collect the flowers by picking them from the stalk one by one. This is time-consuming, but the results are well worth the effort. Macerate the fresh flowers in a bowl and then pour in almond oil to cover them. Almond oil is the best choice as a base, since it is very moisturizing by itself. Cover the bowl and let it stand for one week, then strain and press the excess oil from the flowers. This particular

oil is also good for soothing irritations from infections of the ear.

Making Herbal Salves and Ointments

Herbal salves and ointments, useful for healing cuts and in treating skin ailments, are simple and fun to make. The basic recipe for salves and ointments calls for 2 ounces of the dried herb, or 4 ounces of the fresh herb, per pint of oil. Olive, sesame, and almond oil are good oils to use for salves. Extract the herb's properties by heating the herb in the oil for about one hour as described above for Herbal Oils. Then strain and discard the herb. Add 1 to 1½ ounces of melted beeswax to the herb oil. Stir the mixture as it thickens and cools, and bottle the salve in a wide-mouth jar. If you use your salve very seldom, it is best to store it in the refrigerator, where it will keep for up to a year. If the mixture separates, from heat or long disuse, simply reheat it and allow to cool.

Skin-Healing Salve

A wonderful healing salve can be made using 1 ounce of dried calendula petals, ½ ounce of dried comfrey leaves, and ½ ounce dried plantain leaves. Proceed as described in the general directions for making salves.

Soothing Salve

Chickweed salve is a good medicine to have on hand for soothing itching and rashes. To make it, combine 12 ounces of fresh chickweed with 1 pint of oil in an ovenproof vessel and gently heat it in a low oven (150°F) for three hours. Then strain the chickweed and add the melted beeswax to the oil, as described in the general directions above.

Green Elder Ointment

Elder ointments may have originated with the European gypsies. In addition to soothing cuts and bruises, they are good for rubbing on the back and chest to promote easier breathing and relieve congestion from colds and flu. This old-fashioned remedy is made with the fresh leaves of the green elder. Use 4 ounces of leaves to 1 pint of oil, and prepare according to the general directions above. You can prepare a similar ointment using the green or unripe berries of the elder.

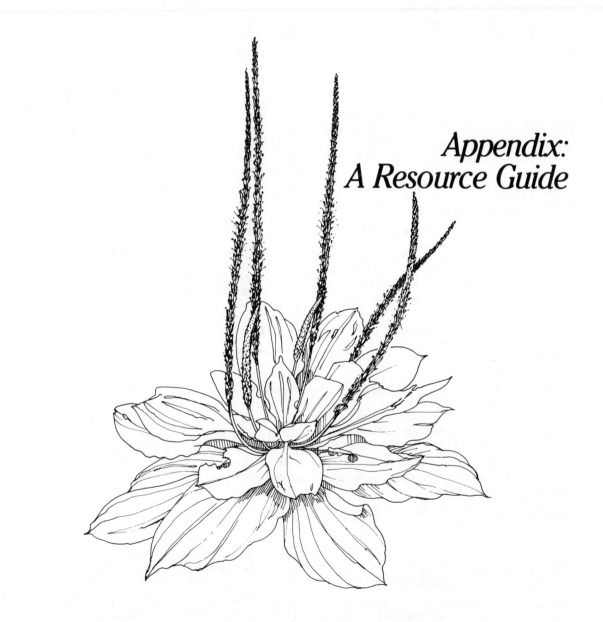

Appendix:
A Resource Guide

Herbal Newsletters

(see also listings below for Gardening Centers,
Schools, and Societies)

The Business of Herbs, P.O. Box 559, Madison, VA
22727. Provides news on herb marketing for the
small grower, classifieds, current market prices for
herbs.

Herb News Herbalgram, P.O. Box 12602, Austin, TX
78711. Covers herb industry news, book reviews,
government rulings, research briefs.

Update on Herbs, Association for the Promotion of
Herbal Healing, 1009 Third St., Santa Cruz, CA
95060. Includes product reviews, articles about
herbal healing and research and education.

Gardening Centers, Schools, and Societies

The Alan Chadwick Society, Green Gulch Farm,
Star Rt. 1, Sausalito, CA 94965. Established to make
available Alan Chadwick's biodynamic teachings
and to help gardeners. Publishes biannual newsletter for members.

Biodynamic Farming and Gardening Association,
Wyoming, RI 02898. Publishes *Bio-Dynamics*, makes
available books and other information about the
biodynamic method.

The Herb Society of America, 191 Sudbury Rd.,
Concord, MA 01742. Publishes annual, as well as
pamphlets on herb growing and use. Slides and
lectures for rent. Please send stamped, self-addressed
envelope with inquiries.

The Maritime Permaculture Institute, 641 Chan-
dler Rd., Chehalis, WA 98532. Offers workshops
and design consultation.

The National Herb Garden, at the U.S. National
Arboretum, Washington, D.C. Contains model herb
gardens and has educational materials and
programs.

Northwest Bio-dynamic Agriculture Society, P.O.
Box 97, Chilliwack, BC, Canada V2P 6H7.

Oak Valley Herb Farm, Star Rt., Camptonville, CA
95922. Offers classes in herb gardening, weekend

workshops on use of herbs, wild herb walks. Hours
by appointment only.

Tilth, 2270 N.W. Irving, Portland, OR 97210. An
association with a dozen chapters in the Pacific
Northwest. Publishes books, pamphlets, newsletters,
conducts workshops and conferences on sustainable agriculture.

Trout Lake Farm, Rt. 1, Box 355, Trout Lake, WA
98650. An organic herb farm, growing high-quality
peppermint, spearmint, clover, alfalfa, and other
herbs on about 55 fertile acres in southern Washington State. Active in the movement to provide
networking for small organic herb farmers, Trout
Lake helped to organize an organic herb growers
and producers cooperative in the Pacific Northwest.
The cooperative recently merged with the American Herb Association.

Herbal Health Centers, Schools, and Societies

American Herb Association, P.O. Box 353, Rescue,
CA 95672. Educational and research organization,
publishes newsletter and journal for members, maintains book department, republishes out-of-print
herbals and other botanical books.

Arura Institute of Buddhist Medicine, 2135 S.E.
76th Ave., Portland, OR 97215. Founded to help
establish the Tibetan Buddhist medical science
in America. Offers instruction, information, and
products related to Tibetan healing.

Association for the Promotion of Herbal Healing,
1009 Third St., Santa Cruz, CA 95060. Publishes
Update on Herbs newsletter, quarterly, serves as
information networking organization in herb
research area.

John Bastyr College of Naturopathic Medicine, 144
N.E. 54th St., Seattle, WA 98104. A degree-granting
naturopathic college.

The Beneficial Plant Research Association, 418
Mission Ave., San Raphael, CA 94901. Educational
organization founded to investigate and promote
use of plants to benefit human life.

California School of Herbal Studies, P.O. Box 350,
Guerneville, CA 95466. Six-month training program

includes study of botany, taxonomy, clinical herbology, Chinese herbology, formulations, etc. Also sponsors herb intensives, retreats, plant walks.

Dominion Herbal College, 7527 Kingsway, Burnaby, BC, Canada V3N 3C1. Offers correspondence courses in herbology.

The Flower Essence Society, P.O. Box 459, Nevada City, CA 95959. Training program in use of flower essences for healing. Practitioner certification available. Publishes *Flower Essence Journal,* available with membership, or separately.

Herb Pharm, P.O. Box 116, Williams, OR 97544. Offers intensive apprenticeship training program in medical herbology, including gardening, harvesting wild plants, cleaning, drying, storing, and preparing herb formulas in the laboratory.

Institute for Traditional Medicine and Preventive Health Care, 215 John St., Santa Cruz, CA 95060. Offers professional training program in Chinese herbology, as well as correspondence course in that area. Maintains research library in Chinese, Tibetan, Ayurvedic medicine, open by appointment. Operates herb clinics in several California cities.

International Tree Crops Institute, P.O. Box 666, Winters, CA 95694. A research organization which provides information on agroforestry and its benefits. The Institute publishes a scientific journal, *Agroforestry Review*, and makes available various scientific papers and books that demonstrate the benefits of tree crops to the environment. These publications also provide information on tree crops' uses as food and fodder.

National College of Naturopathic Medicine, 11231 S.E. Market St., Portland, OR 97216. Oldest of only two colleges in the United States currently granting a doctor of naturopathy degree. Four-year residency program.

The North American Fruit Explorers, 103 Smith Chapel Rd., Mount Olive, NC 28365. A membership organization of fruit growers. Seed and scion wood exchanges are one benefit of membership, and friendship with other "fruit explorers" is another benefit.

The Northern Nut Growers Association, c/o Niagara College, P.O. Box 340, St. Catherines, ON, Canada L2R 6V6. A membership organization of people

interested in nut tree culture. Like the North American Fruit Explorers, it provides benefits of shared information, friendship, and availability of seeds and seedlings.

Oak Valley Herb Farm, Star Rt., Camptonville, CA 95922. Offers instruction in herbology, has a botanical garden.

Oriental Healing Arts Institute, 8820 S. Sepulveda Blvd., Suite 218, Los Angeles, CA 90045. Offers bimonthly bulletin to members, publishes books on Chinese medicine and herb use.

The Platonic Academy of Herbal Studies, Box 409, Santa Cruz, CA 95061. Instruction in growing and using medicinal plants, pharmacognosy, history and practice, medical botany, clinical herbology. One- to four-year program, culminating in professional degree.

Herb Seed and Nursery Companies

Abundant Life Seed Company, P.O. Box 772, Port Townsend, WA 98368. Herb, flower, vegetable, forage crop seeds, catalog available.

Gardens of the Blue Ridge, P.O. Box 10, Pineola, NC 28662. Goldenseal roots, other herbs.

Meadowbrook Herbs and Things, Inc., Whispering Pines Road, Wyoming, RI 02898. Biodynamically grown herbs, seeds, catalog available.

The Naturalists, P.O. Box 435, Yorktown Heights, NY 10598. Catalog of herb seeds available.

Nichol's Garden Nursery, 1190 N. Pacific Hwy., Albany, OR 97321. Herb plants, seeds, products, and books, catalog available.

Sanctuary Seeds, 1913 Yew St., Vancouver, BC, Canada V6K 3G3. Herb and other seeds, catalog available.

Taylor's Herb Garden, 1535 Lone Oak Rd., Vista, CA 92083. Herb plants and seeds, large herb garden, catalog available.

Well-Sweep Herb Farm, 317 Mt. Bethel Rd., Port Murray, NJ 07865. Herb plants and seeds, lectures and tours of garden available, catalog available.

Notes

CHAPTER ONE

Healing Gardens and Herbal Medicine in History

1. Joseph Campbell, *The Masks of God: Occidental Mythology* (New York: Viking Press, 1964), p. 13.

2. Arturo Castiglioni, *A History of Medicine*, trans. E. B. Krumbhaar (New York: Alfred A. Knopf, 1958), p. 172.

CHAPTER TWO

Herbal Healing Traditions in Europe and America

1. *Medical Works*, "Amorphisms," vol. 4 (Cambridge, Mass.: Harvard University Press n.d.), p. 150.

2. Ibid., "The Nature of Man," p. 204.

3. Ibid., p. 208.

4. Ibid., p. 207.

5. Barbara Griggs, *Green Pharmacy: A History of Herbal Medicine* (New York: Viking Press, 1981), p. 229.

6. Black Elk, *Black Elk Speaks*, ed. John G. Neihardt (Lincoln, Nebr.: University of Nebraska Press, 1961), pp. 200–202.

CHAPTER THREE

Herbal Healing Traditions in the East

1. Bhagawan Dash, *Tibetan Medicine, with Special Reference to Yoga Sataka* (Dharamsala, India: Library of Tibetan Works and Archives, 1976), p. 49.

CHAPTER FOUR

An Illustrated Guide to Healing Plants

1. Merritt Lyndon Fernald and Charles Alfred Kinsey, *Edible Wild Plants of Eastern North America*, rev. Reed Collins (New York: Harper and Row, 1958), p. 155.

2. Richard Lucas, *Secrets of the Chinese Herbalists* (New York: Cornerstone Library, 1978), p. 181.

3. Virgil Vogel, *American Indian Medicine* (Norman, Okla.: University of Oklahoma Press, 1970), p. 356.

4. James A. Duke, "Chinese Anti-Cancer Plants," (Beltsville, Md.: USDA Economic Botany Division, 1982), p. 3.

5. Ibid., p. 3.

6. *Herb News*, Spring 1981, p. 18.

7. Ibid., p. 17.

8. Louise Veninga and Benjamin R. Zaricor, *Goldenseal/Etc.* (Santa Cruz, Calif.: Ruka Publications, 1976), p. 29.

9. Charles F. Millspaugh, *American Medicinal Plants* (New York: Dover Publications, 1974), p. 726.

10. Maurice Mességué, *Health Secrets of Plants and Herbs* (New York: William Morrow, 1975), p. 157.

11. Ibid., p. 46.

12. Naboru Muramoto, *Healing Ourselves*, ed. Michel Abehsera (New York: Avon, 1973), p. 94.

13. Mességué, *Health Secrets of Plants and Herbs*, p. 182.

14. Ibid., p. 200.

15. Maude Grieve, *A Modern Herbal* (New York: Dover Publications, 1971), p. 575.

16. Robert Graves, *The White Goddess* (New York: Farrar, Straus and Giroux, 1966), p. 176.

17. Mességué, *Health Secrets of Plants and Herbs*, p. 209.

CHAPTER FIVE

Creating a Garden of Healing Herbs

1. The Mother, *Flowers and Fragrances*, pamphlet (Pondicherry, India: Sri Aurobindo Society, 1979), unpaginated.

2. Ibid.,

3. Ven. Rechung Rinpoche, trans., *Tibetan Medicine* (Berkeley and Los Angeles: University of California Press, 1973), p. 236.

4. Alan Chadwick, interview with the authors, 1976.

5. Rudolph Steiner, *Agriculture* (Shrewsberry, Great Britain: Wilding & Son, 1972), p. 97.

6. Alan Chadwick, *The Dirtman Journal* (Covelo, Calif.: Round Valley Institute for Man and Nature, 1976), p. 8.

7. Masanobu Fukuoka, *The One-Straw Revolution* (Emmaus, Pa.: Rodale Press, 1978), p. 41.

8. Ibid., p. 66.

9. Ibid., p. 147.

10. Bargyla and Glyver Rateaver, *Organic Methods Primer* (Pauma Valley, Calif.: published by the authors, 1975),

11. Fukuoka, *The One-Straw Revolution,* p. 35.

12. John Jeavons, *How to Grow More Vegetables* (Berkeley, Calif.: Ten Speed Press, 1982), p. 52.

13. Becky Burns, "The Healing Power within the Plant Kingdom," *Tilth* 7, no. 3 (Fall 1981):24-25.

14. Francis Adams, trans., *Great Books of the Western World*, "Hippocratic Writings, The Law" (Encyclopedia Britannica, 1952), p. 144.

CHAPTER SIX

Good Things from the Garden: Gathering and Using the Herbal Harvest

1. Maurice Mességué, *Of Men and Plants* (New York: Bantam Books, 1973), p. 10.

2. Ibid., p. 109.

3. Oh Shinnah Fastwolf, interview with the authors, 1977.

4. Michael Tierra, *The Way of Herbs* (New York: Washington Square Press, 1983), p. 485.

5. Mességué, *Of Men and Plants,* p. 2.

6. Naboru Muramoto, *Healing Ourselves*, ed. Michel Abehsera (New York: Avon, 1973), p. 110.

Glossary

Adaptogen: An herb that maintains health by increasing the body's ability to adapt to environmental and internal stress. Adaptogens generally work by strengthening the immune system, nervous system and/or glandular system.

Analgesic: An herb that relieves pain by acting as a nervine, antispasmodic, rubefacient, antiseptic, antibiotic, or counterirritant.

Anesthetic, Local: An agent that reduces pain in an area by desensitizing the nerves.

Anthelmintic: An herb, food, or medicine that expels intestinal worms.

Antibiotic: An organic substance that is capable of killing viruses, bacteria, or other microorganisms and is used to combat infections or diseases.

Antiseptic: A substance that destroys bacteria; usually applied to the skin to prevent infection.

Antispasmodic: A relaxant or nervine that relieves or prevents involuntary muscle contractions, or "spasms," such as those occurring in epilepsy, painful menstruation, intestinal cramping, or muscle "shock."

Aromatic: An herb with a strong, volatile, and fragrant aroma. Sometimes the term is used to denote a general class of herbs in the Umbellifer family (anise, caraway, dill, fennel). But aromatics can also include other herbs that have strong aromas and penetrating oils. In this sense, aromatic is very similar to carminative. Medicinally, aromatics are used to relieve flatulence, open nasal passages, or eliminate phlegm, although many people regard them merely as pleasant scents. The medicinal definition of aromatic is not related to the chemical definition, which refers to a cyclic carbon compound with shared double bonds.

Some constituents of herbs, their essential oils for instance, are also aromatic in the chemical sense of the word.

Astringent: A substance that causes dehydration, tightening, or shrinking of tissues and is used to stop bleeding, close skin pores, tighten muscles, and so on.

Building: A food or herb that is thought to gradually increase some function of the body, generally by supplying nutrients, rather than by stimulation of the nervous or circulatory system.

Calmative: An herb that relaxes, usually a nervine affecting the central nervous system.

Carminative: Medicine that helps to expel gas from the large and/or small intestine.

Cathartic: Substances that strongly evacuate the colon.

Compress: A form of treatment in which a hot or cold herb tea is applied with towels to the skin in order to relieve congestion, soreness, or tension.

Decoction: Preparation of herbal tea made by simmering herbs in water. Herbs and their parts that are woody, waxy, and/or contain nonvolatile oils are usually made into a decoction.

Demulcent: A soothing, moistening herbal property, which helps relieve irritation.

Diaphoretic: An herb or substance taken internally to increase perspiration, usually through expansion of capillaries near the skin.

Diuretic: An herb or food that increases the flow of urine.

Drying: The property of removing or eliminating water, mucus, blood, bile, lymph, or other fluids. When it refers to a process within the body, drying is a relative term: An herb that increases the flow of bile from the liver dries the liver, but moistens the gallbladder and intestines.

Eliminating: The quality or process of removing something from the body, such as heat, fluids, energy, nervous tension, waste products, or toxins.

Emetic: A substance that causes vomiting.

Emmenagogue: Taken internally, a substance that promotes menstruation, or the flow of menses. Some emmenagogues, such as pennyroyal, are so strong that they have been used to induce abortion. The use of emmenagogues as a form of birth control is not recommended.

Emollient: A substance that softens the skin when applied externally.

Expectorant: Taken internally, it helps the body expel phlegm through coughing, sneezing, or spitting.

Extract: A product made by removing essential constituents from herbs through pressing, distilling, or using a solvent.

Holistic: In reference to health, the way of prevention and treatment, which takes into account factors such as diet, attitude, emotions, relationships, activities, and constitution. Holistic therapies aim at treating the whole person. They include herbology, nutrition, fasting, massage, psychotherapy, exercise, creative arts, dreaming, meditation, bathing, acupuncture, and counseling.

Humor: A category of physiological functions and qualities, which also includes nonphysical aspects. Humors are related to subtle element systems. Bile, phlegm, and blood are generally the humors described by the ancient systems of Greece and India.

Infusion: A method of making herbal tea by steeping the herbs in water that has been boiled, but which is no longer boiling when the herbs and water are mixed. Herbs or their parts, which are leaves, flowers, or which contain volatile oils, are usually prepared as infusions.

Laxative: An herb, food, or medicine that causes elimination of the feces. Laxatives work by stimulating peristaltic action of the intestinal wall, by moistening the colon, by increasing the secretion of bile, or by relaxing intestinal cramps.

Moistening: The herbal property of making the body or some part of the body more moist, or encouraging the flow of liquid into a particular part of the body. Like drying, moistening is a relative term when it is used to refer to processes within the body.

Moxa, Moxibustion: A technique used in Tibetan and Chinese medicine, related to acupuncture, in which rolls of dried mugwort are burned above specific points on the body.

Mucilaginous: The herbal property that is soothing to inflammations. These herbs are slippery or slimy.

Nervine: An herb that relaxes the whole body or a part of the body by affecting the nervous system.

Neutral: An herb that gradually strengthens and tones, used by itself or in formulas to balance eliminators and builders. Usually neutrals are also tonics.

Nutritive: see Building.

Plaster: A form of herbal treatment in which herbs are made into a paste or mass and applied to the skin.

Polypharmacy: The branch of herbology in which herbs are combined in formulas in order to increase their synergistic action.

Poultice: An application of fresh or moistened dried herbs to the skin.

Purgative: see Cathartic.

Refrigerant: An herb that is considered cooling. Often, an herb that reduces fever by cooling.

Rubefacient: A substance that increases blood circulation to the area where it is applied, usually on the skin but sometimes internally.

Salve: An ointment or lotion made from herbs and oils, beeswax, lanolin, and similar ingredients, applied externally to the skin.

Sedative: An herb that reduces nervous tension; usually stronger than a calmative.

Simple: An herb used by itself as a complete form of prevention or treatment, called *simpling*. Simples are usually very mild, locally grown, or indigenous plants.

Stimulant: Any substance that increases a physiologic function, as opposed to depressing or decreasing it.

Stomachic: Herbs that tighten or tone the stomach, generally due to bitterness or astringency. Stomachics can also stimulate the secretion of hydrochloric acid.

Styptic: An external remedy that stops the flow of blood from cuts or wounds, usually through astringency.

Suppository: A mixture of herbs and water, oil, or cocoa butter, which is inserted in the rectum in order to induce a bowel movement or to soothe inflammations from piles or hemorrhoids. Herbal suppositories can also be used to treat vaginal infections and inflammations.

Tincture: An alcohol or water/alcohol fluid extraction of medicinal herbs that concentrates herbal properties and can be kept at full potency for years. Tinctures were particularly popular with herbalists during the late nineteenth and early twentieth centuries.

Tisane: see Infusion.

Tonic: An herb usually used by itself to strengthen or tone the body or some part of the body gradually. When tonics are used in formulas they are often referred to as neutrals (see Neutral). Tonics are usually slightly stimulating, as opposed to being only nutritive. Whether an herb is regarded as a tonic, a nutritive builder, or a stimulant often has to do more with the dose or quantity used than with its actual properties.

Vulnerary: Any plant or substance used to treat wounds, usually an antibiotic, antiseptic, styptic, and/or plant that promotes healing through cell regeneration.

Yin/Yang: The feminine/masculine principles of polarity in Oriental philosophy.

Bibliography

The Ambrosia Heart Tantra. Annotations by Yeshe Donden. Translated by Jhampa Kelsang. Dharamsala, India: Library of Tibetan Works and Archives, 1977.

Arano, Luisa Cogliati. *The Medieval Health Handbook, Tacuinum Sanitatis.* New York: George Braziller, 1976.

Badmajew, Peter, Jr.; Badmajew, Vladimir, Jr.; and Park, Lynn. *Healing Herbs: The Heart of Tibetan Medicine.* Berkeley, Calif.: Red Lotus Press, 1982.

Balls, Edward K. *Early Uses of California Plants.* Berkeley and Los Angeles: University of California Press, 1962.

Bauman, Edward; Brint, Armand; Piper, Lorin; and Wright, Amelia. *The Holistic Health Handbook.* Berkeley, Calif.: And/Or Press, 1978.

Birnbaum, Raoul. *The Healing Buddha.* Boulder, Colo.: Shambhala, 1979.

Black Elk. *Black Elk Speaks.* Edited by John G. Neihardt. Lincoln, Nebr.: University of Nebraska Press, 1961.

———. *The Sacred Pipe.* Edited by Joseph Epes Brown. Norman, Okla.: University of Oklahoma Press, 1953.

Campbell, Joseph. *The Masks of God: Occidental Mythology.* New York: The Viking Press, 1964.

Castiglioni, Arturo. *A History of Medicine.* Translated by E. B. Krumbhaar. New York: Alfred A. Knopf, 1958.

Cocannouer, Joseph A. *Weeds: Guardians of the Soil.* New York: Devin Adair, 1950.

Conrow, Robert, and Hecksel, Arlene. *Herbal Pathfinders: Voices of the Herb Renaissance.* Santa Barbara, Calif.: Woodbridge Press, 1983.

Coon, Nelson. *Using Wayside Plants.* New York: Hearthside Press, 1969.

Coulter, Harris L. *Homeopathic Influences in Nineteenth Century Allopathic Therapeutics.* St. Louis: Formur, 1977.

Cram, Jane M., and Donald J. Cram. *The Essence of Organic Chemistry.* Reading, Mass.: Addison-Wesley Publishing Co., 1978.

Culpeper, Nicholas. *Culpeper's Complete Herbal.* London: W. Foulsham & Co., 1959.

Dash, Bhagawan. *Tibetan Medicine, with Special Reference to Yoga Sataka.* Dharamsala, India: Library of Tibetan Works and Archives, 1976.

Davidson, A. K. *The Art of Zen Gardens.* Los Angeles: J. P. Tarcher, 1983.

Dolma, Lobsang. *Ama La: Mother of Tibetan Medicine.* Boulder Creek, Calif.: Vajrapani Institute, n.d.

Eyler, Ellen C. *Early English Gardens and Garden Books.* Ithaca, N.Y.: Cornell University Press, 1963.

Fernald, Merritt Lyndon, and Kinsey, Charles Alfred. *Edible Wild Plants of Eastern North America.* Revised by Reed Collins. New York: Harper and Row, 1958.

Fukuoka, Masanobu. *The One-Straw Revolution.* Emmaus, Pa.: Rodale Press, 1978.

Gerard, John. *Leaves from Gerard's Herball.* Edited by Marcus Woodward. New York: Dover Publications, 1969.

Gibbons, Euell. *Stalking the Healthful Herbs.* New York: David McKay Company, 1966.

———. *Stalking the Wild Asparagus.* New York: David McKay Company, 1962.

Grieve, Maude. *A Modern Herbal.* vol. 1 and 2. New York: Dover Publications, 1971.

Griggs, Barbara. *Green Pharmacy: A History of Herbal Medicine.* New York: Viking Press, 1981.

Grossinger, Richard. *Planet Medicine.* Garden City, N.Y.: Anchor Press/Doubleday, 1980.

Halpin, Anne M., ed. *Rodale's Encyclopedia of Indoor Gardening.* Emmaus, Pa.: Rodale Press, 1980.

Heffern, Richard. *The Complete Book of Ginseng.* Millbrae, Calif.: Celestial Arts, 1976.

Hippocrates. *The Genuine Works of Hippocrates.* Translated by Francis Adams. Baltimore: Williams and Wilkins Co., 1939.

———. "Hippocratic Writings, The Law." In *Great Books of the Western World.* Encyclopedia Britannica, 1952.

Holme, Brian. *The Enchanted Garden.* New York: Oxford University Press, 1982.

Howard, Sir Albert. *The Soil and Health.* New York: Schocken Books, 1947.

Hsu, Hong-yen. *How to Treat Yourself with Chinese Herbs.* Los Angeles: Oriental Healing Arts Institute, 1980.

Hyatt, Richard. *Chinese Herbal Medicine.* New York: Schocken Books, 1978.

Hylton, William H., ed. *The Rodale Herb Book.* Emmaus, Pa.: Rodale Press, 1974.

Jeavons, John. *How to Grow More Vegetables.* Berkeley, Calif.: Ten Speed Press, 1982.

Kaptchuk, Ted J. *The Web That Has No Weaver.* New York: Congdon and Weed, 1983.

Kaufman, Martin. *Homeopathy in America: The Rise and Fall of a Medical Heresy.* Baltimore and London: Johns Hopkins Press, 1971.

Kervran, Louis C. *Biological Transmutations.* Translated by Michel Abehsera. Binghamton, N.Y.: Swan House Publishing Co., 1972.

King, F. H. *Farmers of Forty Centuries.* 1911. Reprint. Emmaus, Pa.: Rodale Press, 1977.

Kloss, Jethro. *Back to Eden.* New York: Benedict Lust Publications, 1971.

Koepf, Herbert H.; Pettersson, Bo D; and Schaumann, Wolfgang. *Bio-Dynamic Agriculture: An Introduction.* Spring Valley, N.Y.: Anthroposophic Press, 1976.

Korn, Larry; Snyder, Barbara; and Musick, Mark, eds. *The Future Is Abundant.* Arlington, Wash.: Tilth, 1982.

Krochmal, Arnold, and Connie Krochmal. *A Guide to the Medicinal Plants of the United States.* New York: New York Times Book Co., 1973.

Kunz, Jeffrey R. M., ed. *The American Medical Association Family Medical Guide.* New York: Random House, 1982.

Lao Tzu. *Tao Teh Ching.* Translated by Gia-Fu Feng and Jane English. New York: Vintage Books, 1972.

The Lawrence Review of Natural Products. Vol. 2. No. 19, 15 May 1981.

Li, C. P. *Chinese Herbal Medicine.* U.S., Department of Health, Education and Welfare, Public Health Service, National Institutes of Health (NIH) 75-732. Washington D.C.: Government Printing Office, 1974.

Lighthall, J. I. *Indian Household Medicine.* Hammond, Ind.: Hammond Book Co., 1940.

Logsdon, Gene. *Organic Orcharding.* Emmaus, Pa.: Rodale Press, 1981.

————. *Wildlife in Your Garden.* Emmaus, Pa.: Rodale Press, 1983.

Lucas, Richard. *Common and Uncommon Uses of Herbs for Healthful Living.* New York: Arco Publishing, 1969.

McHarg, Ian L. *Design with Nature.* Garden City, N.Y.: Doubleday/Natural History Press, 1969.

Matsumoto, Kosai. *Traditional Herbs for Natural Healing.* 1977. Kosai Matsumoto Office c/o Plum Research, Box 1705, Sausalito, CA 94965.

Mességué, Maurice. *Health Secrets of Plants and Herbs.* New York: William Morrow, 1975.

———. *Of Men and Plants.* New York: Bantam Books, 1973.

Millspaugh, Charles F. *American Medicinal Plants.* New York: Dover Publications, 1974.

The Mother. *Flowers and Fragrances.* Pamphlet. Pondicherry, India: Sri Aurobindo Society, 1979.

———. *Flowers and Their Messages.* Pondicherry, India: Sri Aurobindo Society, 1979.

Muramoto, Naboru. *Healing Ourselves.* Edited by Michel Abehsera. New York: Avon, 1973.

Nash, Roderick. *Wilderness and the American Mind.* New Haven, Conn.: Yale University Press, 1967.

Neumann, Erich. *The Great Mother.* Translated by Ralph Manheim. Princeton, N.J.: Princeton University Press, 1963.

Palos, Stephen. *The Chinese Art of Healing.* New York: Herder & Herder, 1971.

Pandit Shiv Sharma, ed. *Realms of Ayurveda.* New York: Arnold-Heinemann, 1979.

Paracelsus. *Selected Writings.* Edited by Jolande Jacobi. Translated by Norbert Guterman. New York: Pantheon Books, 1958.

———. *The Hermetic and Alchemical Writings of Paracelsus.* Edited by Arthur Edward Waite. Vols. 1 and 2. Boulder, Colo.: Shambhala Publications, 1976.

Philbrick, Helen, and Gregg, Richard B. *Companion Plants and How to Use Them.* Old Greenwich, Conn.: Devin-Adair Co., 1976.

Philbrick, John, and Helen Philbrick *The Bug Book.* Charlotte, Vt.: Garden Way, 1974.

Platt, Rutherford. *The Green World.* New York: Dodd Mead & Co., 1942.

Rateaver, Bargyla, and Glyver Rateaver. *Organic Methods Primer.* Pauma Valley, Calif.: Published by the authors, 1975.

Ven. Rechung Rinpoche, trans. *Tibetan Medicine.* Berkeley and Los Angeles: University of California Press, 1973.

Robinette, Gary O. *Plants/People/and Environmental Quality.* U.S., Department of the Interior, National Park Service, with the American Society of Landscape Architects Foundation. Washington, D.C.: Government Printing Office, 1972.

Rodale, J. I. and the Staff of *Organic Gardening and Farming* Magazine. *The Encyclopedia of Organic Gardening.* Emmaus, Pa.: Rodale Books, 1959.

———. *How to Landscape Your Own Home.* Emmaus, Pa.: Rodale Press, 1963.

Rose, Jeanne. *Jeanne Rose's Herbal Body Beauty Book*. New York: Grosset and Dunlap, 1976.

Seymour, John. *The Self-Sufficient Gardener*. Garden City, N.Y.: Doubleday & Company, 1978.

Shoffner, Charles P. *The Bird Book*. New York: Frederick A. Stokes Co., 1932.

Silverstein, Martin; I-Lok Chang; and Macon, Nathaniel, trans. *Acupuncture and Moxibustion*. New York: Schocken Books, 1975.

Smyser, Carol A. and the Editors of Rodale Press Books. *Nature's Design*. Emmaus, Pa.: Rodale Press, 1982.

Thomson, William A. R., ed. *Medicines from the Earth*. New York: McGraw-Hill Book Co., 1978.

Thoreau, Henry David. *The Maine Woods*. New York: Bramhall House, 1950.

————. *Walden & Civil Disobedience*. New York: Washington Square Press, 1967.

Thorwald, Jurgen. *Science and Secrets of Early Medicine*. Translated by Richard and Clara Winston. New York: Harcourt, Brace & World, 1962.

Tibetan Medical Center. Booklet about the Tibetan Medical Center, Dharamsala, India. n.d.

Tierra, Michael. *The Way of Herbs*. New York: Washington Square Press, 1983.

Tobey, Peter. *Pirating Plants*. New Canaan, Conn.: Tobey Publishing Co., 1975.

Tsarong, T. J., ed., trans. *Fundamentals of Tibetan Medicine*. Dharamsala, India: Tibetan Medical Center, 1981.

Veith, Ilza, trans. *Nei Chung: The Yellow Emperor's Classic of Internal Medicine*. Berkeley, Calif.: University of California Press, 1972.

Veninga, Louise, and Zaricor, Benjamin R. *Goldenseal/Etc*. Santa Cruz, Calif.: Ruka Publications, 1976.

Vogel, Virgil. *American Indian Medicine*. Norman, Okla.: University of Oklahoma Press, 1970.

Weiner, Michael A. *Earth Medicine-Earth Foods*. New York: Collier Books, Macmillan Publishing Co., 1972.

Wheelwright, Edith Grey. *Medicinal Plants and Their History*. New York: Dover Publications, 1974.

Wood, Magda Ironside, and Wickham, Cynthia. *Herbs*. London and New York: Marshall Cavendish Publications, 1976.

Wright, Richardson. *The Story of Gardening*. New York: Dodd, Mead and Co., 1934.

Yepsen, Roger, ed. *The Encyclopedia of Natural Insect and Disease Control*. Emmaus, Pa.: Rodale Press, 1984.

Index

Page numbers in italic indicate illustrations.

Rodale Press, Inc., publishes PREVENTION®, the better health magazine.
For information on how to order your subscription,
write to PREVENTION®, Emmaus, PA 18049.